The Dentist's Quick Guide to Medical Conditions

The Dentist's Quick Guide to Medical Conditions

Mea A. Weinberg, DMD, MSD, RPh

Diplomate, American Board of Periodontology
Clinical Professor
Department of Periodontology and Implant Dentistry
New York University College of Dentistry
New York, NY, USA

Stuart L. Segelnick, DDS, MS

Diplomate, American Board of Periodontology
Diplomate, International Congress of Oral Implantologists
Clinical Associate Professor
Department of Periodontology and Implant Dentistry
New York University College of Dentistry
New York, NY, USA

Section Chief of Periodontics
Brookdale University Hospital and Medical Center
Brooklyn, NY, USA

Joseph S. Insler, MD

Fellow, Addiction Psychiatry
Department of Psychiatry
Boston University
Boston, MA, USA

with Samuel Kramer, DDS

Clinical Assistant Professor
Department of Endodontics
New York University College of Dentistry
New York, NY, USA

WILEY Blackwell

Library of Congress Cataloging-in-Publication Data

Weinberg, Mea A., author.

The dentist's quick guide to medical conditions / Mea A. Weinberg, Stuart L. Segelnick, Joseph S. Insler.

    p. ; cm.

Includes bibliographical references and index.

ISBN 978-1-118-71011-1 (pbk.)

I. Segelnick, Stuart L., author. II. Insler, Joseph S., author. III. Title.

    [DNLM: 1. Signs and Symptoms. 2. Dental Care. 3. Therapeutics. WB 143]

    RK61

    617.6–dc23

                       2014027086

A catalogue record for this book is available from the British Library.

Dedication

We would like to dedicate this book to our family
Dr. Mea Weinberg: Adam, Nina, & Nigel
Dr. Stuart Segelnick: Tina & Noah
Dr. Joseph Insler: Suzanne & Jacob
Dr. Samuel Kramer: Cynthia & Harry
for without their love and support this wonderful work would not be possible.

Contents

Contributors   x
Foreword   xi
Preface   xii

1   Gastrointestinal disorders   **1**
    A.   Peptic ulcer disease   1
    B.   Gastroesophageal reflux disease   4
    C.   Irritable bowel syndrome   6
    D.   Inflammatory bowel disease   7
         a.   Crohn's disease   7
         b.   Ulcerative colitis   10
    E.   Diverticular disease   11
    F.   Acute pancreatitis   12
    G.   Celiac sprue   13
    H.   Pseudomembranous colitis   13

2   Medical conditions of the respiratory system   **17**
    A.   Respiratory diseases   17
         a.   Asthma   17
         b.   Chronic obstructive pulmonary diseases   23
         c.   Pulmonary tuberculosis   24
         d.   Obstructive sleep apnea   27

3   Disorders of the urinary system   **30**
    A.   Acute renal injury and chronic kidney disease   30
    B.   Kidney dialysis   37
    C.   Kidney transplant   39
    D.   Polycystic kidney disease   42
    E.   Benign prostatic hypertrophy   42

4   Diseases of the endocrine system   **46**
    A.   Diabetes   46
    B.   Thyroid diseases   50
    C.   Adrenal gland disorders   53

5   Disorders of the cardiovascular system   **59**
   A. Hypertension   59
   B. Angina Pectoris   68
      Clinic   68
   C. Myocardial infarction   70
   D. Heart failure   73
   E. Arrhythmias   75
   F. Valvular heart disease   78
   G. Epinephrine in cardiac patients   79

6   Pregnancy, lactation, and oral contraceptives   **82**
   A. Pregnancy and lactation   82
   B. Oral contraceptives   89

7   Disorders of the liver and gallbladder   **93**
   A. Liver disease   93
      a. Alcoholic liver disease and cirrhosis   98
      b. Hepatitis   99
      c. Liver transplant   103
   B. Gallstones   105

8   Diseases of the neurological system   **109**
   A. Parkinson's disease   109
   B. Multiple sclerosis   113
   C. Seizures   116

9   Psychiatric disorders   **125**
   Introduction   125
   A. Antipsychotics   126
      a. Typical antipsychotics   127
      b. Atypical antipsychotics   128
      c. Anticholinergic medications   128
   B. Antidepressants   132
      a. Monoamine oxidase inhibitors   133
      b. Tricyclics and tetracyclics   134
      c. Selective serotonin reuptake inhibitors   135
      d. Selective serotonin norepinephrine reuptake
         inhibitors (SNRIs)   136
      e. Others   136
      f. Summary: Dental interactions and
         side effects   136
   C. Mood stabilizers   138
      a. Lithium   139
      b. Valproic acid (Depakote)   140
      c. Lamotrigine (Lamictal)   140
      d. Carbamazepine (Tegretol)   141
      e. Oxcarbazepine (Trileptal)   141

	D.	Alcohol and other drugs with addictive potential	142
		a. Alcohol	142
		b. Sedatives and hypnotics	143
		c. Opioids	143
		d. Cocaine	145

10 Hematologic disorders and drugs that cause bleeding — **149**
	A.	Brief overview of the coagulation process	149
		a. Thrombocytopenia	152
		b. Thrombocytopathy	153
		c. Antiplatelet medications	153
	B.	Bleeding disorders: Coagulation disorders	154
		a. von Willebrand disease	154
		b. Hemophilias	155
		c. End-stage liver disease	156
		d. Anticoagulation medications	157

11 Blood dyscrasias — **171**
	A.	Red blood cell disorders	174
		a. Anemia	174
		b. Myeloproliferative disorders	181
	B.	White blood cell disorders	182
		a. Leukemia	182
		b. Lymphoma	186
		c. Multiple myeloma	187

12 Musculoskeletal and connective tissue disorders — **193**
	A.	Osteoporosis	193
	B.	Osteoarthritis	197
	C.	Rheumatoid arthritis	198
	D.	Gout	201
	E.	Fibromyalgia syndrome	203
	F.	Systemic lupus erythematosus	205
	G.	Sjögren's syndrome	208

13 HIV and oral health care — **214**

14 Radiation and chemotherapy — **237**

Appendices
Appendix A	Antibiotic prophylaxis of the dental patient	252
Appendix B	Common dental drug interactions	255
Appendix C	Summary of tables/boxes	266
Appendix D	Interpretation of common laboratory values	270

Index — 274

Contributors

Cheryl A. Barber, MPH, MS
Senior Research Scientist
Department of Basic Sciences
HIV/AIDS Research Program
New York University College of Dentistry
New York, NY, USA

Floyd L. Dussetschleger, DDS
Clinical Professor
Cariology & Comprehensive Care
New York University College of Dentistry
New York, NY, USA

David H. Hershkowitz, DDS
Clinical Assistant Professor; Associate Chairperson
Cariology & Comprehensive Care
New York University College of Dentistry
New York, NY, USA

Joseph S. Insler, MD
Fellow
Addiction Psychiatry
Department of Psychiatry
Boston University
Boston, MA, USA

Foreword

People are living longer. According to "The State of Aging and Health in America 2013," the increase in the number of Americans aged 65 years and older is unparalleled in the history of the USA.

Chronic conditions present a major modification in the principal causes of death for all age groups from infectious diseases and acute conditions to chronic diseases and degenerative illnesses. Many Americans, including the older population, present with numerous chronic medical conditions. Treatment of this section of the population makes up a good majority of the country's healthcare allocation.

Dentists will be seeing more people with medical issues that will have to be treated differently than in a healthy individual. The *The Dentist's Quick Handbook of Medical Updates* is a must-have to help dentists navigate treatment for these patients.

The book is detailed yet easy to read. The dental notes for each condition located by system are a handy quick reference that will help make precise treatment decisions.

Charles N. Bertolami
Professor and Herman Robert Fox Dean
College of Dentistry
New York University

Preface

The Dentist's Quick Guide to Medical Conditions is a manual designed to provide practicing dental clinicians with a comprehensive review of the latest information on treatment of dental patients with common medical disorders. The information in this book is primarily concerned with the clinical practical aspects of different medical conditions, pharmacologic management, and dental management of these conditions.

The book is structured around the clinical synopsis of the medical condition, specific diagnostic/laboratory values that are important for the dentist to know, significant drug–drug and drug–disease interactions, and key dental notes needed to treat the medically complex dental patient. Each chapter's discussion of medical and pharmacological treatment relies heavily on the clinical experience of the authors and therefore addresses many of the problems that the dentist encounters in daily practice.

Most chapters contain easy-to-follow tables and bullets denoting important facts. Features of *The Dentist's Quick Guide to Medical Conditions* include the following.

- At the end of each chapter are easy-to-follow dental notes on management of the medically complex patient.
- Drug tables: many tables are provided that summarize the main medical/pharmacologic/dental features of the different medical conditions.
- Many appendices: Appendix A, antibiotic prophylaxis of the dental patient; Appendix B, common dental drug interactions; Appendix C, summary guide to dental management of systemic diseases; Appendix D, interpretation of common laboratory values.
- Comprehensive up-to-date references with each chapter.

The authors are deeply grateful for the opportunity to write this book, and hopefully it will meet the needs of the dentist in practice.

Mea A. Weinberg
Stuart L. Segelnick
Joseph S. Insler

I will have been a clinical instructor of endodontics at New York University College of Dentistry for almost 20 years at the time of this publication.

One day it dawned upon me that the very students I was mentoring in the clinic had greater medical knowledge than myself. To mention a few instances, the students had knowledge of new medical tests for disease entities and their corresponding normal values, better disease diagnosis with probable treatment outcomes, and knowledge of newer pharmacologic agents including their indications, contraindications, and side effects. Most of this information was not part of my original dental school program as medical advances had left me and albeit some older graduates deficient in the newer procedures.

A graduate of the University of Buffalo Dental School (1979), I desired to update my medical knowledge; this was the inspiration for the first edition of this book.

It is with great pride and humility that we bring this book into the medical literature.

Samuel Kramer, DDS
SUNY Buffalo 1979-DDS
New York University College of Dentistry 1991-Certificate in Endodontics

Chapter 1

Gastrointestinal disorders

A. Peptic ulcer disease 1
B. Gastroesophageal reflux disease 4
C. Irritable bowel syndrome 6
D. Inflammatory bowel disease (CD and UC) 7
   a. Crohn's disease 7
   b. Ulcerative colitis 10
E. Diverticular disease 11
F. Acute pancreatitis 12
G. Celiac sprue 13
H. Pseudomembranous colitis 13
References 14

A. Peptic ulcer disease

Clinical synopsis

Peptic ulcer disease (PUD) is a general term describing a group of acid-peptic disorders of the upper gastrointestinal (GI) tract including the esophagus, stomach, and duodenum. A peptic ulcer is defined as a circumscribed loss of tissue or break that occurs in the GI mucosa extending through the GI tract smooth muscle. There is an imbalance between gastric acid and pepsin and mucosal defense factors, including prostaglandins, which protect the stomach by increasing the production of gastric mucus and reducing the production of gastric acid.

There are three types of peptic ulcers: gastric ulcer, which occurs in the stomach; duodenal ulcer, which occurs in the duodenum; and esophageal ulcer, which occurs in the esophagus. Most peptic ulcers are asymptomatic; however, the more commonly seen symptoms in symptomatic ulcers are midepigastric pain, dyspepsia (indigestion), nausea, fullness, nocturnal pain, anorexia, and weight loss. One of the distinguishing features of gastric ulcer is the presence of stomach pain after eating. When pain occurs hours after eating or on an empty stomach accompanied with pain at night, it is duodenal ulcer (Peters *et al.* 2010). The classical epigastric pain in a duodenal ulcer occurs when acid is produced and secreted in the absence of food in the stomach.

The Dentist's Quick Guide to Medical Conditions, First Edition. Mea A. Weinberg, Stuart L. Segelnick, Joseph S. Insler, with Samuel Kramer.
© 2015 John Wiley & Sons, Inc. Published 2015 by John Wiley & Sons, Inc.

Table 1.1   Medications for peptic ulcer disease and gastroesophageal reflux disease.

Generic drug	Brand name
Proton pump inhibitors (PPI)	
Dexlansoprazole	Dexilant
Esomeprazole	Nexium
Lansoprazole	Prevacid
Omeprazole	Prilosec
Pantoprazole	Protonix
Rabeprazole	AcipHex
Histamine-2 receptor antagonists (H2RAs)	
Cimetidine	Tagamet
Famotidine	Pepcid
Nizatidine	Axid
Ranitidine	Zantac
Prostaglandin supplements	
Misoprostol (prevention of gastric and duodenal ulcers due to nonsteroidal anti-inflammatory drugs)	Cytotec
Protective barrier drug	
Sucralfate (for healing of duodenal ulcers, not gastric ulcers)	Carafate
Gastrointestinal stimulant drug	
Metoclopramide	Reglan

The two most common causes of PUD are chronic nonsteroidal anti-inflammatory drugs (NSAIDs) use and *Helicobacter pylori* (*H. pylori*), a Gram-negative bacterium, which resides in the GI mucosal lining and in certain individuals can erode the mucosa resulting in ulceration. Even though the majority of duodenal ulcers are caused by *H. pylori*, only 5–10% will develop ulcers (Malfertheiner *et al.* 2009; Peters *et al.* 2010). The definitive diagnosis of PUD is generally made by an upper GI endoscopy (Peters *et al.* 2010).

Diagnostics/lab values

If it is certain that the ulcer is not caused by chronic NSAID use, a blood test to detect the presence of *H. pylori* antibodies is a noninvasive test. Although the test has high sensitivity and specificity when lab serology is used, it cannot discriminate if it is a current infection or previous exposure. Additionally, IgG testing may be positive for many years after treatment and eradication of the bacteria. Saliva can also be used but there is low sensitivity and specificity (Meurer and Bower 2002). Urea breath test (UBT) and fecal antigen test are the other preferred methods for diagnosing the presence of *H. pylori* before administration of antibiotic and antisecretory drugs (Peters *et al.* 2010). The UBT is utilized to confirm the eradication of *H. pylori*. Recurrence of *H. pylori* infection usually is defined by a positive result on urea breath or stool antigen testing six or more months after documented successful eradication therapy (Ables *et al.* 2007).

Medications

Management of PUD can differ depending upon whether the etiology is NSAID use or *H. pylori* infection. Antibiotics are used to eradicate *H. pylori* infection. Proton pump inhibitors (PPIs) and histamine-2 receptor antagonists (H$_2$RAs) provide quick pain relief and accelerated healing of the ulcer (Table 1.1). H2 receptor blockers reduce histamine-stimulated gastric acid secretion by competitively inhibiting

H_2 receptors on the parietal cells in the stomach. These agents have a limited effect on gastric acid secretion after food ingestion and are effective in healing ulcers in 6–12 weeks. Antacids are used for the treatment of dyspepsia. PPIs provide rapid symptomatic relief with accelerated healing of duodenal ulcers, thus providing the most rapid symptom relief and highest percentage of esophageal healing of all agents used in gastroesophageal reflux disease (GERD) management. They are the drug of choice for patients with frequent daily symptoms, patients with moderate to severe GERD symptoms, patients not responding to H_2RAs, and patients with complicated disease, including Barrett's esophagus and esophagitis.

For NSAID-induced peptic ulcer, an H_2 antagonist or PPI is prescribed. Antacids are recommended for the epigastric pain. Antibiotics are not prescribed.

Management of non–NSAID-induced peptic ulcer that is positive to *H. pylori* includes systemic antibiotics and H_2 antagonists or PPIs. Over the years, resistance to antibiotics is emerging. The goal of treating ulcers is the elimination of *H. pylori*, which will increase healing of the ulcer, improve symptoms, and reduce recurrence. Although the management of *H. pylori* is being continuously investigated, currently, the accepted protocol for *H. pylori* eradication (Box 1.1) is quadruple or triple therapy; usually, it is triple therapy. The drawback of therapy is low adherence because of the vast number of medications that have to be taken for 14 days; *H. pylori* cannot be eradicated with just one antibiotic or medication.

Helicobacter pylori has been found in dental biofilms, and its appearance varies from one site to another in the oral cavity (Kilmartin 2002). Individuals with gastric *H. pylori* were positive for oral *H. pylori* also (Anand *et al.* 2006). Other studies have found that patients with the presence of *H. pylori* in dental plaque had a greater prevalence of gastric infection (Lui *et al.* 2009). It has been theorized that antibiotics used to eliminate gastric *H. pylori* do not eliminate *H. pylori* in dental plaque and can be a source of future reinfection (Anand *et al.* 2006).

Dental drug–drug interactions/adverse reactions

Common dental drug-peptic ulcer disease drug interactions are listed in Table 1.2.
Oral adverse reactions of medications/disease (McGrath *et al.* 2008)
   Common oral adverse reactions of medications/disease are:

- Antacids and bismuth can cause black hairy tongue.
- Metronidazole can cause a metallic taste in the mouth.
- Clarithromycin can cause a metallic taste in the mouth.
- Tetracycline can cause black hairy tongue.
- GERD can cause erosion of enamel.

Box 1.1   Therapy for *H. pylori* Management (http://www.fpnotebook.com/GI/ID/HlcbctrPylr.htm; Ables *et al.* 2007; Chey and Wong, 2007; Peters *et al.* 2010).

Quadruple Therapy
- Metronidazole (Flagyl) 250 mg four times a day +
- Tetracycline 500 mg four times a day +
- Bismuth subcitrate (Pepto-Bismol) 525 mg four times a day +
- Antisecretory drug (up to 6 weeks): omeprazole (Prilosec) 20 mg twice a day OR esomeprazole 20–40 mg daily OR lansoprazole (Prevacid) 20 mg twice a day OR pantoprazole (Protonix) 40 mg twice a day OR rabeprazole (Aciphex) 20 mg twice a day

Triple Therapy
- Amoxicillin 500 mg twice a day
- Clarithromycin (Biaxin) 1000 mg twice a day
- Metronidazole (Flagyl) 500 mg twice a day (only use if allergic to penicillin)
- Prevpac is a combination product containing pantoprazole, clarithromycin, and amoxicillin.

Table 1.2   Dental drug–drug interactions (www.rxlist.com; Peters *et al.* 2010).

Prescribing dental drug	Peptic ulcer disease drug	Management
Ketoconazole	Proton pump inhibitors, histamine-2 receptor antagonists	Not as effective in a less acidic stomach environment
Doxycycline, tetracycline (if it is not being prescribed as quadruple therapy)	Antacids (e.g., Mylanta, Maalox, and Gelusil contain aluminum hydroxide), calcium tablets, zinc, iron	Antacids that contain di- or trivalent ions (Mg^{2+}, Ca^{2+}, Al^{3+}) bind to and form an insoluble complex with tetracyclines, which will decrease the absorption *rate* of these antibiotics. Thus, antacids should not be given concurrently with these antibiotics but 1–2 h before or after taking the antibiotics. Kaolin (in Kaopectate) binds to the tetracycline molecule and decreases the absorption rate of the antibiotic. Do not take Kaopectate together with tetracycline. It is best to wait 1–2 h before or after taking kaolin or the antibiotic.
Ciprofloxacin (Cipro)	Antacids, calcium tablets, zinc, iron	Di- or trivalent ions (Mg^{2+}, Ca^{2+}, Al^{3+}) containing antacids bind to and form an insoluble complex with fluoroquinolones, which will decrease the absorption *rate* of these antibiotics. Thus, antacids should not be given concurrently with these antibiotics but 1–2 h before or after taking the antibiotics.

B.   Gastroesophageal reflux disease

Clinical synopsis

GERD is one of the most common chronic conditions of the upper GI tract. In GERD, there is a reflux or "backing up" of gastric contents from the stomach into the esophagus, which generally occurs in many individuals without causing any complications and damage to the mucosal lining of the esophagus. The most common complaint or symptom is heartburn, but the individual may also complain of epigastric pain.

If the acidic gastric contents stay in contact for prolonged periods of time with the mucosal tissue of the esophagus, a form of GERD called reflux esophagitis will develop, which is characterized by inflammation of the esophagus due to excessive acid reflux. Acid reflux into the oral cavity may cause the development of tooth erosion, particularly on the palatal surfaces of the maxillary incisors. Esophagitis results from excessive reflux of gastric juices rather than excessive acid secretion in the stomach as seen in PUD. Other complications from GERD include dysphagia (difficulty in swallowing) and esophageal ulcers.

Medications

Antacids are primarily used in the treatment of dyspepsia (indigestion or heartburn). Antacids are basic salts that dissolve in gastric acid secretions and neutralize some but not all gastric hydrochloric acid and have a greater effect of increasing the pH in the duodenum than in the stomach. Antacids neutralize or reduce the *acidity* of gastric juices, but they do not affect the rate or amount of gastric acid secretion by the stomach cells and do not prevent ulcer recurrence. Rather, antacids are usually used to relieve occasional duodenal ulcer symptoms or GERD on an as-needed basis by the patient.

The first-line drug therapy for GERD is antacids and a nonprescription H_2RA such as famotidine (Pepcid) or a PPI such as omeprazole (Prilosec). Given the chronic nature of GERD and the high recurrence rates if acid suppressive therapy is discontinued, long-term maintenance therapy is appropriate and indicated for most patients.

Lab tests

There are no specific laboratory tests for GERD that dentists need to know for dental treatment.

Medications: Drugs used to treat GERD include the following

- Antacids
- H_2RAs
- PPIs

Dental notes: PUD and GERD

1. There are no precautions or contraindications with epinephrine and antacids, H_2RAs, or PPIs.
2. Note all drug–drug interactions that can occur with medications used for PUD/GERD.
3. If a patient requires an antibiotic for a dental infection and since the patient is already taking amoxicillin and clarithromycin, the dose of these antibiotics should not be increased but rather a different class of antibiotic should be prescribed such as clindamycin.
4. Question the patient regarding the use of OTC and prescription NSAIDs (e.g., Advil and Aleve) and antacids. Avoid recommending or prescribing NSAIDs in patients with a previous history or current history of peptic ulcers/GERD.
5. Avoid prescribing steroids in patients with PUD.
6. Remember to ask patients if they are taking any OTC medications for their ulcer or GERD. Many of these medications are available OTC (e.g., antacids, Tagamet, and Prilosec).
7. Patients that have GERD and are taking only antacids should not take tetracycline or doxycycline concurrently with the antacid; wait for 1–2 h.
8. Black hairy tongue due to antacids, bismuth subsalicylate, and tetracycline is temporary and will disappear when the medications are stopped.
9. Patients with gastroesophageal reflux may present with oral symptoms, including burning mouth and tooth erosion. In fact, GERD is a differential diagnosis for burning mouth symptoms.
10. Place the patient in a semi-supine position in the dental chair.
11. Recommend reducing acid content in the mouth with sodium bicarbonate mouthrinse.
12. Recommend to apply in-office fluoride and possible prescription for home-applied fluoride for GERD patients.

C.   Irritable bowel syndrome

Clinical synopsis

Irritable bowel syndrome (IBS) is a noninflammatory condition that consists of chronic or recurrent GI symptoms that are diagnosed only clinically without any specific laboratory test or any biological cause. IBS causes a dysregulation in the functions of the intestinal motor, sensory and central nervous systems resulting in altered bowel habit (American Gastroenterology Association 2002). The main GI and non-GI symptoms include diarrhea, bloating, constipation, and increased urinary frequency. Irritable bowel symptoms can also be associated with other conditions such as ulcerative colitis (UC) or Crohn's disease (CD) (Ringel and Drossman 2000).

The clinical diagnosis of IBS is usually based on the Rome criterion, which requires the presence of abdominal pain or discomfort to make a definitive diagnosis of IBS (Thompson *et al.* 2000). Additionally, the biopsychosocial approach melds the physiologic and psychosocial aspects to the overall diagnosis (Drossman *et al.* 1997; Ringel and Drossman 2000).

There is also a rating for the severity of pain, and management is based on this severity. For example, if the symptoms are mild, then only dietary and lifestyle changes and patient education are recommended. Moderate symptoms most likely will require medications and psychological therapy. Severe symptoms may require the addition of antidepressants (Olden and Schuster 1997; Engstrom and Goosenberg 1999).

Medications

The pharmacologic management of IBS poses a therapeutic challenge since there are multiple symptoms, sometimes nonspecific, that cannot be managed with just a single drug. Most of the medications used to manage IBS have not changed in the past few decades and are aimed at controlling the abdominal pain and bloating, constipation, and diarrhea (Engstrom and Goosenberg 1999). The following are the medications indicated for IBS:

- Antimotility drugs such as loperamide (Imodium) and adsorbents such as bismuth salicylate (Pepto-Bismol, Kaopectate) indicated for diarrhea
- Bile acid sequestrant such as cholestyramine (Questran powder) indicated for diarrhea from excess bile acids and could cause constipation
- Laxatives for constipation. Chronic laxative use may lead to hypokalemia.
- Antispasmodic/anticholinergics: dicyclomine (Bentyl), chlordiazepoxide/clidinium bromide (Librax), phenobarbital, hyoscyamine, atropine, scopolamine (Donnatal), and hyoscyamine (Levsin) indicated for abdominal cramping pain and bloating
- Tricyclic antidepressants (TCAs) such as amitriptyline (Elavil) or selective serotonin reuptake inhibitors are for the psychological component of the IBS
- Nonnarcotic analgesics are indicated for pain relief as narcotic analgesics increase the incidence of constipation.

Probiotics are live organisms formulated from bacteria found in the GI tract. The rationale for its use is based on the theory that endogenous intestinal microflora play a crucial role in the pathogenesis of disorders such as IBS and UC (Quigley 2007). Probiotics are intended to restore the normal intestinal flora that may have been altered in the disease state due to stasis and reduced colonic transit time (Boynton and Floch 2013). Common encountered dental drug interactions are listed in Table 1.3.

Table 1.3   Dental drug–drug interactions (www.drugs.com; www.rxlist.com).

Dental drug prescribed	Irritable bowel syndrome drug	Management
Acetaminophen/ hydrocodone; acetaminophen/ codeine; acetaminophen/ oxycodone	Bismuth subsalicylate (Kaopectate; Pepto-Bismol)	Can increase blood levels or adverse reaction of either medication. Severe abdominal cramps or bloating can occur. Use with caution or substitute another analgesic.
Doxycycline, tetracycline	Bismuth subsalicylate (Kaopectate; Pepto-Bismol)	May decrease the effect of doxycycline; space dosing 2–3 h apart.
Penicillins	Cholestyramine (Questran)	When administered concurrently reduces rate of absorption. Separate doses 1–2 h apart.
Epinephrine in local anesthetic	Tricyclic antidepressants (TCAs)	TCAs inhibit the reuptake of norepinephrine via the NE reuptake pump allowing NE to stay in the synapse helping to relieve antidepressant symptoms. Epinephrine works similar to TCAs, through the reuptake pump. So, when the reuptake pump is not working, there will be enhanced accumulation of epinephrine (EPI) and norepinephrine (NE) in the synapse resulting in hypertension and cardiac arrhythmias. Epinephrine is NOT contraindicated but just the amount has to be limited to two cartridges of 1:100,000. Levonordefrin is CONTRAINDICATED. This drug–drug interaction DOES NOT occur with selective serotonin reuptake inhibitors

Dental notes

- Since patients with IBS may be taking numerous medications for their symptoms, it is important to ask at every dental visit what prescription and OTC drugs they are taking.
- Remember to limit the amount of epinephrine to two cartridges of 1:100,000 if the patient is taking a TCA.
- Avoid codeine and derivatives including hydrocodone and oxycodone if the patient is already constipated from IBS.

D.   Inflammatory bowel disease (CD and UC)

a.   Crohn's disease

Medical synopsis

CD is a chronic condition that can occur anywhere in the entire GI tract from the oral cavity to the rectum; however, the lower part of the small intestine is mostly affected (Ganda 2013). Chronic inflammation occurs with increased number of white blood cells (WBCs) in the lining of the duodenum resulting in ulceration. Chronic blood loss can lead to the development of anemia. Symptoms of CD include chronic diarrhea, abdominal pain, weight loss, fever, and nausea/vomiting.

Oral features (Engstrom and Goosenberg 1999)

- The oral cavity especially the gingiva and buccal mucosa may appear to be swollen. In severe attacks, there may be oral candidiasis (thrush) and aphthous ulcerations.
- Patients may be deficient in vitamin B12 due to malabsorption. Orally this may manifest as glossitis, oral candidiasis, erythematous mucositis, and pale oral mucosa (Pontes *et al.* 2009).
- Bleeding may be a problem due to abnormal liver function; evaluate the patient's CBC and liver function test profile before dental treatment (Ganda 2013).

Diagnosis/lab tests

Diagnosis of CD is based on signs and symptoms, computed tomography (CT) or MRI, and endoscopy with biopsy. The disease severity is categorized into mild to moderate, moderate to severe, or severe to fulminant (American College of Gastroenterology *et al.* 1997).

Medications

Medications indicated in the treatment of CD include anti-inflammatories and antibiotics (American College of Gastroenterology *et al.* 1997).

For mild to moderate CD:

1. Oral 5-aminosalicylate (e.g., mesalamine, sulfasalazine) is a bowel-specific anti-inflammatory class of drugs that are metabolized by the normal flora in the bowel, which allows for the drug to work at the site of inflammation.
2. Metronidazole is prescribed when patients do not respond to oral aminosalicylate drugs. Metronidazole is antibacterial as well as anti-inflammatory and is recommended in the treatment of *Clostridium difficile* infections.

For moderate to severe CD:

1. Systemic corticosteroids (e.g., prednisone and methylprednisolone)
2. Immunosuppressant or immunomodulator drugs (e.g., 6-mercaptopurine, azathioprine, and cyclosporine). The CBC and absolute neutrophil count should be reviewed before starting dental treatment (Ganda 2013).
3. Anti–tumor necrosis factor (anti-TNF) drugs [e.g., adalimumab (Humira), infliximab (Remicade), and certolizumab (Cimzia)] reduce the synthesis of elevated TNF, thus reducing inflammation. Indicated for patients that do not respond to other drugs.
4. Antibiotics such as tetracycline, clarithromycin, ciprofloxacin, or metronidazole for intestinal infection.
5. Antidiarrheal medications [e.g., loperamide (Imodium), diphenoxylate (Lomotil), and bismuth subsalicylate (Kaopectate)]
6. Hydration: The patient may need to use the restroom frequently.

For severe to fulminant CD:

1. Hospitalization
2. Parenteral steroids and antibiotics

Dental notes

- Patients on long-term systemic steroids may present with steroid-induced diabetes mellitus, which is a risk factor for periodontal diseases. The patient's periodontal condition should be closely monitored.
- Epinephrine is synthesized and secreted by the adrenal medulla and can safely be used in patients taking a systemic steroid such as prednisone.
- Cyclosporine, an immunomodulator, may cause gingival enlargement. As long as the patient is taking this drug, there will be gingival enlargement. Meticulous plaque control is important. In severe cases, periodontal surgery may be indicated to excise the gingival overgrowth; however, it will recur as long as the patient continues to take cyclosporine.
- Avoid prescribing codeine or derivatives including hydrocodone and oxycodone if the patient is taking an antidiarrheal medication.
- Some patients may take omega-3 fatty acids, which may increase the risk of bleeding. Caution should be used when performing invasive dental procedures.
- Metronidazole may cause a metallic taste in the mouth. Do not prescribe an alcoholic mouthrinse while the patient is taking metronidazole.
- A significant adverse reaction to anti-TNF drugs is *oral tuberculosis* and oral candidiasis (thrush)/oral ulcers (www.rxlist.com). The oral cavity infrequently becomes a site for extrapulmonary tuberculosis; however, if it happens clinically it may show ulcerated lesions on the tongue, gingiva, and palate. Diagnosis is confirmed by biopsy, histopathology, sputum, and immunology (Nanda *et al.* 2011). Treatment of extrapulmonary tuberculosis is the same as for pulmonary tuberculosis (Ferguson and McCormack 1993).
- If the patient is taking tetracycline, clarithromycin, ciprofloxacin, or metronidazole and concurrently has a dental infection and requires an antibiotic, do not increase the dose of the current antibiotic but rather prescribe a different antibiotic. Remember that tetracycline and clarithromycin are bacteriostatic, so prescribing clindamycin would be appropriate since it is also bacteriostatic. If the patient is taking metronidazole, which is bactericidal, then penicillin, which is also bactericidal, would be appropriate. Hence, if the patient is taking a bacteriostatic antibiotic, it is contraindicated to prescribe a bactericidal antibiotic and vice versa.
- The adrenal cortex normally produces and secretes cortisol, an endogenous hormone, in the body. When exogenous steroids (e.g., prednisone and methylprednisolone) are taken, the adrenal gland shuts off. In the normal, nonstressed person, about 20–30 mg of cortisol is produced per day, which is equivalent to about 5–7 mg of prednisone. Cortisol is released in a highly irregular manner with peak secretion in the early morning, which then tapers out in the late afternoon and evening. When a person is stressed, cortisol production is increased to about 50–300 mg/day. Cortisol functions to regulate energy by selecting the right type and amount of substrate (carbohydrate, fat, or protein) that is needed by the body to meet the physiological demands that are placed upon it. Cortisol mobilizes energy by moving the body's fat stores (in the form of triglycerides) from one area to another or delivering it to hungry tissues such as working muscles. During stressful times, higher levels of cortisol are released, which has been associated with several medical conditions including suppressed thyroid function and hyperglycemia; however, when taking exogenous steroids, the person's endogenous production is stopped and there may not be enough endogenous cortisol to handle the body's stressful demands. For this reason, in the past, patients on long-term systemic steroid have been advised to take supplemental glucocorticoids. *A medical consultation is necessary before any additional steroids are prescribed.*
- An "older" theory concerning the need for steroid supplementation in patients taking steroids was called the "rule-of-twos," which stated that if the patient was currently on 20 mg of cortisone (equivalent to 5 mg prednisone) daily for 2 weeks or longer within the past 2 years, then it was necessary to give supplemental steroids to prevent an adrenal crisis.

Adrenal crisis is associated with a stressful event that is caused by the failure of cortisol levels to meet the body's increased requirements for cortisol and is primarily a mineralocorticoid steroid deficiency, not a glucocorticoid deficiency. Mineralocorticoids (e.g., aldosterone) maintain the level of sodium and potassium in the body. Adrenal crisis, a medical emergency that oc*curs very rarely in dental patients,* is characterized by abdominal pain, weakness, hypotension, dehydration, and nausea and vomiting (Khalaf *et al.* 2013). It has been concluded in clinical studies that *patients on long-term steroid drugs do not require supplemental "steroid coverage"* for routine dentistry, including minor surgical procedures under profound local anesthesia with adequate postoperative pain control (Miller *et al.* 2001). The low incidence of significant adrenal insufficiency precludes the addition of supplemental steroids (Gibson and Ferguson 2004). For major oral/periodontal surgery under general anesthesia, supplemental steroids may be required depending upon the dose of steroid and duration of treatment. It is important to obtain a medical consultation from the patient's physician.

The final conclusion is that adrenal crisis is a rare event in dentistry, especially for patients with secondary adrenal insufficiency who develop this condition from taking steroids for common medical conditions. Most routine dental procedures, including nonsurgical periodontal therapy (scaling and root planing) and restorative procedures, can be performed without glucocorticoid supplementation.

• See Tables 1.2 and 1.3 for dental drug interactions.

b. Ulcerative colitis

Clinical synopsis

UC is a chronic condition causing inflammation and ulceration of the mucosa of the colon. It usually begins in the rectum and may involve various lengths of the colon over time or at the same time (Engstrom and Goosenberg 1999). The etiology is unclear, and it is diagnosed by positive WBC and bacteria in the stool, sigmoidoscopy, colonoscopy, barium enema, and X-rays. If the patient has recently taken antibiotics, the stool should be tested for the presence of *Clostridium difficile.* Stress, NSAIDs, and some antibiotics (e.g., penicillin, erythromycin, and quinolones such as ciprofloxacin) have been reported to cause inflammatory bowel disease (Singh *et al.* 2009).

Lab tests

UC is diagnosed based on the presence of WBCs and bacteria in stool samples. UC can occur as a result of recent antibiotic exposure with the development of *Clostridium difficile* (Engstrom and Goosenberg 1999). Additionally, a signoidoscopy or colonoscopy is performed to determine the extent of the colitis (Engstrom and Goosenberg 1999). Other diagnostic tools include X-rays and barium enema.

There are no laboratory values that are important for dentistry. Iron deficiency may result from the chronic blood loss. Additionally, hypokalemia and hypoalbuminemia may occur. Also, there may be abnormal liver function tests.

Medications

Management of UC depends on the severity of the disease and is very similar to the drugs prescribed for CD (Lichenstein *et al.* 2009; Lichenstein 2011). There is no curative pharmacological treatment, and drugs are used to induce and maintain remission (Gledhill and Bodger 2013). The following drugs are used in the management of mild to moderate UC (American College of Gastroenterology *et al.* (1997); Kornbluth and Sachar 2010).

1. Oral 5-aminosalicylate (e.g., mesalamine and sulfasalazine) is a bowel-specific anti-inflammatory class of drugs that are metabolized by the normal flora in the bowel, which allows for the drug to work at the site of inflammation.
2. Topical mesalamine enema (foam or suppository) or hydrocortisone (enema or foam)
3. Oral corticosteroids (e.g., prednisone and methylprednisolone)
4. Immunosuppressant or immunomodulator drugs (e.g., 6-mercaptopurine, azathioprine, and cyclosporine)
5. Metronidazole is prescribed when patients do not respond to oral aminosalicylate drugs. Metronidazole is antibacterial as well as anti-inflammatory and is recommended in the treatment of *Clostridium difficile* infections.
6. Omega-3 fatty acids have an anti-inflammatory action and are used in the management of active UC but not when the patient is in remission.
7. Anti-TNF drugs [e.g., adalimumab (Humira), infliximab (Remicade), and certolizumab (Cimzia)] reduce the synthesis of elevated TNF thus reducing inflammation. These drugs are indicated in severe refractory CD.
8. Newest therapy: Integrin antagonists (e.g., vedolizumab) inhibit leukocyte adhesion which inhibits inflammation. This drug is used to induce remission in UC (Gledhill and Bodger 2013).

Dental drug–drug interactions

- Mesalamine + NSAIDs [e.g., ibuprofen and naproxen sodium (Aleve)] may increase the risk of renal reactions. It is best to avoid both the drugs. Recommend or prescribe another analgesic.

Oral features

- The oral cavity especially the gingiva and buccal mucosa may appear to be swollen. In severe attacks, there may be oral candidiasis (thrush) and aphthous ulcerations. Oral aphthous ulcers occur in about 10% of patients with UC and usually will disappear when the disease is in remission.
- Patients may be deficient in vitamin B12 due to malabsorption. Orally this may manifest as glossitis, oral candidiasis, erythromatous mucositis, and pale oral mucosa (Pontes *et al.* 2009).
- Bleeding may be a problem due to abnormal liver function; evaluate the patient's CBC and liver function test profile before dental treatment (Ganda 2013).

Key notes

Key notes are the same as for CD. See the dental notes given earlier.
1. In addition, clindamycin should be prescribed with caution in patients with colitis or regional enteritis.

E. Diverticular disease

Clinical synopsis

Diverticular disease is divided into diverticulitis and diverticulosis. Diverticular disease is a condition where herniation of the mucosa of the colon occurs communicating with the muscle layer of the colon rather than the entire layers of the bowel wall, which is a congenital condition (Wilkins *et al.* 2013). It usually occurs in individuals over the age of 50 (Engstrom and Goosenberg 1999). Diverticular disease includes diverticulosis and diverticulitis, which are the same except that inflammation and diverticulum perforation are present in the latter and it is usually a more severe condition than diverticulosis. In the USA, by the age of 80, approximately 70% of individuals have diverticulosis (Shaheen *et al.* 2006).

Diverticulosis is usually asymptomatic, and individuals go through life maybe not even knowing that they have the disease, but some clinical signs and symptoms that can occur include constipation, abdominal pain in lower left abdomen, and flatulence. In about 15–40% of patients, there is an accompanied diverticular (lower GI) bleeding (Engstrom and Goosenberg 1999).

Dental features

There are no corresponding oral lesions associated with diverticular diseases.

Diagnosis/lab values

CT is recommended for the diagnosis of diverticulosis and determining the extent and severity of the disease. Colonoscopy is recommended 4–6 weeks after resolution of symptoms for patients with complicated disease (Wilkins *et al.* 2013).

Medications

Treatment for diverticular disease is based on the presence of symptoms (Boynton and Floch 2013). For uncomplicated or asymptomatic diverticular disease, the only treatment is to increase fiber in the diet, which increases the bulk of stool, lowers colonic pressure, and increases transit time through the colon (Engstrom and Goosenberg 1999). For symptomatic diverticulitis, additional therapy includes bowel rest, antibiotics, analgesics, anticholinergic and antispasmodic agents (for some patients), and surgery (for selected cases) (Boynton and Floch 2013).

In colonic diverticulosis, the content of the colon is static, which can ultimately cause a bacterial overgrowth and result in a chronic mucosal inflammation (Ventrucci *et al.* 1994; Colecchia *et al.* 2003; Boynton and Floch 2013). Rifaximin (Xifaxan), a poorly absorbed antibiotic, is recommended for this condition. Since it is poorly absorbed into the bloodstream, it remains in the GI tract longer which allows for its efficacy. Rifaximin can also be used in IBS. There are no documented dental drug interactions with rifaximin. Mesalamine is prescribed for the anti-inflammatory effect.

Dental drug–drug interactions

- Mesalamine+NSAIDs [e.g., ibuprofen and naproxen (Aleve)] may increase the risk of renal reactions. It is best to avoid both the drugs. Recommend or prescribe another analgesic.

Dental notes

1. Avoid prescribing codeine in patients with diverticular disease to prevent further constipation.
2. Avoid recommending or prescribing NSAIDs to patients taking mesalamine.

F. Acute pancreatitis

Clinical synopsis

Acute pancreatitis is primarily caused by alcoholism and alcohol abuse and gallstones. Other factors include genetic, autoimmune, damage or injury to the pancreas, Reyes syndrome, cystic fibrosis, hyperparathyroidism, and hypertriglyceridemia (Banks and Freeman 2006). Most cases are treated in the hospital and will probably not be seen in the dental office.

G. Celiac sprue

Clinical synopsis

Celiac sprue or celiac disease is a genetic/autoimmune disease of the small intestine.

Medications

None. Gluten-free diet is the only effective treatment.

Dental drug–drug interactions

Since treatment is solely through change of diet with a gluten-free diet, there are no drug–drug interactions relating to dentistry.

Dental notes

- There may be affected dental enamel defects in patients, especially children, with celiac disease. Enamel defects include tooth discoloration (white, yellow, or brown), enamel pitting, and a mottled or translucent appearance to the teeth. These tooth defects are usually seen on the incisors and molars. If all other systemic diseases are ruled out, referral to a gastroenterologist is recommended (Malahias *et al.* 2009)
- Celiac disease may be associated with an increased incidence of recurrent aphthous ulcers, atrophic glossitis, dry mouth, and squamous cell carcinoma.

H. Pseudomembranous colitis

Clinical synopsis

Clostridium difficile-associated diarrhea (CDAD) or pseudomembranous colitis has been reported with the use of nearly all antibacterial agents, not only clindamycin but almost any broad-spectrum antibiotic, and may range in severity from mild diarrhea to fatal colitis. CDAD may or may not be due to antibiotic usage. Antibiotic-associated diarrhea may be constant and watery/bloody diarrhea (new onset of more than three partially formed or watery stools per 24 h period). Treatment with antibacterial agents alters the normal flora of the colon leading to the overgrowth of *C. difficile*, which produces toxins A and B. There is an increased morbidity and mortality, as these infections can be refractory to antimicrobial therapy and usually require hospitalization. CDAD must be considered in all patients who present with diarrhea following antibiotic use; however, not all diarrhea associated with antibiotic use are positive for *C. difficile* (McFarland *et al.* 1994; Fordtran 2006). Careful medical history is necessary since CDAD has been reported to occur over 2 months after the administration of antibacterial agents. If CDAD is suspected or confirmed, the offending antibiotic is discontinued and appropriate fluid and electrolyte management, protein supplementation, antibiotics, or surgical intervention may be required. The most important first step in the treatment of mild cases is to immediately discontinue the antibiotic. Treatment of more severe cases involves the administration of antibiotics. The choice of initial antibiotic therapy depends on the severity of the presenting disease and whether the GI tract is functioning. Primary treatment will usually be with oral metronidazole or oral vancomycin; vancomycin is reserved to hospital patients who do not respond to metronidazole. Vancomycin is actually the only treatment that is FDA approved (Fekety 1997; Fordtran 2006; Gerding *et al.* 2008).

Lab values

Patients with *C. difficile* colitis often have elevated WBC counts and, in severe colitis, the WBC counts can be very high (20,000–40,000).

Management to prevent antibiotic-associated Clostridium difficile *infection*

- To help avoid antibiotic-related diarrhea, it is recommended to all patients to eat yogurt (containing live and active cultures such as Kefir, Dannon, or Yoplait). *Approximately 4–8 ounces of yogurt should be taken twice daily while on the antibiotic. Yogurt should be taken at least 2 h before or 2 h after the antibiotic.* If diarrhea does not stop, the patient should discontinue the antibiotic and call emergency services.
- The patient should not take antidiarrheal medications because it is advantageous to eliminate the bacterial toxins. *Pseudomembranous colitis symptoms could appear after a few doses or from 2 to 9 days or even months after the start of antibiotic therapy; it could happen at any time while taking the antibiotic.*
- If a patient has reported on their past medical history and hospitalization due to pseudomembranous colitis (*C. difficile*), caution should be used in the antibiotic prescribed. Most likely the patient has already been on antibiotics. In dentistry, in most cases, a broad-spectrum antibiotic is unnecessary; always start with a narrow-spectrum antibiotic such as penicillin V rather than amoxicillin in non–penicillin-allergic patients. Consultation with the patient's physician is recommended.

References

Ables, A.Z., Simon, I., & Melton, E.R. (2007) Update on *Helicobacter pylori* treatment. *American Family Physician*, **75 (3)**, 351–358.

American College of Gastroenterology, Hanauer, S.B., & Meyers, S. (1997) Keys to the diagnosis and treatment of Crohn's disease in adults, Arlington, VA. *American Journal of Gastroenterology*, **92**, 559–566.

American Gastroenterology Association (2002) American Gastroenterological Association medical position statement: irritable bowel syndrome. *Gastroenterology*, **123**, 2105.

Anand, P.S., Nandakumar, K., & Shenoy, K.T. (2006) Are dental plaque, poor oral hygiene, and periodontal disease associated with Helicobacter pylori infection? *Journal of Periodontology*, **77**, 692–698.

Banks, P.A. & Freeman, M.L. (2006) Practice parameters committee of the American College of Gastroenterology. Practice guidelines in acute pancreatitis. *American Journal of Gastroenterology*, **101**, 2379–2400.

Boynton, W. & Floch, M. (2013) New strategies for the management of diverticular disease: insights for the clinician. *Therapeutic Advances in Gastroenterology*, **6 (3)**, 205–213.

Chey, W.D. & Wong, B.C. (2007) Practice parameters Committee of the American College of Gastroenterology. American College of Gastroenterology guideline on the management of Helicobacter pylori infection. *American Journal of Gastroenterology*, **102**, 1808–1825.

Colecchia, A., Vestito, A, Pasqui, F. *et al.* (2007) Efficacy of long-term cyclic administration of the poorly absorbed antibiotic rifaximin in symptomatic, uncomplicated colonic diverticular disease. *World Journal of Gastroenterology*, **13**, 264–269.

Drossman, D.A., Whitehead, W.E., & Camilleri, M. (1997) Irritable bowel syndrome: a technical review for practice guideline development. *Gastroenterology*, **112**, 2120–2137.

Engstrom, P.F. & Goosenberg, E.B. (1999) *Diagnosis and Management of Bowel Diseases*. Professional Communications, INC., Philadelphia, PA.

Fekety, R. (1997) Guidelines for the diagnosis and management of Clostridium difficile-associated diarrhea and colitis. American College of Gastroenterology, Practice Parameters Committee. *American Journal of Gastroenterology*, **92**, 739–750.

Ferguson, K.A. & McCormack, D.G. (1993) Tuberculosis involving the oral cavity. *The Canadian Journal of Infectious Diseases*, **4**, 12–14.

Fordtran, J.S. (2006) Colitis due to *Clostridium difficile* toxins: underdiagnosed, highly virulent, and nosocomial. *Proceedings Baylor University Medical Center*, **19**, 3–12.

Ganda, K. (2013) *Dentist's Guide to Medical Conditions and Complications*, 2nd ed. Wiley-Blackwell, IA.

Gerding, D.N., Muto, C.A., & Owens, R.C. Jr. (2008) Treatment of *Clostridium difficile* infection. *Clinical Infectious Diseases*, **46 (Suppl. 1)**, S32–S42.

Gibson, N. & Ferguson, J.W. (2004) Steroid cover for dental patients on long-term steroid medication: proposed clinical guidelines based upon a critical review of the literature. *British Dental Journal*, **197**, 681–685.

Gledhill, T & Bodger, K. (2013) New and emerging treatments for ulcerative colitis: a focus on vedolizumab. *Biologics* **7**, 123–130.

Khalaf, M.W., Khader, R., Cobetto, G. *et al.* (2013) Risk of adrenal crisis in dental patients. *Results of a systematic search of the literature. Journal of the American Dental Association*, **144**, 152–160.

Kilmartin, C.M. (2002) Dental implications of Helicobacter pylori. *Journal of the Canadian Dental Association*, **68**, 489–493.

Kornbluth, A. & Sachar, D.B. (2010) Practice Parameters Committee of the American College of Gastroenterology. Ulcerative colitis practice guidelines in adults: American College Of Gastroenterology, Practice Parameters Committee. *American Journal of Gastroenterology*, **105**, 501.

Lichenstein, G.R. (2011) Inflammatory bowel disease. In: L. Goldman & A.L. Schafer (eds). *Cecil Medicine*, 24th ed, Chapter 143. Saunders Elsevier, Philadelphia, PA.

Lichenstein, G.R., Hanauer, S.B., & Sandborn, W.J. (2009) Practice Parameters Committee of American College of Gastroenterology. Management of Crohn's disease in adults. *American Journal of Gastroenterology*, **104**, 465–483.

Lui, Y., Yue, H., Li, A. *et al.* (2009) An epidemiologic study on the correlation between oral *Helicobacter pylori* and gastric *H. pylori*. *Current Microbiology*, **58**, 449–453.

Malahias, T., Cheng, J., Brar, P. *et al.* (2009) The association between celiac disease, dental enamel defects and aphthous ulcers in a United States cohort. *Journal of Clinical Gastroenterology*, **44**, 191–194.

Malfertheiner, P., Chan, F.K., & McColl, K.E. (2009) Peptic ulcer disease. *Lancet*, **374**, 1449–1461.

McFarland, L.V., Surawicz, C.M., Greenberg, R.N. *et al.* (1994) A randomized placebo-controlled trial of *Saccharomyces boulardii* in combination with standard antibiotics for *Clostridium difficile* disease. *Journal of the American Medical Association*, **271**, 1913–1918.

McGrath, E., Bardsley, P., & Basran, G. (2008) Black hairy tongue: what is your call? *Journal Canadian Medical Association MAJ*, **178**, 1137–1138.

Meurer, L.N. & Bower, D.J. (2002) Management of Helicobacter pylori infection. *American Family Physician*, **65 (7)**, 1327–1336.

Miller, C.S., Little, J.W., & Falace, D.A. (2001) Supplemental corticosteroids for dental patients with adrenal insufficiency. Reconsideration of the problem. *Journal of the American Dental Association*, **132**, 1570–1570.

Nanda, K.D.S., Mehta, A., & Nanda, J. (2011) A disguised tuberculosis in oral buccal mucosa. *Dental Research Journal (Isfahan)*, **8**, 154–159.

Nasrolahel, M., Maleki, I., & Emadian, O. (2003) *Helicobacter pylori* colonization in dental plaque and gastric infection. *Romanian Journal of Gastroenterology*, **12**, 293–299.

Olden, K.W. & Schuster, M.M. (1997) Irritable bowel syndrome. In: M. Feldman, B.F. Scharschmidt, & M.H. Sleisenger (eds). *Sleisenger and Fordtran's Gastrointestinal and Liver Disease: Pathophysiology, Diagnosis, and Management*, 6th ed. WB Saunders, Philadelphia, PA.

Peters, G.L., Rosselli, J.L., & Kerr, J.L. (2010) Overview of peptic ulcer disease. *U.S. Pharmacist*, **12**, 29–43.

Pontes, H.A., Neto, N.C., Ferreira, K.B. *et al.* (2009) Oral manifestations of vitamin B12 deficiency: a case report. *Journal of the Canadian Dental Association*, **75**, 533–537.

Quigley E. (2007) Probiotics in the management of colonic disorders. *Current Gastroenterology Reports* **9**, 434–440.

Ringel, Y. & Drossman, D.A. (2000) Toward a positive and comprehensive diagnosis of irritable bowel syndrome. *Medscape Gastroenterology* **2 (6)**, 1–8.

Shaheen N., Hansen R., Morgan D. *et al.* (2006) The burden of gastrointestinal and liver disease. *American Journal of Gastroenterology*, **101**, 2128–2138.

Singh, S, Graff, L.A., & Bernstein, C.N. (2009) Do NSAIDs, antibiotics, infections, or stress trigger flares in IBD? Etiological agents to treat IBD. *American Journal of Gastroenterology*, **104**, 1298–1313.

Thompson, W.G., Longstreth, G., Drossman, D.A. *et al.* (2000) Functional bowel disorder and functional abdominal pain. In: D.A. Drossman, E. Corazziari, N.J. Tally *et al.* (eds) *Rome II. The Functional Gastrointestinal Disorders. Diagnosis, Pathophysiology and Treatment: A Multinational Consensus*, 2nd ed, pp. 351–432. Degnon Associates, McLean, VA.

Ventrucci, M., Ferrieri, A., Bergami, R. *et al.* (1994) Evaluation of the effect of rifaximin in colon diverticular disease by means of lactulose hydrogen breath test. *Current Medical Research Opinion*, **13**, 202–206.

Wilkins, T., Embry, K., & George, R. (2013) Diagnosis and management of acute diverticulitis. *American Family Physicians*, **87**, 612–620.

Chapter 2

Medical conditions of the respiratory system

A. Respiratory diseases	17
a. Asthma	17
b. Chronic obstructive pulmonary diseases	23
c. Pulmonary tuberculosis	24
d. Obstructive sleep apnea	27
References	28

A. Respiratory diseases

The dental management of patients with severe pulmonary problems continues to be an important challenge to the dental practitioner. The majority of these patients can be treated safely; however, there are some important key points that must be addressed and followed (Hupp 2006).

a. Asthma

Condition synopsis

An expert panel of the National Institutes of Health National Asthma Education and Prevention Program Report 3 (National Heart, Lung, and Blood Institute 2007) defines asthma as a chronic inflammatory condition due to reversible bronchial constriction. Additionally, many inflammatory and immune cells and cellular elements are involved. Triggers for asthma include pollen, dander, food, dust, physical activity, respiratory infections, and some medications such as beta blockers. Signs and symptoms of an acute attack are diverse including wheezing, tightness in the chest, breathlessness (dyspnea), and coughing.

The three features of bronchial asthma include airway obstruction (constriction), hyperresponsiveness to stimuli, and inflammation. Asthma is ordinarily an allergic condition in which an extrinsic or intrinsic precipitating excitant is superposed upon a fundamental hypersensitivity. This hypersensitivity or increased bronchial responsiveness is the hallmark of asthma and causes inflammation and mucous hypersecretion. The airways become obstructed by the excess mucous and swelling of airway linings. This results in the contraction of the airway smooth muscle or bronchospasm, which leads to further airway obstruction and limitation of airflow. Inflammation of the airways causes the release of inflammatory mediators such as histamine, eosinophils, prostaglandins, leukocytes, and neutrophil chemotactic factors (e.g., leukotrienes), which are responsible for the maintenance of bronchial hyperreactivity and the production of high-viscosity mucous secretions. Loss of lung elasticity occurs due to air sac enlargement. Treatment to reverse this is more difficult and requires long-term, high-dose medications.

Asthma is classified according to the frequency of symptoms and the severity: intermittent or mild asthma, moderate persistent asthma, or severe persistent asthma. Treatment is based on this classification.

Diagnostic tests/lab results

The spirometry test is the most commonly used pulmonary function test performed to measure and monitor lung function (e.g., volume of flow of inhaled and exhaled air). There are no lab results that dental practitioners require from the patient's physician for dental treatment.

Medications prescribed

Besides controlling the triggers for asthma, different medications are also used depending on the severity of the condition. Medications for asthma are classified as rescue inhalers prescribed for an acute attack (bronchospasm) and long-term control medications, which mainly control airway inflammation.

In 2007, Expert Panel Report 3: Guidelines for the Diagnosis and Management of Asthma summarized the step-by-step treatment of asthma (Table 2.1) (Global Strategy for Asthma Management and Prevention, Global Initiative for Asthma, 2012). Step-by-step treatment refers to the method wherein the number and frequency of medications increase (step up) as the severity of asthma increases and decrease (step down) when asthma is under control. When starting treatment, the recommendation is to begin with the highest appropriate drug and step down as the patient improves. Inhaled medications are preferred because of their high therapeutic ratio, with high concentrations of the drug being delivered directly to the airways with few systemic adverse effects (Weinberg 2013).

Rescue medications are intended to cause bronchodilation and are used to prevent or treat an asthmatic attack. Rescue medications are primarily short-acting beta-agonists that cause dilation of the bronchial muscles and reverse the bronchospasm. It is recommended to prescribe a selective $beta_2$ receptor agonist, which targets the receptors on/in the lungs, to avoid any cardiac involvement that would occur if a nonselective beta-agonist were used ($beta_1$ receptors are found on/in the heart muscle, and stimulation of these receptors results in increased heart rate and contraction force). Since bronchospasm is mediated through the $beta_2$ receptors located on the bronchioles, it is rapidly relieved by inhaled bronchodilators or short-acting $beta_2$ agonists. Table 2.2 lists the commonly prescribed asthma medications.

The objective of long-term prevention medications is to reduce the airway inflammation; however, inflammation may be controlled, with anti-inflammatory corticosteroids, but not completely eradicated. Long-term control medications consist of inhaled corticosteroids (ICSs), long-acting beta-agonists, and leukotriene modifiers (Table 2.2).

Common dental drug–drug interactions *are reviewed in Box* 2.1.

Dental notes: Management of the asthmatic patient

(Steinbacher and Glick 2001; Coke and Karaki 2002; Sandor 2004; Weinberg *et al.* 2013)

1. Take a thorough medical history at each visit.
2. Ask the patient when their last attack was and what the trigger was. There can be concern regarding an increased frequency of emergency visits; patient is most likely uncontrolled and should be immediately seen by their physician, and any dental treatment should be postponed.

Table 2.1   Step-by-step treatment of asthma in adults (National Heart, Lung, and Blood Institute 2008, 2007; Global Strategy for Asthma Management and Prevention, Global Initiative for Asthma (GINA) 2010).

Long-term prevention		Rescue inhaler
Classification	Treatment of choice	Alternative treatment
Step 1 Intermittent asthma	No medications	No medications	Short-acting inhaled beta$_2$ agonist as needed for symptom control (bronchodilator) (e.g., albuterol)
Step 2 Mild persistent	Low-dose inhaled corticosteroid (ICS)	Sodium cromolyn, nedocromil, or a leukotriene receptor antagonist (LTRA)	Short-acting inhaled beta$_2$ agonist as needed for symptom control (bronchodilator) e.g., albuterol)
Step 3 Moderate persistent	Either a low-dose ICS plus a long-acting beta-agonist (combination medication preferred choice to improve compliance)	Inhaled a low-dose ICS plus either a leukotriene receptor agonist, theophylline, or zileuton (Zyflo)	Short-acting inhaled beta$_2$ agonist as needed for symptom control (bronchodilator) (e.g., albuterol)
Step 4 Moderate to severe persistent	Medium-dose ICS + long-acting β2 agonist or medium-dose ICS	Medium-dose ICS + either a leukotriene modifier or theophylline	Short-acting inhaled beta$_2$ agonist as needed for symptom control (bronchodilator) (e.g., albuterol)
Step 5 Severe persistent	Inhaled medium-dose corticosteroid plus a LTRA (combination therapy)	Inhaled medium-dose corticosteroid plus either a LTRA, theophylline, or zileuton	Short-acting inhaled beta$_2$ agonist as needed for symptom control (bronchodilator) (e.g., albuterol)
Step 6 Severe persistent	High-dose ICS plus a leukotriene receptor agonist plus an oral corticosteroid	—	Short-acting inhaled beta$_2$ agonist as needed for symptom control (bronchodilator) (e.g., albuterol)

Table 2.2   Rescue and long-term control medications for asthma (Weinberg *et al.* 2013).

Drug		
Rescue (quick-relief) medications	**Generic name**	**Brand name**
Short-acting β-agonists (inhalers)	• Albuterol Sulfate	Ventolin, Proventil, AccuNeb (nebulizer)
	• Pirbuterol	Maxair
	• Levalbuterol HCl	Xopenex
Systemic β-agonists	• Epinephrine 1:1000 (1 ml)	Adrenalin
Long-term control medications	**Generic name**	**Brand name**
Inhaled corticosteroids	• Beclomethasone propionate HFA	QVAR inhalation aerosol
	• Budesonide	Pulmicort Flexhaler
	• Flunisolide	Aerobid aerosol
	• Fluticasone propionate	Flovent Diskus/HFA
	• Fluticasone in combination with salmeterol (bronchodilator)	Advair Diskus/HFA
	• Mometasone	Asmanex
	• Mometasone in combination with formoterol (bronchodilator)	Dulera
	• Triamcinolone Acetonide	Azmacort
Systemic corticosteroids (also considered as first-line treatment for acute asthma exacerbations, especially severe exacerbations)	• Prednisone • Prednisolone	Many products Many products
Long-acting beta-agonists (LABA) (Note: The FDA has recommended that LABAs be used only in conjunction with inhaled steroids due to severe adverse effects of LABAs)	• Albuterol sulfate • Salmeterol xinafoate	VoSpire ER Serevent Diskus
Cromolyn and theophylline	• Cromolyn sodium • Theophylline	Intal Many products
Leukotriene modifiers	• Montelukast • Zafirlukast • Zileuton	Singulair Accolate Zyflo CR
Immunomodulators	• Omalizumab	Xolair

Box 2.1   Common Dental Drug–Drug Interactions.

Interactions with antibiotics:

- Erythromycin + **theophylline** = increased theophylline blood levels leading to toxicity due to inhibition of hepatic cytochrome enzyme metabolism. Avoid this combination and prescribe an alternative antibiotic.
- Azole antifungals (e.g., fluconazole) + **theophylline** = increased theophylline serum levels; monitor levels of theophylline. Consult with physician.
- Erythromycin + **albuterol** = may increase the risk of QT prolongation and cardiac arrhythmias (hypokalemia). Either monitor drug effects or modify treatment using an alternative antibiotic.
- Erythromycin + inhaled **levalbuterol** or **pirbuterol** = may increase the risk of QT prolongation and cardiac arrhythmias. Monitor therapy or use alternative antibiotic.
- Erythromycin + **zafirlukast, zileuton,** or **montelukast** = may increase blood levels of asthmatic drugs due to inhibition of hepatic metabolism. Caution is advised.
- Erythromycin + **systemic corticosteroids** = may increase the risk of QT prolongation and cardiac arrhythmias (hypokalemia). Either monitor drug effects or modify treatment using an alternative antibiotic.
- Azithromycin + **Dulera** = increased risk of QT prolongation and cardiac arrhythmias; monitor potassium levels. Best to prescribe an alternative antibiotic.
- Azithromycin/clarithromycin + **levalbuterol** or **pirbuterol** = may increase the risk of QT prolongation and cardiac arrhythmias. Monitor or use alterative antibiotic.
- Azithromycin + **systemic corticosteroids** = may increase the risk of QT prolongation and cardiac arrhythmias. Monitor or use alterative antibiotic.
- Clarithromycin + **Dulera** = may increase steroid levels and the risk of developing Cushing syndrome and adrenal suppression; may increase the risk of QT prolongation and cardiac arrhythmias. Best to prescribe an alternative antibiotic.
- Clarithromycin + **systemic corticosteroids** = may increase the risk of QT prolongation and cardiac arrhythmias. Monitor or use alterative antibiotic.

Interactions with aspirin and nonsteroidal anti-inflammatory drugs (NSAIDs):

- Samter's triad [also referred to as aspirin-exacerbated respiratory disease (AERD)] is a condition that occurs when aspirin or NSAIDs trigger an asthmatic attack in about 3–5% of individuals with asthma. Exacerbated respiratory disease is a clinical condition consisting of a combination of nasal polyps, chronic hypertrophic eosinophilic sinusitis, asthma, and sensitivity to any medication that inhibits cyclooxygenase-1 enzymes, namely, aspirin and other NSAIDs (Lee and Stevenson 2011). AERD affects approximately 0.3–0.9% of the general population; however, the prevalence rises to 10–20% in asthmatics and up to 30–40% in asthmatics with nasal polyps (Berges-Gimeno *et al.* 2002). Symptoms that usually appear within 30 min to 3 h after taking aspirin or NSAIDs include bronchoconstriction and nasal congestion. It is probably best to avoid recommending or prescribing NSAIDs and aspirin to asthmatic patients (Samter and Beers 1968; Berges-Gimeno *et al.* 2002; Fahrenholz 2003; Lee and Stevenson 2011).

Interactions with narcotics:

- Codeine may precipitate an asthmatic attack in an asthmatic due to respiratory depression; codeine should not be taken if the patient is having an asthmatic attack.

Interactions with epinephrine:

- Local anesthetics that contain epinephrine as the vasoconstrictor require an antioxidant to prevent its breakdown. This antioxidant is sodium metabisulfite, which may induce allergic

(continued)

asthma in sulfite-susceptible patients. These patients may also be sensitive to sulfites present in red wine (during fermentation) and other foods to prevent microbial spoilage (25–200 mg sulfites) (Perusse *et al.* 1992). This reaction may have a small incidence of occurrence in nonsteroid-dependent asthmatics because the amount of sodium metabisulfite in local anesthetics is relatively low (e.g., 0.15–2.0 mg/mL) and may not cause this reaction; however, the practitioner must be prudent that it is still a possibility especially in asthmatics taking steroid medications (Perusse *et al.* 1992; Budenz 2008). Otherwise, there are no interactions with asthmatic medications and epinephrine. It must be emphasized that epinephrine in low doses used in dentistry primarily effects beta$_2$ adrenergic receptors. Stimulation of beta$_2$ receptors results in bronchodilation and vasodilation of skeletal muscle and organs. In fact, epinephrine 1:1000 solution (1/2 to 1 cc) is used in the treatment of an immediate asthmatic attack to reverse the bronchospasm.

3. The primary concern with asthmatic dental patients is to prevent an acute asthmatic attack during dental treatment. Pain and stress are two factors that could precipitate an asthmatic attack. Asking the patient when the last attack was and the precipitating factor is important and should be documented in the chart. Being aware of how to handle a patient having an attack is of utmost importance.

4. Before starting dental treatment, the severity of the patient's asthma should be determined. Dental treatment in a patient with mild intermittent asthma can usually be started, but the patient with severe and frequent bronchospasms most likely will require a medical consult before dental treatment (Eversole 2002).

5. If the patient is symptomatic (e.g., wheezing and coughing), they are not considered controlled and elective dental treatment should be postponed until they are well controlled.

6. Sedative drugs with anticholinergic effects should not be prescribed to an asthmatic patient. Additionally, narcotics can cause an attack.

7. If the patient is prescribed an inhaler, it must be within the reach of the patient during dental treatment. If the patient forgot the inhaler at home, the inhaler from the emergency kit can be placed within reach or it is probably best to postpone treatment or place your own emergency kit inhaler within reach). A beta$_2$ agonist bronchodilator inhaler is used for an acute attack.

8. Have a current emergency kit with oxygen and bronchodilator available.

9. Patients with severe asthma may be taking a corticosteroid. A recent article states that the risk of adrenal crisis in dental patients is rare (Khalaf *et al.* 2013). Patients taking long-term systemic corticosteroids should be properly monitored and proper preventive measures must be followed. ICSs are not absorbed systemically into the bloodstream, so there is no worry about adrenal crisis. Medical literature has suggested that it may be most appropriate to take systemic corticosteroids in the morning as a daily dose when endogenous cortisol is at its peak, which reduces the negative feedback effect on the hypothalamic–pituitary–adrenal axis (Lewis and Cochrane 1986). Also, patients on corticosteroids may be more prone to developing an infection.

10. Patients on long-term systemic corticosteroids are at an increased risk of diabetes mellitus. Steroid-induced diabetic dental patients should be monitored carefully for periodontal diseases and dental caries.

11. Consider nitrous oxide in patients with mild to moderate asthma. Nitrous oxide is a bronchodilator that is helpful in these patients; however, *nitrous oxide is contraindicated in severe asthma*. In any event, always obtain a physician's consult before administering nitrous oxide.

12. Use local anesthetics with epinephrine cautiously.

13. Anything in the dental office including sealants, methyl methacrylate, suction tips, and aerosol irritants from the handpiece can precipitate an attack (Marez *et al.* 1993; Harrel 2003; Harrel and Molinari 2004). Make sure the rubber dam is positioned effectively to help avoid harmful irritants.

14. Be careful when using the ultrasonic devices; aerosols can be irritants (Harrel *et al.* 1998).
15. Avoid having the patient lying in supine position for long periods of time, as it results in more trouble for breathing.
16. Many asthmatic medications (e.g., anticholinergics and bronchodilator inhalers) can cause xerostomia. Monitor patient for dental caries and periodontal disease. Increasing water intake or the use of salivary substitutes and fluoride application can be helpful.
17. To avoid the development of oral candidiasis, especially in the oropharynx, from the use of ICSs, instruct patients to rinse and brush teeth after use.
18. Reinforce oral hygiene care to help prevent gingivitis.
19. Avoid aspirin and nonsteroidal anti-inflammatory drugs (NSAIDs) in sensitive patients: Always interview your patient thoroughly about allergies. For example, a patient with asthma who is allergic to aspirin may experience an acute bronchospasm after taking an NSAID such as ibuprofen (Advil, Nuprin) or naproxen sodium (Aleve). This reaction is called Samter's triad, and it is a condition consisting of asthma, aspirin sensitivity, and nasal polyps (Samter and Beers 1968). This occurs because NSAIDs block the production of prostaglandins, allowing arachidonic acid cascade to shut entirely the production of leukotrienes, chemical substances involved in the inflammatory response, resulting in severe allergy-like symptoms.
20. Acetaminophen is the analgesic of choice in asthmatic patients. Caution should be taken with the maximum amount used.

b. Chronic obstructive pulmonary diseases

Condition synopsis

Chronic obstructive pulmonary diseases (COPDs) comprises bronchitis and emphysema that cause chronic obstruction of airflow and irreversible loss of lung function. Chronic bronchitis is irritation and inflammation in the bronchi which is characterized by excessive mucous resulting in a productive cough. Bronchitis can be acute or chronic, especially in smokers, lasting years.

Emphysema is an irreversible destruction of the elastic fibers of the alveolar walls with dilation of air spaces that is characterized by shortness of breath or breathlessness. Other symptoms in emphysema include expiratory wheezing and a "smokers" dry cough. Treatment may slow the progression of emphysema, but the damage is permanent. Some patients may have an oxygen tank. Smoking cessation therapy should be a part of dental treatment.

Diagnostic tests/lab results

There are no important lab results that are necessary to know before treating a patient with COPD. Emphysema is diagnosed by chest X-ray and CT scan. Blood tests determine lung performance in transferring oxygen into and removing carbon dioxide from the bloodstream. Also, lung functioning tests are used. The results of these tests are not important for dental procedures.

Medications prescribed

There is no cure for COPD. Medication management consists of a variety of step-by-step treatment regimens similar to those for asthma (bronchodilators and inhaled steroids) and over-the-counter expectorant medicines. Other drugs used for the long-term control of COPD include the following:

- Formoterol fumarate inhalation solution (Perforomist): Long-term control of COPD.
- Arformoterol tartrate inhalation solution (Brovana): To prevent bronchoconstriction (bronchospasm) in patients with COPD.
- Formoterol + budesonide (Symbicort): To prevent bronchospasm in patients with COPD.

Dental drug interactions

In addition to the drug interactions listed above,

- Azithromycin + **formoterol, arformoterol** may increase the risk of QT prolongation and cardiac arrhythmias. Monitor or use alterative antibiotic.

Dental notes: Management of the COPD patient

1. Patients with chronic obstructive respiratory disease already have compromised respiratory function, making it of upmost importance that the dental practitioner takes all precautions to prevent further depression. This means that any drugs that cause respiratory depression such as narcotics and barbiturates should not be prescribed to these patients.
2. At every visit, ask the patient about medications; this should be done for all patients.
3. At every visit, assess the patient's breathing pattern. If the patient presents with an upper respiratory infection, breathlessness at rest (dyspnea), productive cough, or looks cyanotic, postpone any elective dental treatment.
4. There are no contraindications for the use of dental therapeutic doses of local anesthetics in these patients.
5. Patients with emphysema may have comorbidities including hypertension and heart failure.
6. Patients with emphysema and low oxygen levels may come to the dental office with an oxygen tank; have adequate space in the dental unit.
7. In smokers, recommend a smoking cessation program.
8. Patients with COPD and a compromised airway may have difficulty breathing in a supine position. To avoid orthopnea, it is recommended to avoid the supine position if the patient is uncomfortable. Sit the patient in an upright position or semi-supine position. Oxygen should be made readily available; however, forcing oxygen into a patient with emphysema may cause respiratory arrest (Eversole 2002). If it is necessary to administer oxygen, use a low flow rate of ≤3 L/min.
9. General anesthetic must be used with caution in COPD patients, especially moderate to severe disease because of respiratory depression (Eversole 2002).
10. Nitrous oxide with low oxygen can be used in mild to moderate emphysema but not in severe cases; consult with physician.
11. Many COPD medications (e.g., anticholinergerics and bronchodilator inhalers) can cause xerostomia. Monitor patient for dental caries and periodontal disease. Increasing water intake or the use of salivary substitutes and fluoride application can be helpful.
12. To avoid the development of oral candidiasis, including the oropharynx, from the use of ICSs, instruct patients to rinse and brush teeth after use.

c. Pulmonary tuberculosis

Clinical synopsis

Tuberculosis (TB) is a bacterial infection caused by *Mycobacterium tuberculosis (MTB)*, a tubercle bacillus that can affect any organ in the body including the larynx, brain, kidneys, lymph nodes but most commonly the lungs. TB is contracted by aerosol (e.g., coughing and sneezing) spread during close contact with an infected person. MTB can remain aerosolized for up to 8 h and is slow growing. A person may be exposed to MTB but may not show clinical signs of the disease (Blumberg *et al.* 2005). This primary infection can become quiescent and becomes a secondary active infection when there is reinfection or reactivation of the tubercle bacillus (Diaz-Guzma 2001; Weinberg *et al.* 2013; Araujo and Andreana

2002). In 2011, 8.7 million new cases of active TB were diagnosed worldwide. Thirteen percent of these cases involved coinfection with the human immunodeficiency virus (HIV) (Zumla *et al.* 2013).

Many times, just from the patient's symptoms, TB can be suspected. About 4–6 weeks after the first contact with the bacillus, symptoms including fever, chills, gastrointestinal upset, loss of appetite, night sweats, and later a productive cough producing odorless, green-yellow sputum with blood (hemoptysis) may develop. If active TB is suspected, all elective dental treatment should be postponed, and the patient should be referred to a physician or hospital immediately.

Diagnostic tests/lab results

Screening for TB is done using the tuberculin skin test, which indicates only exposure to the infection and does not differentiate between infection (the presence of organisms; normal chest X-ray and no symptoms) and actual disease. The tuberculin skin test is based on a skin reaction to the intradermal injection of purified protein derivative (PPD) tuberculin, which is a protein fraction of the bacillus. Latent infection can also be diagnosed with an interferon-gamma release assay (Zumla *et al.* 2013). In the USA, a sputum culture is recommended for diagnosing active TB.

If a patient has a positive PPD skin test, they should have a subsequent chest X-ray. If the X-ray is negative, the individual may have just been exposed to the bacteria (past exposure) and not be infectious. A definitive diagnosis of TB requires sputum culture; however, typical signs and symptoms with a positive chest X-ray and positive PPD are enough to begin drug therapy.

Medications prescribed

Patients with active TB will be on a long-term regimen of antibiotics and most likely be in the hospital; however, there are many people that have active TB and are not being treated due to either nonadherence to the medications or failure to report to a physician. Elective dental treatment should be postponed in any patient with active TB.

Patients that have only the primary *latent* infection (positive PPD, no symptoms, and negative chest X-ray) will be on a prophylaxis drug regimen (Table 2.3). Treatment of those with latent TB infection helps eliminate a large reservoir of individuals at risk for progression to TB and the spread of the disease. The goals of antituberculosis drug therapy are to cure the disease without relapse, prevent death, stop the spread of the disease, and prevent the emergence of drug-resistant TB. To help avoid the development of resistance, more than one drug is used to kill the tubercle bacilli rapidly.

Table 2.3 Drug regimens for latent tuberculosis infection (prophylaxis): Patients with positive purified protein derivative but negative chest X-ray and no symptoms; patients were exposed but did not develop the infection (Munsiff *et al.* 2005).

Drug	Adverse side effects	Notes
Isoniazid	Hepatitis, elevated liver enzymes, neuropathy, and CNS	The most effective drug for TB therapy. Supplemental vitamin B6 may reduce peripheral and CNS effects. Obtain serum liver enzyme levels.
Rifampin (rifapentine)	Hepatitis, fever, thrombocytopenia, flu-like syndrome, and orange discoloration of secretions, urine, tears, and contact lenses	Liver toxicity is the most significant adverse effect, so it is important to obtain serum liver enzyme levels.

Table 2.4   Drug regimens for active tuberculosis (Two or more drugs are needed to treat active TB to reduce emergence of resistant bacteria).

Initial phase (four-drug regimen) Isoniazid Rifampin Pyrazinamide Ethambutol
Continuous phase Isoniazid Rifampin

According to the NYC Department of Health & Mental Hygiene, Bureau of Tuberculosis Control, these drugs are recommended to be taken for 9 months (Munsiff *et al.* 2005; Zumla *et al.* 2013). Isoniazid is the drug of choice for the treatment of latent TB infection; however, recently literature has suggested a combination of isoniazid and rifampin results in less adverse reactions (Zumla *et al.* 2013). Table 2.4 lists drugs used in the treatment of *active* TB infection (Munsiff *et al.* 2005; Blumberg *et al.* 2005).

Common dental drug–drug interactions

Interactions with analgesics:
- Acetaminophen + **isoniazid** = increased risk of hepatotoxicity; not contraindicated but caution is advised.

Interactions with antibiotics:
- Clarithromycin and erythromycin + **isoniazid** = may increase clarithromycin levels and there is increased risk for prolongation of QT interval and arrhythmias; caution advised —best to use azithromycin if a macrolide is recommended.

Interactions with epinephrine
- There are no interactions with epinephrine.

Dental notes

1. Get a thorough medical history including medication conditions (e.g., HIV infection, IV drug abuser, and people working or living in close quarters) that increase the risk for TB.
2. Be aware of any past TB infection and treatments.
3. In certain states (e.g., New York), any person that has been diagnosed with active TB and treated must be recorded with the health department and before treatment of these patients, a copy of the letter from the health department should be required before dental treatment is started.
4. Adults presenting to the dental office who are currently taking isoniazid should have a physician's consultation regarding liver function tests. Some patients will develop hepatitis. Liver function tests should be checked every month.
5. Patients with active TB should not have elective dental treatment. Consultation with the patient's physician is necessary.
6. If emergency treatment is necessary for a patient suspected of having or who has been diagnosed with active TB, care should be provided in a facility such as a hospital with airborne infection

isolation and fit-tested disposable N-95 respirators; standard surgical face masks do not provide enough protection (Robbins 2009).

7. Patients with positive PPD and positive chest X-ray; if asymptomatic and finished isoniazid course and follow-up with negative X-ray, then treat as normal.

8. Otherwise, standard precautions should be taken including the use of aerosols.

9. A past history of active TB requires a consultation with the physician.

10. There is an association between obstructive sleep apnea and nonarteritic anterior ischemic optic neuropathy. If necessary, refer patient to an ophthalmologist (Archer & Pepin 2013).

d. Obstructive sleep apnea

Clinical synopsis

Obstructive sleep apnea (OSA), which is common in both children and adults, is defined as repeated episodes of airway obstruction for more than 10 seconds during sleep which causes gaps in breathing (Verma *et al.* 2010).

Sleep apnea should be suspected in patients who are obese, hypertensive, habitual snorers, hypersomnolent, and have adenotonsillar hypertrophy (in children). In a primary care setting, patients with a high risk of sleep apnea were those who met two of the following three criteria: snoring, persistent daytime sleepiness or drowsiness while driving, and obesity or hypertension. Additionally, the patient may have diabetes or gastroesophageal reflux disease (Kratt 2010).

Medications prescribed

There are no medications for the treatment of OSA. Treatment of sleep apnea is empirical consisting of continuous positive airway pressure therapy with a specific device (treatment of choice), surgery (for severe cases), changing sleeping position, avoiding alcohol, and weight loss if overweight (Flemons 2002). The American Academy of Sleep Medicine (AAOSM) recommends oral appliances for use in patients with primary snoring and mild to moderate OSA (Padma *et al.* 2007). There are two types of devices: mandibular advancement appliance (moves mandible to an anterior and forward position to aid in patency of the airway) and tongue-retaining devices (move the tongue forward) (National Heart, Lung and Blood Institute 1995).

Dental notes

1. The dental practitioner should do an intra- and extraoral examination (including the size of the tongue, tonsils, and adenoids), which would help to determine if the patient has OSA.

2. The AAOSM has stated that therapeutic nonsurgical interventions for OSA with oral appliances are within the scope of dentistry (Padma *et al.* 2007).

3. Patients with OSA may have xerostomia, TMJ problems, periodontal problems, bruxism, and narrow palates with crowding of anterior teeth (usually in children) (Bencome and Castellanos 2011).

4. OSA may also be suspected in a patient that falls asleep in the dental chair or in the waiting room due to sleepiness and lack of sleep (Dort 2003).

5. Avoid the supine position in the dental chair.

6. In certain states (e.g., New York), a sleep study by a physician is necessary for diagnosis before a dentist can treat OSA.

7. Every dentist should do active screening for sleep apnea.

8. Never make snore appliance without prior testing for sleep apnea.

References

Araujo, M.W. & Andreana, S. (2002) Risk and prevention of transmission of infectious diseases in dentistry. *Quintessence International*, **33**, 376–382.

Archer, E.L. & Pepin, S. (2013) Obstructive sleep apnea and nonarteritic anterior ischemic optic neuropathy: evidence for an association. *Journal of Clinical Sleep Medicine*, **9**(6):613–618.

Bencome, J. & Castellanos, S. (2011) Sleep apnea syndrome. *Registered Dental Hygienist*, **31**, 76–77, 115.

Berges-Gimeno, M.P., Simon, R.A., & Stevenson, D.D. (2002) The natural history and clinical characteristics of aspirin-exacerbated respiratory disease. *Annals of Allergy Asthma Immunology*, **89**, 474–478.

Blumberg, H.M., Leonard Jr., M.K., & Jasmer, R.M. (2005) Update on the treatment of tuberculosis and latent tuberculosis infection. *Journal of the American Medical Association*, **293**, 2776–2784.

Budenz, A.W. (2008) Local anesthetics and medically compromised patients. *Journal of the California Dental Association*, **28**, 611–619.

Coke, J.M. & Karaki, D.T. (2002) The asthma patient and dental management. *General Dentistry*, **50**, 504–507.

Diaz-Guzman, L.M. (2001) Management of the dental patient with pulmonary tuberculosis. *Medicina Oral*, **6**, 124–134.

Dort, L.C. (2003) When patients fall asleep in the dental chair—a wake-up call for dentists. *Journal of the Canadian Dental Association*, **69**, 14–15.

Dye, C., Watt, C.J., Bleed, D.M. *et al.* (2005) Evolution of tuberculosis control and prospects for reducing tuberculosis incidence, prevalence, and deaths globally. *Journal of the American Medical Association*, **227**, 1794–2801.

Eversole, L.R. (2002) Respiratory diseases. In: S. Silverman, L.E. Eversole, E.L. Truelove (eds). *Essentials of Oral Medicine*. Becker, Inc., Ontario.

Fahrenholz, J.M. (2003) Natural history and clinical features of aspirin-exacerbated respiratory disease. *Clinical Reviews of Allergy and Immunology*, **24**, 113–124.

Flemons, W.W. (2002) Obstructive sleep apnea. *The New England Journal of Medicine*, **347**, 498–504.

Global Strategy for Asthma Management and Prevention, Global Initiative for Asthma (GINA) (2012) http://www.ginasthma.org [accessed April 10, 2013].

Harrel, S.K. (2003) Contaminated dental aerosols: the risks and implications for dental hygienists. *Dimensions of Dental Hygiene*, **1 (6)**, 16–20.

Harrel, S.K. & Molinari, J. (2004) Aerosols and splatter in dentistry: a brief review of the literature and infection control implications. *The Journal of the American Dental Association*, **135**, 429–437.

Harrel, S.K., Barnes, J.B., & Rivera-Hidalgo, F. (1998) Aerosol and splatter contamination from the operative site during ultrasonic scaling. *Journal of American Dental Association*, **129**, 1241–1249.

Hupp, W.S. (2006) Dental management of patients with obstructive pulmonary disease. *Dental Clinics of North America*, **50**, 513–527.

Khalaf, M.W., Khader, R., Cobetto, G. *et al.* (2013) Risk of adrenal crisis in dental patients. *Journal of the American Dental Association*, **144 (2)**, 152–160.

Kratt, M. (2010) The relationship between sleep apnea and dentistry. *Dentistry IQ Network*. http://www.dentistryiq.com/articles/2010/06/the-relationship-between.html [accessed April 10, 2013].

Lee, R.U. & Stevenson, D.D. (2011) Aspirin-exacerbated respiratory disease: evaluation and management. *Allergy Asthma and Immunology Research*, **3**, 3–10.

Lewis, L.D. & Cochrane, G.M. (1986) Systemic steroids in chronic severe asthma. *British Medical Journal*, **292**, 1289.

Lozano, A.C., Sarrión Perez, M.G., & Esteve, C.G. (2011): Dental considerations in patients with respiratory problems. *Journal Clinical Experimental Dentistry*, **3 (3)**, e222–e227.

Marez, T., Edmé, T.L., Boulenguez, C. *et al.* (1993) Bronchial symptoms and respiratory function in workers exposed to methylmethacrylate. *British Journal of Indian Medicine*, **50**, 894–897.

Munsiff, S., Nilsen, D., & Dworkin F. (2005) Guidelines for Testing and Treatment of Latent Tuberculosis Infection. NYC Department of Health & Mental Hygiene, Bureau of Tuberculosis Control.

National Heart, Lung and Blood Institute (1995) *Sleep Apnea. Is Your Patient at Risk*. NIH publication 95-3803. National Institute of Health (NIH), Washington, DC.

National Heart, Lung, and Blood Institute (2007) National Asthma Education and Prevention Program: Expert panel report III: Guidelines for the diagnosis and management of asthma. National Heart, Lung, and Blood Institute, Bethesda, MD, July 2007. (NIH publication no. 08-4051). www.nhlbi.nih.gov/guidelines/asthma/asthgdln.htm [accessed April 10, 2013).

National Heart, Lung, and Blood Institute (2008) *Global Strategy for Asthma Management and Prevention*. NIH Publication, Washington, DC.

Padma, A., Ramakrishnan, N., & Narayanan, V. (2007) Management of obstructive sleep apnea: a dental perspective. *Indian Journal of Dental Research* **18**, 201–209.

Perusse, R., Goulet, J.P., & Turcotte, J.-Y. (1992) Contraindications to vasoconstrictors in dentistry: Part II. *Oral Surgery Oral Medicine Oral Pathology*, **74**, 687–691.

Robbins, M.L. (2009) Tuberculosis in your dental practice: can it happen? *Journal of the Tennessee Dental Association*, **89**, 22–25.

Samter, M. & Beers, R.F., Jr. (1968) Intolerance to aspirin. Clinical studies and consideration of its pathogenesis. *Annals of Internal Medicine*, **68**, 975.

Sandor, G. (2004) Point of care. *Journal of the Canadian Dental Association*, **70** (7), 481–482.

Steinbacher, D.M. & Glick, M. (2001) The dental patient with asthma. *An update and oral health consideration. Journal of the American Dental Association*, **132** (9), 1229–1239.

Verma, S.K., Maheshwari, S., Kumar, N. *et al.* (2010) Role of oral health professional in pediatric obstructive sleep apnea. *National Journal of Maxillofacial Surgery*, **1**, 35–40.

Weinberg, M.A. (2013) Antibacterial agents. In: M.A. Weinberg, C. Westphal Tiele, & J. Fine (eds). *Oral Pharmacology*, pp. 110–139. Pearson Publications, Upper Saddle River.

Weinberg, M.A., Westphal Thiele, C., & Fine, J.B. (2013) Respiratory drugs. In: M.A. Weinberg, C. Westphal Tiele, & J. Fine (eds). *Oral Pharmacology*. Pearson Publications, Upper Saddle River, NJ.

Zumla, A., Raviglione, M., Hafner, R. *et al.* (2013) Current concepts of tuberculosis. *The New England Journal of Medicine*, **368**, 745–755.

Chapter 3

Disorders of the urinary system

A. Acute renal injury and chronic kidney disease	30
B. Kidney dialysis	37
C. Kidney transplant	39
D. Polycystic kidney disease	42
E. Benign prostatic hypertrophy	42
References	43

A. Acute renal injury and chronic kidney disease

Clinical synopsis

It should be noted that there has been a change in medical terminology of kidney diseases. Acute renal failure has been changed to acute renal injury and chronic renal failure to chronic kidney disease (CKD) because patients may have kidney insufficiency but not failure (Lameire *et al.* 2005; Zhang *et al.* 2005). Renal injury occurs when there is a decreased blood flow to the kidneys from severe dehydration, shock, kidney disease, or trauma.

Acute kidney disease versus CKD is determined according to how quick the rise in serum creatinine concentration or glomerular filtration rate (GFR) occurs (Levey and Coresh 2012). Acute renal disease is the sudden inability of both kidneys to perform their function. It is a serious medical condition resulting in a reduction or cessation of urine flow.

CKD, characterized as kidney damage or decreased kidney function and occurring for 3 months or more with or without decreased GFR, is a life-threatening condition with a poorer prognosis than acute renal injury (Eckardt *et al.* 2009). Individuals with CKD with loss of kidney function may have numerous comorbidities including diabetes, hypertension, anemia, hyperlipidemia, glomerulonephritis, secondary hyperparathyroidism, and electrolyte imbalances (Brockmann and Badr, 2010; Álamo *et al.* 2011; http://www.kdigo.org/clinical_practice_guidelines/pdf/CKD/KDIGO_2012_CKD_GL.pdf). The two most common conditions that cause CKD/ end-stage renal disease (ESRD) are diabetes and hypertension and are associated with a high death rate from cardiovascular disease (Kasiske and Cosio 2003; Johnson *et al.* 2004). Dental patients should be monitored in the dental office for early signs of cardiovascular disease. The patient's blood pressure must be regularly taken.

The Dentist's Quick Guide to Medical Conditions, First Edition. Mea A. Weinberg, Stuart L. Segelnick, Joseph S. Insler, with Samuel Kramer.
© 2015 John Wiley & Sons, Inc. Published 2015 by John Wiley & Sons, Inc.

Table 3.1 Chronic kidney disease: severity and staging (National Kidney Foundation, https://www.kidney.org/professionals/KDOQI/guidelines_commentaries).

Stage	Severity	Glomerular filtration rate (GFR) (ml/min/1.73 mm²)	Blood creatinine (mg/dl)
Stage 1	Kidney damage with normal or increased GFR	≥90	0.5–1.3
Stage 2	Mild	60–89	1.7–3.4
Stage 3	Moderate	30–59	3.4–7.9
Stage 4	Severe	15–29	>7.9
Stage 5	Kidney failure	<15 (or dialysis)	>7.9

Eventually, CKD, which is irreversible, may result in ESRD with complete or almost complete kidney failure; however, it could take many years after the development of CKD before ESRD occurs. ESRD does not describe renal failure or the severity of the disease but rather ESRD is an administrative/insurance term designating that the CKD patient is at the point where they require either dialysis or renal transplantation (Johnson *et al.* 2004). The kidneys function to help to maintain the acid–base balance allowing it to be kept in equilibrium, which maintains the pH of the arterial blood at about 7.4. In addition, the kidneys are important in excreting metabolic waste products. When the kidneys cannot effectively function in the excretion of waste products, the nephrons lose function with the development of uremia and uremic bleeding (increased bleeding due to decreased function of platelets) (Brockmann and Badr 2010). http://www.kdigo.org/clinical_practice_guidelines/pdf/CKD/KDIGO_2012_CKD_GL.pdf). In addition, the immune system is impaired as well, increasing the risk of infection (Sulejmanagic *et al.* 2005). All these features are important when treating the dental patient with kidney disease.

The appearance of signs and symptoms depends on the extent and duration of renal insufficiency. Symptoms usually do not appear until complications occur. The degree and severity of kidney dysfunction/disease are generally reflected in the decline of GFR. A medical consult must be obtained before commencing dental therapy. It should not be assumed that all patients with earlier stages of CKD will likely progress to ESRD. Stages 1 through 3 CKD are present in ≥10% of the population (Gansevoort and de Jong 2009). Table 3.1 describes the classification and staging of chronic renal disease based on GFR.

Uremia, a complication of kidney diseases, occurs when urea and other waste products accumulate in the body when the kidneys cannot efficiently eliminate them. With high serum levels of urea, many complications occur including abnormal bleeding, heart arrhythmias, seizures, and pleural effusion. This uremic syndrome has been linked to further complications in these patients including leukopenia, insulin resistance, and decreased platelet function (Caster *et al.* 2010).

Secondary hyperparathyroidism (high parathyroid hormone [PTH]), which occurs in most patients with CKD, starts early in the disease process and steadily progresses as GFR declines (Al-Badr and Martin 2008). Vitamin D comes from the diet and sunlight. Sunlight converts 7-dehydrocholesterol to vitamin D3 (cholecalciferol) (Dusso *et al.* 2005; Holick 2005). Cholecalciferol can also be obtained naturally from diet. Vitamin D–binding protein carries vitamin D3 to the liver, which converts it to 25-hydroxy vitamin D (calcidiol), the major circulating form of vitamin D that is measured by routine laboratory testing (Kestenbaum 2008). The enzyme 1-alpha hydroxylase, which is expressed primarily in the proximal tubule of the kidney, then converts 25-hydroxy vitamin D to 1,25-dihydroxy vitamin D (calcitriol), the biologically active form of the molecule (Al-Badr and Martin 2008; Kestenbaum 2008). PTH stimulates 1-alpha hydroxylase activity, whereas phosphate and fibroblast growth factor 23 inhibit activity (Al-Badr and Martin 2008; Kestenbaum 2008).

The failing kidney cannot maintain levels of 1,25-dihydroxy vitamin D despite increasing levels of PTH resulting in abnormalities in bone and mineral metabolism. Treatment consists of administration of activated vitamin D and monitoring of serum calcium and phosphate levels (Andress 2005; Holick 2005; Al-Badr and Martin 2008; Kestenbaum 2008).

Diagnostic tests/lab results

Measurement of the GFR is used to assess the severity of renal disease and shows the ability of the kidney to clear creatinine, a nitrogenous waste blood product produced by the muscles. The plasma concentration of creatinine depends on the rate of excretion by the kidneys. When the GFR is impaired, the serum creatinine level increases while the creatinine clearance (CrCl) rate decreases. Essentially, the assessment of renal function is done by determining the GFR, via measurement of the serum creatinine concentration. CrCl is defined as the rate of removal of creatinine from the blood and measures the filtering capacity of the kidneys. Because mild and moderate kidney injury is poorly diagnosed from serum creatinine alone, *GFR is a more accurate method to measure how efficiently your kidneys filter waste from the blood* and must be obtained from the patient's physician before any medications are prescribed in the dental office. Recent research has found that serum cystatin C, a new kidney function marker, alone or in combination with estimated GFR can estimate kidney function and may be important in predicting mortality in patients with CKD/ESRD (Rule and Glassock 2013; Shlipak *et al.* 2013). Table 3.2 lists specific medications that the dentist may prescribe to a patient with chronic renal disease. Drug prescribing may be altered in patients with compromised liver function. As such, either the dosage or the dosing interval of the drug may need to be adjusted according to the patient's most recent GFR values. Additionally, it is necessary to obtain complete blood count (CBC) with coagulation tests before dental treatment.

Blood urea nitrogen, which is a component of the waste products of protein metabolism removed by the kidneys, represents kidney function and increases in progressive kidney failure.

Oral features of CKD

Up to 90% of patients with CKD will show some oral signs/symptoms affecting the soft tissues and bone (Álamo *et al.* 2011). The most commonly reported oral symptoms in CKD patients are xerostomia, halitosis, soft tissue pallor (due to anemia), "uremic frost" (due to urea crystal on epithelial surfaces of the skin), uremic stomatitis (erythematous ulcerations of ventral surface of tongue and mucosal tissues), and altered taste disturbances that can be due to metabolic disturbances owing to declining renal function (De Rossi and Glick 1996; Cervero *et al.* 2008; Patil *et al.* 2012). Uremic patients have increased levels of urea in the blood as well as in the saliva by bacterial ureases, where it is changed into ammonia and presents with a characteristic halitosis and a reduction in salivary pH that may increase the incidence of caries (Dibdin and Dawes 1998; Álamo *et al.* 2011). These patients may also complain of altered tastes especially with sweet and acidic flavors (Álamo *et al.* 2011).

In addition, studies have shown that poor oral health is frequently seen in CKD patients and may be more advanced than in the normal population. Poor dentition and poor oral health may be early signs of kidney disease (Akar *et al.* 2011)

Medications prescribed

Most likely the CKD patient, rather than the acute kidney injury patient, will present to the dental office.

- Patients with CKD are usually taking medications for hypertension that will help curtail further kidney damage. Angiotensin-converting enzyme inhibitors (ACEIs) or angiotensin II receptor

Table 3.2 Common dental drugs that require dose adjustment (dosing or dosing interval) in end-stage renal disease.

Drug prescribed	Glomerular filtration rate (ml/min)		
	>50	10–50	<10
Antibiotics			
Amoxicillin	250–500 mg every 8 h	250–500 mg every 8–12 h	q24 h
Amoxicillin/ clavulanate (Augmentin)	250–500 mg every 8 h; 875 mg every 12 h	250–500 mg every 12 h	q24 h
Azithromycin	500 mg once a day	No adjustment	Use with caution (manufacturer)
Clarithromycin	250–500 mg every 12 h	Decrease dose 50%	Decrease dose 50%
Ciprofoxacin	500–700 mg every 12 h	50–75%	50%
Clindamycin	300 mg three times a day	No adjustment (eliminated through liver)	No adjustment
Metronidazole	500 mg every 8 h	No adjustment	No adjustment
Doxycycline (hepatic elimination)	100 mg twice a day	No adjustment	No adjustment
Tetracycline	250 mg every 6–8 h	250 mg every 12–24 h	Avoid
Penicillin VK	250–500 mg every 6 h	No adjustment	No adjustment
Antivirals			
Acyclovir, oral	No adjustment; normal dose 200–800 mg every 4–12 h	No adjustment	200 mg q12 h
Valacyclovir	No adjustment; normal dose 500 mg every 12 h	500 mg q12–24 h	500 mg q24 h
Antifungals			
Fluconazole (Diflucan)	200–400 mg every 24 h	50% of dose	50% of dose
Analgesics			
Acetaminophen	500 mg every 4 h	Every 6 h	Every 8 h
Aspirin	q4–6 h	q4–6 h	Avoid
Ibuprofen	50–75% of normal dose; best to avoid	No adjustment but take caution with long-term use	Avoid
Naproxen	50–75% of normal dose; best to avoid	Avoid	Avoid
Diflunisal (Dolobid)	No change	Decrease dose 50%	Decrease dose 50%
Codeine/ acetaminophen	30–60 mg every 4–6 h	Not defined: consider 50% of normal dose or avoid	Avoid
Hydrocodone (combination with acetaminophen)	50–100% of normal dose	Not defined: consider 50–75% of normal dose—use with caution	25% of normal dose—use with caution

(*continued*)

Table 3.2   *(cont'd)*

Drug prescribed	Glomerular filtration rate (ml/min)		
	>50	10–50	<10
Oxycodone (combination with acetaminophen)	No change; normal dose	50–75% of normal dose—use with caution	Avoid
Fentanyl	100% of normal dose	75% of normal dose	Avoid
Tramadol (Ultram)	Normal dose	Immediate-release form: 50–100 mg every 12 h or avoid; extended-release form: avoid	Avoid
Local anesthetics			
Lidocaine	No adjustment	No adjustment	No adjustment
Carbocaine (Mepivacaine)	No adjustment	Not defined: caution advised with repeated doses	Caution advised since there are no data
Septocaine (Articaine)	No precautions except in hypoxia	Not defined: no precautions except in hypoxia	No precautions except in hypoxia
Oral, sedatives			
Diazepam	No change	Start lower dose with chronic use; use caution	Start lower dose and titrate with chronic use; use caution
Midazolam (versed)	0.5–2 mg IV over 2 min; then titrate	No adjustment; use with caution	Use with caution

Adapted from National Kidney Foundation 2002; Johnson 2007; Munar and Singh 2007; Cervero *et al.* 2008; Brockmann and Badr 2010; Nizharadze *et al.* 2011; King 2013; www.epocrates.com

blockers (ARBs) are primarily prescribed in these patients because they affect kidney function the most. The combination of an ACEI or an ARB with a diuretic is particularly effective in lowering blood pressure (Sic 2002). The incremental reduction in blood pressure during combination therapy with either an ACEI or an ARB and a diuretic is related to the degree of diuresis and therefore may be more significant when a more potent loop diuretic is being administered (Sic 2002).

- Diuretics will help to reduce fluid retention which causes high blood pressure and swelling of arms and legs (peripheral edema). Common diuretics include thiazides such as hydrochlorothiazide and loop diuretics such as furosemide (Lasix). Patient will also be taking a potassium supplement. Diuretic therapy enhances the antihypertensive effect of most antihypertensive agents.
- Many CKD patients have anemia which is treated by erythropoietin (increases production of new red blood cells [RBCs]) plus iron.
- Many CKD patients also have high blood cholesterol which is primarily treated with HMG-CoA reductase inhibitors or "statin" drugs including simvastatin (Zocor), atorvastatin (Lipitor), and rosuvastatin (Crestor).
- Diabetes is a common cause for CKD. Patients may be controlled with diet, oral medications, or insulin.
- Microalbuminuria or proteinuria can predict ESRD and progressive decline in renal function in patients with diabetes, hypertension, and even in the general population (Gansevoort and de Jong

2009; Glassock 2010). Microalbuminuria occurs when the kidney leaks small amounts of albumin into the urine and is an important prognostic marker for kidney damage in patients with kidney disease and diabetes, hypertension, or glomerulonephritis and is an independent risk factor for cardiovascular mortality (Gansevoort and de Jong 2009; Rivera *et al.* 2012).

- As kidney function declines, there will be an increase in serum phosphate (retention of phosphate due to secondary hyperparathyroidism), especially in ESRD, which potentially increases the risk for cardiovascular disease and even death. These patients may be taking phosphate binders, calcium carbonate (TUMS) antacids or calcitriol, a form of vitamin D, which increases levels of vitamin D. Phosphate binders are approved for use in individuals with ESRD but not in patients with nondialysis CKD. More clinical studies are required to determine the safety and efficacy of these drugs (Weaver 2012).

When comorbidities are present, the patient most likely will be taking specific medications. For example, when prescribing an antihypertensive drug to a patient with ESRD, it is ideal to choose a drug that preserves renal function, maintains renal blood flow, and reduces glomerular pressure such as ACEIs. Calcium channel blockers (CCBs) are also preferred since they increase renal blood flow and reduce renal vasoconstriction and increase GFR. Both these antihypertensive medications have been shown to slow the progression of renal failure, which is the goal of medications used to treat ESRD.

Dental notes

Dental management is important in patients with CKD because complications from declining kidney function may have an impact on dental care. The dentist should be aware of a greater bleeding tendency, hypertension, anemia, changes in drug elimination, and increased incidence to developing infections (Alamo *et al.* 2011). Obtain a current CBC including white blood cell (WBC) count, differential and platelet count, hemoglobin, hematocrit, RBC indices, serum ferritin (for iron), and absolute reticulocyte count.

- Altered drug dosing: In CKD, there is altered drug pharmacokinetics including absorption, distribution, metabolism, and renal excretion. These features must be taken into consideration when prescribing dental drugs to CKD patients. Essentially, every patient with chronic renal disease must be individually assessed for GFR (the best measure of overall kidney function) and subsequent medication prescribing. NSAIDs (e.g., ibuprofen and naproxen) can safely be prescribed in patients who are well hydrated with good renal function and *no* comorbidities such as hypertension, diabetes, or heart failure (Munar and Singh 2007). Long-term use should be avoided (Munar and Singh 2007). It is best to avoid codeine in patients with renal failure or on dialysis (Johnson 2007). Lidocaine can be used safely in the renal-impaired dental patient but carbocaine is extensively excreted by the kidney and in patients with renal insufficiency toxic reaction may occur, especially in the older adult with already-decreased renal function (www.rxlist.com/carbocaine). Table 3.2 lists dental medications prescribed that may need adjustments in dose or dosing interval. Dosing adjustments depend on the severity of renal impairment and patient size (Munar and Singh 2007).
- Increased bleeding tendencies: As kidney function gets worse, there is an increased bleeding due to anemia, decreased RBC maturation, abnormality in platelets (thrombocytopenia), defect in platelet vessel wall, and accumulation of uremic toxins (Brockmann and Badr 2010). Obtain current platelet counts. Anticipate bleeding during and after invasive dental procedures (Carpenter 2012). To establish normal bleeding time, the hematocrit has to increase to ≥30%. Obtain current hematocrit levels. Consult with the patient's nephrologist and hematologist for invasive dental procedures. Local measures can help to control mild bleeding but for major bleeding patients may need to have a platelet transfusion or be administered preoperatively with intranasal

desmopressin acetate (DDAVP) or other medications. Consult with the patient's hematologist (Carpenter 2012). Any elective dental procedures should be delayed until normal levels are attained.

- Increased incidence of anemia: Normocytic anemia is a classic early symptom of CKD that occurs when GFR is <60 mL/min (Carpenter 2012). Anemia occurs due to a decrease in the production of erythropoietin by the endothelial cells in the kidney. Erythropoietin is necessary for stimulation of bone marrow production of RBCs. Additionally, patients may be taking vitamin B_{12}, folic acid supplements, and recombinant human erythropoietin (epoetin alfa; Procrit®) injections, which reverses the anemia and prevents the development of cardiovascular problems (Brockmann and Badr 2010). Darbepoetin, a hyperglycosylated derivative of epoetin, has a longer half-life and is administered less frequently than epoetin (Brockmann and Badr 2010). Many patients become iron deficient and require iron supplementation. If patients are taking iron, caution is used when prescribing tetracycline and doxycycline (space the two medications at least 2 h apart). Hematocrit or hemoglobin should be determined before starting invasive dental procedures with anticipated blood loss (Carpenter 2012).
- Increased risk for infections: Decrease in WBCs (leukopenia). Intraoral exam and monitor for oral infections. Consult with patient's nephrologist/hematologist for the need of antibiotic prophylaxis.
- Hypertension: CKD can be either a risk factor for CKD or a result of CKD. The kidney regulates blood pressure through the release of renin which activates angiotensin, a hormone that causes the wall of the arteries to constrict and increases blood pressure. Angiotensin also causes the release of aldosterone, a hormone that causes the kidneys to retain sodium and water, expanding blood volume and blood pressure. Medications that cause vasodilation and excretion of excess fluid by the kidneys will reduce blood pressure. In any case, blood pressure should be monitored at least before and after dental procedures. A majority of patients will be taking a diuretic (e.g., furosemide and thiazide) ACEIs and ARBs, which has oral adverse effects including xerostomia (monitor patient) and orthostatic hypotension (allow patient to remain in an upright position in the dental chair before dismissing).
- Diabetes: Diabetic neuropathy is extremely common in patients with CKD and who may be already taking insulin or oral hypoglycemic drugs (e.g., repaglinide, nateglinide, pioglitazone, and rosiglitazone) (Brockmann and Badr 2010).
- Periodontal diseases (relationship between periodontal inflammation and kidney disease): Moderate to severe inflammatory periodontal diseases can be a possible source of inflammation

Table 3.3   Dental drug–drug interactions in chronic kidney disease patients (www.epocrates.com).

Dental drug	Drug for CKD	Management
Clarithromycin/ erythromycin	Ezetimibe/simvastatin, niacin/ simvastatin, niacin/lovastatin, and all statins	Avoid. Increase "statin" blood levels. Best to avoid and prescribe azithromycin or clindamycin if the patient is allergic to penicillin or stop the statin while on the antibiotic.
Clarithromycin/ erythromycin	Angiotensin-converting enzyme inhibitor/thiazide combos (e.g., benazepril, captopril, enalapril, fosinopril, lisinopril, moexipril, quinapril + hydrochlorothiazide)	Monitor potassium. Increased risk of QT prolongation and cardiac arrhythmias. Either monitor treatment or prescribe azithromycin or clindamycin instead.
Clarithromycin/ erythromycin	Amlodipine/angiotensin II receptor blocker combos	Combination with amlodipine may increase risk of hypotension. Monitor or prescribe alternative antibiotic
Clarithromycin/ erythromycin	Calcium channel blockers	May increase risk of hypotension. Monitor or prescribe alternative antibiotic

in ESRD patients and could also contribute to the chronic inflammatory condition in CKD (Ismail *et al*. 2013). In addition, studies have found increased levels of plaque, calculus, and gingival inflammation in ESRD patients; however, it is still debatable if there is an increased prevalence of periodontal disease in ESRD patients (Craig *et al*. 2002; Craig 2008). If a kidney patient presents with periodontal disease, then the disease should be treated.

- Dental caries: Increased incidence for dental caries; monitor patient and provide possible fluoride supplements.
- Monitor the patient for vitamin D deficiency, which some studies have shown to be related to the development of periodontal diseases (Yao and Fine 2012).

Table 3.3 lists potential drug interactions that could occur between drugs taken by patients with CKD and dental drugs prescribed.

B. Kidney dialysis

Clinical synopsis

Once the patient has advanced to a GFR below $15\,ml/min/1.73\,m^2$, usually with signs and symptoms of uremia, there will be a need to start kidney replacement therapy, either dialysis, which removes toxic substances from the blood, or kidney transplantation. There are two types of dialysis: hemodialysis, performed in a dialysis center, and peritoneum dialysis, performed in the home by the patient. Dialysis normalizes blood pressure in about 60% of patients with CKD by controlling total body sodium. Eventually, if dialysis is not successful in controlling blood pressure the patient may be started on medications. Patients with irreversible renal failure are candidates for a kidney transplant. Everything mentioned in the CKD section of this chapter including dental evaluation involves the patient on hemodialysis also. Everything mentioned in the CKD section including oral signs/symptoms occurs in the patient on dialysis since they do have CKD/ESRD.

Many articles have been published in dental and medical journals linking poor oral health with hemodialysis (Klassen and Krasko 2012; de Souza *et al*. 2013). Poor oral hygiene resulting in gingivitis/periodontitis is seen in ESRD patients undergoing hemodialysis, and periodontal therapy may affect the mortality of these patients (de Souza *et al*. 2013). Patients on long-term hemodialysis may also develop secondary hyperparathyroidism. Early clinical studies found specific radiographic features (e.g., loss of lamina dura and loss of alveolar bone) in hemodialysis patients with secondary hyperparathyroidism (Houston *et al*. 1968; Fletcher *et al*. 1977); however, a more current study found no relationship of secondary hyperparathyroidism with alveolar bone loss and periodontitis (Frankenthal *et al*. 2002).

The most commonly used method to attach the patient to the hemodialysis machine for permanent access is via an arteriovenous (AV) fistula, which is surgically created by connecting an artery to a vein in the arm. The arm that has the fistula should not be used for measuring blood pressure (Konner 2005). AV shunts are used but they provide only temporary access, and they need to be premedicated with antibiotics.

During hemodialysis, heparin, an anticoagulant, is generally administered to allow blood cycling (extracorporeal blood flow) through the dialyzer without forming thrombosis (Cervero *et al*. 2008). To reduce the risk of hemorrhaging, low-dose heparin or fast-flow "no-heparin" technique has been implemented (Lohr and Schwab 1991). This is important because patients with advanced renal failure also have platelet dysfunction, which enhances the risk for bleeding (www.uptodate.com/contents/hemodialysis-anticoagulation). An international normalized ratio is required for warfarin only, not heparin. Dental patients may be more prone to bleeding due to the anticoagulant and vascular access maintenance (De Rossi and Glick 1996). Bleeding may also be due to decreased platelet count and increased capillary fragility (Buckley *et al*. 1986; De Rossi and Glick 1996).

A frequent adverse reaction of hemodialysis is hypotension and orthostatic hypotension (referred to as "dialysis hypotension"), which manifests as either episodic hypotension occurring during the later dialysis procedure or chronic persistent hypotension occurring in long-term dialysis patients with an already-low systolic blood pressure of <100 mm Hg. Symptoms include light-headedness, muscle cramps, nausea/vomiting, and dyspnea (Dheenan and Henrich 2001; www.uptodate.com/ Hemodynamic instability during hemodialysis: Overview).

Medications prescribed

Drugs prescribed to patients on dialysis include the following:

- Most patients with CKD and ESRD have anemia which is treated with erythropoietin, a hormone responsible for RBC production. Both dialysis and nondialysis patients will also be receiving iron, which is needed for erythropoietin to function properly.
- Phosphate binders, calcium binders, or calcium carbonate antacids to maintain serum phosphate levels.
- Dialysis removes important vitamins, so patients may be taking supplemental water-soluble vitamins, including vitamin C, B-complex vitamins, and folic acid.
- HMG-CoA reductase inhibitors or "statins."
- Antidiabetic medications: oral or insulin.

Dental notes

1. Obtain a consult from the nephrologist to know the status of the patient's kidney functions.
2. Major considerations to pay attention to in the patient undergoing hemodialysis are bleeding, infection, and medication use (De Rossi and Glick 1996).
3. Patients on hemodialysis may require antibiotic prophylaxis following the American Heart Association (AHA) guidelines because they are more prone to developing infections, including dental infections, infections of the artery lining, and infective endocarditis; mortality due to infective endocarditis is very high (De Rossi and Glick 1996). Patients having peritoneal dialysis usually do not require antibiotic prophylaxis (Tong and Walker 2004).
4. Obtain current lab values including CBC to determine bleeding risk.
5. Uremic bleeding usually occurs if the patient is not adequately dialyzed (hemodialysis), at day 2 (Weigert and Schafer 1998; Carpenter 2012). However, many patients will not have uremic bleeding in the dental office since they would have undergone dialysis before clinical manifestations (Carpenter 2012).
6. Before prescribing any medications have the patient's current GFR values and adjust dosing interval/dose accordingly.
7. Certain antibiotics are dialyzable, which means that they can be taken if the patient is on dialysis but they must be taken on the day of the dialysis after the session. These antibiotics that are dialyzable include amoxicillin, amoxicillin/clavulanate, and metronidazole (King 2013).
8. Evaluate, monitor, and treat accordingly the periodontal condition of hemodialysis patients.
9. Patients may be prone to developing candidiasis infections and herpes infection due to immunosuppression.
10. Incidence of hepatitis B and C may be higher among dialysis patients.
11. Most patients are dialyzed on alternate days. It is recommended to schedule dental appointments 24 h after hemodialysis because $t^{1/2}$ of heparin is about 1 h (i.e., at 1 h, 50% of heparin is eliminated), which means that by a day after dialysis heparin is out of the body (Hirsh *et al.* 2001). The arm that has the AV fistula should not be used for measuring blood pressure.

C. Kidney transplant

Clinical synopsis

Kidney transplant is the ultimate treatment for ESRD (Suthanthiran and Strom 1994). Patients on an organ transplant list require close follow-up before and after transplantation since they are taking multiple medications including immunosuppressive drugs which increase the risk to infection, malignancy, and cardiovascular disease. Patients usually have comorbidities (e.g., hypertension and diabetes) which are most likely related to their ESRD. Having a kidney transplant versus dialysis may increase long-term survival for the patient (Wolfe *et al.* 1999; Weinberg *et al.* 2013). However, there are certainly many risks as well as benefits with kidney, as well as any organ, transplantation including infection, graft rejection and failure, and adverse reactions of the immunosuppressive medications taken. Patients with ESRD usually have comorbidities including diabetes, hypertension, glomerulonephritis, and polycystic kidney disease (PKD) that make them candidates for renal transplantation (Georgakopoulou *et al.* 2011).

The oral health of these patients must be emphasized by the dentist. Usually, there is a healthcare transplant team consisting of physicians, nephrologists, nurses, and dentists. Dentists in the transplant team play a pivotal role in dental care of the transplant patient before as well as after the transplant (Weinberg *et al.* 2013). It is extremely important to maintain the patient inflammation and infection free as far as possible to prevent graft rejection and failure (Segelnick and Weinberg 2009). Therefore, the transplant patient should be seen by the dentist during all phases of transplantation (Segelnick and Weinberg 2009). Treatment of dental caries, abscesses, necessary extractions, and periodontal diseases is important before transplantation since postoperative immunosuppression reduces a patient's ability to fight off systemic infection.

It is definitely important to have the patient return after transplantation to the dental office for regular maintenance appointment. Usually, the patient should not have any dental care for at least 3 months but up to 6 months after transplantation because this is the time period of the highest risk of organ rejection and the high dosage of immunosuppressant agents taken during this time puts the patient at risk for systemic infections.

Medications prescribed

Patients who had a major organ transplant are most likely taking a cocktail of immunosuppressant drugs such as azathioprine (Imuran), cyclosporine, tacrolimus (Prograf, FK506), sirolimus (Rapamune), mycophenolate, and prednisone.

Azathioprine is an antimetabolite indicated as an adjunct for the prevention of rejection in renal transplantation. It has a mechanism of action to reduce inflammation and interfere with the growth of rapidly dividing cells. There is a warning about chronic immunosuppression with an increased risk of malignancy. It functions to prevent organ rejection by inhibiting the production of blood cells in the bone marrow. Serious infections are a constant concern for patients receiving azathioprine and any other immunosuppressive drug. The medical consultation from the patient's physician should address the potential for severe infections occurring while the patient is taking azathioprine. The dentist should have the most recent results of the CBC before dental treatment is started. Also, there could be bleeding; oral sores; or swelling of the face, lips, tongue, or throat. There are no drug interactions that would be of concern in dentistry.

Tacrolimus is an immunosuppressive drug used to prevent rejection of liver and kidney organ transplant. There is a warning about *increased susceptibility to infection* and the possible development of lymphoma. The medical consultation from the patient's physician should address the potential for severe infections occurring while the patient is taking tacrolimus. Since hypertension is a common adverse effect, patients may be taking a CCB which could cause gingival enlargement.

Cyclosporine is a potent immunosuppressive agent that prolongs survival of many transplants such as kidney, liver, and heart. Patients taking cyclosporine usually have hypertension and those taking a CCB such as nifedipine (Adalat, Procardia) can have gingival enlargement. Meticulous oral home care and maintenance/recare appointments every 3 months are important in these patients. Cyclosporine can cause nephrotoxicity (including structural kidney damage) and hepatotoxicity.

Table 3.4 lists drugs prescribed by the dentist that may have an interaction with immunosuppressant drugs taken by the kidney transplant patient.

Table 3.4   Dental drug–drug interactions in the kidney transplant patient (http://www.medscape.com/viewarticle/726344_6; www.rxlist.com; www.epocrates.com; Saad *et al.* 2006).

Dental drug	Kidney drug	Management
Clarithromycin/ erythromycin	Cyclosporine, tacrolimus	AVOID. Increase levels of immunosuppressant drugs and possible toxicity. May increase risk of QT prolongation and cardiac arrhythmias. Best to prescribe azithromycin or clindamycin instead.
Ciprofloxacin (Cipro)	Cyclosporine	AVOID. Increase cyclosporine levels with risk of nephrotoxicity.
Clindamycin	Mycophenolate	Caution advised; may decrease mycophenolate levels.
"Azole" antifungals (e.g., clotrimazole, fluconazole, and ketoconazole)	Cyclosporine, tacrolimus, sirolimus	Increased blood concentrations of the immunosuppressants resulting in increased potential for adverse events because of excessive immunosuppression and toxicity (e.g., nephrotoxicity, neurotoxicity). Consult with patient's nephrologist; may require a dosage reduction of the immunosuppressant.
"Azole" antifungals (e.g., clortrimazole, fluconazole, and ketoconazole)	Statins	Azoles can increase plasma concentrations of statins that are Cytochrome (CYP)3A4 substrates (e.g., atorvastatin, lovastatin, and simvastatin). AVOID
Systemic corticosteroids	Cyclosporine, tacrolimus, sirolimus	All azole antifungal agents have been associated with development of adrenal insufficiency. This may be potentiated by coadministration with high-dose corticosteroids. Consult with patient's nephrologist
Metronidazole	Mycophenolate	Caution advised; may increase mycophenolate levels.
Tetracycline	Mycophenolate	Caution advised; may decrease mycophenolate levels.
Azithromycin, clarithromycin, erythromycin	Mycophenolate	Caution advised; may decrease mycophenolate levels
Acyclovir, valacyclovir	Mycophenolate	Caution advised; may increase levels and risk of toxicity with both drugs.
Corticosteroids	Mycophenolate	Combination may increase risk of immunosuppression and infections. Caution advised.

Dental notes: Summary: Patients with all stages of kidney disease

1. Any patient with acute renal injury, CKD, or ESRD must have a nephrology consult.
2. Be in constant contact, e-mails, and documented phone calls with the transplantation team, especially the nephrologist.
3. Monitor blood pressure; hypertension is a major cause of kidney disease and worsens in patients with kidney disease.
4. Important questions that must be asked when treating a patient with kidney disease include the following:
   a. What is the patient's GFR/CrCl?
   b. What medications is the patient taking?
   c. What is the platelet count; the patient may require a platelet transfusion on the day of tooth extraction or periodontal/implant surgery?
   d. Is the patient undergoing dialysis?
   e. Is the patient on a kidney transplant list and if so, where; is dental treatment important to eliminate any oral infection?
5. Polypharmacy is common in drug prescriptions of patients with CKD. Be prudent in suspected drug–drug interactions.
6. The main concern of dental patients with kidney disease is bleeding tendencies due to altered platelet function; obtain CBC and coagulation tests results. Patients may require platelet transfusion for invasive bleeding dental procedures such as extractions or periodontal/implant surgery. Uremia causes decreased platelet function resulting in prolongation of bleeding time.
7. The renal clearance of local anesthetics is not reduced in patients with CKD because the amide anesthetic is inactivated either in the liver or in the plasma with ester anesthetics. In addition, the synthesis of the local anesthetic-binding protein, alpha 1-acid glycoprotein, is stimulated in CKD which gives some protection against systemic toxicity (Cox *et al.* 2003).
8. Prophylactic antibiotics may be prescribed due to immunosuppression; medical consult required.
9. Dental treatment is best carried out on the day after dialysis.
10. Patients have altered drug elimination; tetracycline should be avoided in chronic renal failure because it can exacerbate uremia; however, doxycycline is appropriate to prescribe.
11. Azithromycin, clindamycin, doxycycline, and penicillin VK can be prescribed in patients with CKD without adjustments in dose or dosing interval.
12. The safest nonnarcotic analgesic is acetaminophen.
13. NSAIDs can compromise existing renal function, and renal toxicity can occur in patients with impaired renal function. Aspirin and NSAIDs should be avoided because both affect renal function; however, short-term NSAID use is well tolerated if patient is well hydrated and has good renal function and absence of heart failure, diabetes, or hypertension (Barclay 2007; http://www.medscape.org/viewarticle/557381). It is recommended to consult with the patient's nephrologist.
14. The risk of acute renal failure is three times higher in NSAID users (Munar and Singh 2007).
15. Diflunisal, a nonacetylated salicylate, inhibits renal prostaglandins to a lesser extent than NSAIDs, but still there are precautions.
16. The safest opioid is fentanyl. Codeine dose should either be reduced by 50–75% if GFR <50 mL/min or totally avoided. Codeine should be avoided in ESRD and patients undergoing dialysis.
17. Patients on the organ transplant list waiting for an organ must be treated for oral inflammation and infection before the transplant. Close contact with the transplant team is important.
18. Maintenance of good oral hygiene is important for the transplant patient.
19. More than likely the patient will require antibiotic prophylaxis before dental treatment; consult with the nephrologist.

20. Before and after transplantation, patients may be on corticosteroids, cyclosporine, tacrolimus, azathioprine, or mycophenolate mofetil. Check for drug–drug interactions.

21. Monitor and manage gingival enlargement with cyclosporine and CCBs. Maintain meticulous oral hygiene with the patient. Gingival surgery may be indicated if gingival enlargement interferes with proper oral hygiene care.

D. Polycystic kidney disease

PKD is an autosomal dominant kidney disorder characterized by numerous clusters of enlarged cysts in the kidneys. The etiology of cyst formation is unknown (Torres and Grantham 2007). Patients with PKD may also present with anemia, CKD, ESRD, hypertension, and liver disease. As such, patients may be taking antihypertensive medications and diabetic medications (Amaout 2011) (Refer to Section A). Long-term PKD may result in the patient undergoing dialysis or kidney transplant. About one-half of the people with autosomal dominant PKD progress to kidney failure or ESRD (Amaout 2011).

E. Benign prostatic hypertrophy

Clinical synopsis

The prostate gland surrounds the neck of the bladder and the urethra. Benign prostatic hyperplasia (BPH) is a condition where there is obstruction of urinary flow due to proliferation or enlargement of prostatic tissue around the urethra leading to a problem with either storage or voiding urine. Bacterial infections can occur when the urine is not completely voided. BPH is one of the most common neoplastic conditions.

Diagnosis/lab values

There are no lab values that are important for dental care. Besides a clinical examination, prostate-specific antigen screening and serum creatinine measurements are performed (McVary 2003).

Medications

There are mainly two types of medications used to treat BPH, which are as follows:

α-blockers: Alpha-adrenergic blockers are considered to be the drug of choice in treating moderate-to-severe BPH. The mechanism of action is to relax the smooth muscles of the neck of the bladder and prostate thereby inhibiting the active part of the obstruction (Tahmatzopoulos *et al.* 2004). These drugs are indicated for males with prostates that are not severely enlarged to increase urinary flow.

Nonselective α-adrenergic blockers target all alpha receptors in the body, resulting in more adverse effects including low blood pressure and orthostatic hypotension. Examples of nonselective α-blockers include terazosin (Hytrin) and doxazosin (Cardura). Selective α-adrenergic blockers are selective for the prostate but also affect the eyes. Examples of selective α-adrenergic blockers include tamsulosin (Flomax), alfuzosin (Uroxatral), and silodosin (Rapaflo).

5-Alpha-reductase inhibitors are drugs that block 5-alpha-reductase, an enzyme found in the prostate gland that converts testosterone to dihydrotestosterone, thereby reducing the enlarged prostate and inhibiting further tissue proliferation. It may take many months for a reduction of symptoms to occur. These drugs include finasteride (Proscar) and dutasteride (Avodart).

Dental notes

1. α-Blockers can cause orthostatic hypotension and dizziness and light-headedness. Allow the patients to sit in an upright position in the dental chair for a few minutes before dismissing them.
2. Otherwise, there are no changes in dental care for patients taking these medications.

References

Akar, H., Akar, G.C., Carrero, J.J. *et al.* (2011) Systemic consequences of poor oral health in chronic kidney disease patients. *Clinical Journal of the American Society of Nephrology,* **6,** 218–226.

Álamo, S.A., Esteve, C.G., & Pérez, M.G.S. (2011) Dental considerations for the patient with renal disease. *Journal of Clinical Experimental Dentistry,* **3,** e112–e119.

Al-Badr, W. & Martin, K.J. (2008) Vitamin D and kidney disease. *Clinical Journal of the American Society of Nephrology,* **3,** 1555–1560.

Amaout, M.A. (2011) Cystic kidney diseases. In: L. Goldman & D. Ausiello (eds). *Cecil Medicine,* 24th ed, Chapter 128. Saunders Elsevier, Philadelphia, PA.

Andress, D.L. (2005) Vitamin D treatment in chronic renal disease. *Seminars in Dialysis,* **18,** 315–324.

Barclay, L. (2007) Guidelines for drug dosing regimens in chronic kidney disease. Medscape Medical News. http://www.medscape.org/viewarticle/557381 (accessed on July 14, 2014).

Brockmann, W. & Badr, M. (2010) Chronic kidney disease. Pharmacological considerations for the dentist. *The Journal of the American Dental Association,* **141 (11),** 1330–1339.

Buckley, D.J., Barrett, A.P., Koutta, J. *et al.* (1986) Control of bleeding in severely uremic patients undergoing oral surgery. *Oral Surgery Oral Medicine Oral Pathology,* **61,** 546–549.

Carpenter, W. (2012) Chapter 5 Renal and urinary tract disease. In: L.L. Patton (ed). *The ADA Practical Guide to Patients with Medical Conditions,* 1st ed, pp. 95–112. Wiley-Blackwell, Ames, IA.

Caster, D.J., Loughran, J.H., & Kinane, D.F. (2010) Dental and medical comanagement of osteoporosis, kidney disease, and cancer. In: R.J. Genco & R.C. Williams (eds), 1st ed, Chapter 17, pp. 270–287. *Periodontal Diseases and Overall Health: A Clinician's Guide.* Professional Audience Communications, Inc., Yardley, PA.

Cervero, A.J., Bagan, J.V., Sorian, J.Y. *et al.* (2008) Dental management in renal failure: patients on dialysis. *Medicina Oral Patologia Oral y Cirugia Bucal,* **13 (7),** E419–E426.

Cox, B., Durieux, M.E., & Marcus, M.A.E. (2003) Toxicity of local anesthetics. *Best Practice & Research Clinical Anaesthesiology,* **17,** 111–136.

Craig, R. (2008) Interactions between chronic renal disease and periodontal disease. *Oral Diseases,* **14,** 1–7.

Craig, R., Spittle, M.A., & Levin, N.W. (2002) Importance of periodontal disease in the kidney patient. *Blood Purification,* **20,** 133–119.

De Rossi, S.S. & Glick, M. (1996) Dental considerations for the patient with renal disease receiving hemodialysis. *Journal of the American Dental Association,* **127,** 211–219.

De Souza, C.M., Braosi, A.P.R., Luczyszyn, S.M. *et al.* (2014) Association between oral health parameters, periodontitis and its treatment and mortality in hemodialysis patients. *Journal of Periodontology,* **85(6),** e169–e178.

Dheenan, S. & Henrich, W.L. (2001) Preventing dialysis hypotension: a comparison of usual protective maneuvers. *Kidney International* **59 (3),** 1175–1181.

Dibdin, G.H. & Dawes, C. (1998) A mathematical model of the influence of salivary urea on the pH of fasted dental plaque and on the changes occurring during a cariogenic challenge. *Caries Research,* **32,** 70–74.

Dusso, A.S., Brown, A.J., & Slatopolsky, E. (2005) Vitamin D. *American Journal of Physiology—Renal Physiology,* **289 (1),** F8–F28.

Eckardt, K., Berns, J.S., Rocco, M.V. *et al.* (2009) Definition and classification of CKD: the debate should be about patient prognosis—a position statement from KDOQI and KDIGO. *American Journal of Kidney Diseases,* **53,** 915–920.

Fletcher, P.D., Scopp, I.W., & Hersch, R.A. (1977) Oral manifestations of secondary hyperparathyroidism related to long-term hemodialysis therapy. *Journal of Oral Surgery,* **43,** 218–226.

Frankenthal, S., Nakhoul, F., Machtei, E.E. *et al.* (2002) The effect of secondary hyperparathyroidism and hemodialysis therapy on alveolar bone and periodontium. *The Journal of Clinical Periodontology*, **29**, 479–483.

Gansevoort, R.T. & de Jong, P.E. (2009) The case for using albuminuria in staging chronic kidney disease. *The American Society of Nephrology*, **20**, 465–468.

Georgakopoulou, E.A., Achtari, M.D., & Afentoulide, N. (2011) Dental management of patients before and after renal transplantation. *Stomatologija, Baltic Dental and Maxillofacial Journal*, **12**, 107–112.

Glassock, R.J. (2010) Is the presence of microalbuminuria a relevant marker of kidney disease? *Current Hypertension Reports* **12**, 364–368.

Hirsh, J., Anand, S.S., Halperin, J.L. *et al.* (2001) AHA Scientific Statement. Guide to anticoagulant therapy: heparin. *Circulation*, **103**, 2994–3018.

Holick, M.F. (2005) Photobiology of vitamin D. In: D. Feldman, J. Pike, F. Glorieux (eds). *Vitamin D*, 2nd ed, pp. 37–46. Elsevier Academic Press, New York.

Houston, J.B., Dolan, K.B., Appleby, R.C. *et al.* (1968) Radiography of secondary hyperparathyroidism. *Journal of Oral Surgery*, **26**, 746–750.

Ismail, G., Dumitriu, H.T., Dumitriu, A.S. *et al.* (2013) Periodontal disease: a convert source of inflammation in chronic kidney disease patients. *International Journal of Nephrology*, **2013**, 515796.

Johnson, C.A., Levey, A.S., Coresh, J. *et al.* (2004) Clinical practice guidelines for chronic kidney disease in adults. Part I. Definition, disease stages, evaluation, treatment, and risk factors. *American Family Physician*, **70**, 869–876.

Johnson, R.J. *Opioid safety in patients with renal or hepatic dysfunction.* www.pain-topics.com. Updated: November 30, 2007 [accessed on July 31, 2014].

Kasiske, B. & Cosio, F.G. (2003) K/DOQI clinical practice guidelines for managing dyslipidemias in chronic kidney disease. *American Journal of Kidney Disease*, **41 (Suppl. 3)**, S8–S91.

KDIGO (2013) Chapter 1: Definition and classification of CKD. *Kidney International Suppl*, **3**, 19. http://www.kdigo.org/clinical_practice_guidelines/pdf/CKD/KDIGO_2012_CKD_GL.pdf [accessed on July 14, 2014].

Kestenbaum, B.R. (2008) Vitamin D metabolism and treatment in chronic kidney disease: vitamin D metabolism in chronic kidney disease. *Medscape Nephrology*, http://www.medscape.org/viewarticle/571558_2 [accessed January 21, 2014].

King, E. (2013) Dental management of patients in end stage renal failure on dialysis. *Journal of the Michigan Dental Association*, **59**, 42–45.

Klassen, J.T. & Karsko, B.M. (2009) The dental health status of dialysis patients. *The Journal of the Canadian Dental Association*, **68**, 34–38.

Konner, K. (2005) History of vascular access for haemodialysis. *Nephrology Dialysis Transplantation*, **20**, 2629–2635.

Lameire, N., Van Biesen, W., & Vanholder, R. (2005) Acute renal failure. *Lancet*, **365** (9457), 417–430.

Levey, A.S. & Coresh, J. (2012) Chronic kidney disease. *Lancet*, **379**, 165–180.

Lohr, J.W. & Schwab, S.J. (1991) Minimizing hemorrhagic complications in dialysis patients. *Journal of the American Society of Nephrology*, **2** (5), 961–975.

McVary, K.T. (2003) Clinical evaluation of benign prostatic hyperplasia. *Reviews in Urology*, **5** (**Suppl.** 4), S3–S11.

Munar, M.Y. & Singh, H. (2007) Drug dosing adjustments in patients with chronic kidney disease. *American Family Physicians* **75** (10), 1487–1496.

National Kidney Foundation. https://www.kidney.org/professionals/KDOQI/guidelines_commentaries [accessed on July 14, 2014].

National Kidney Foundation (2002) K/DOQI clinical practice guidelines for chronic kidney disease: evaluation, classification, and stratification. *American Journal of Kidney Disease*, **39** (**2 Suppl. 1**), S1–S266.

Nizharadze, N., Mamaladze, M., Chipashvill, N. *et al.* (2011) Articaine—the best choice of local anesthetic in contemporary dentistry. *Georgian Medical News*, **190**, 15–23.

Patil, S., Khaandelwal, S., Doni, B. *et al.* (2012) Oral manifestations in chronic renal failure patients attending two hospitals in North Karnataka, India. *Oral Health and Dental Management*, **11**, 100–106.

Rivera, J.A., O'Hare, A. M., & Harper, G.M. (2012) Update on the management of chronic kidney disease. *American Family Physician*, **86**, 749–754.

Rule, A.D. & Glassock, R.J. (2013) Chronic kidney disease: classification of CKD should be bout more than prognosis. *Nature Reviews Nephrology*, **9**, 697–698.

Saad, A.H., DePestel, D.D., & Carver, P.L. (2006) Factors influencing the magnitude and clinical significance of drug interactions between azole antifungals and select immunosuppressants. *Pharmacotherapy*, **26**, 1730–1744.

Segelnick, S.L. & Weinberg, M.A. (2009) The periodontist's role in obtaining clearance prior to patients undergoing a kidney transplant. *Journal of Periodontology*, **80**, 874–877.

Shlipak, M.G., Matsushita, K., Ärnlöv, J. *et al.* (2013) Cystatin C versus creatinine in determining risk based on kidney function. *New England Journal of Medicine*, **369**, 932–943.

Sic, D.A. (2002) Rationale for fixed-dose combinations in the treatment of hypertension: the cycle repeats. *Drugs*, **62**, 443–462.

Sulejmanagic, H., Sulejmanagic, N., Prohic, S. *et al.* (2005). Dental treatment of patients with kidney diseases—review. *Bosnian Journal of Basic Medical Sciences*, **5 (1)**, 52–56.

Suthanthiran, M. & Strom, T.B. (1994) Renal transplantation. *New England Journal of Medicine*, **331** (6), 365–376.

Tahmatzopoulos, A., Rowland, R.G., & Kyprianou, N. (2004) The role of alpha-blockers in the management of prostate cancer. *Expert Opinion on Pharmacology*, **5**, 1279–1285.

Tong, D.C. & Walker, R.J. (2004) Antibiotic prophylaxis in dialysis patients undergoing invasive dental procedures. *Nephrology*, **9**, 167–170.

Torres, V.E. & Grantham, J.J. (2007) Cystic diseases of the kidney. In: B.M. Brenner (ed). *Brenner and Rector's the Kidney*, 8th ed, Chapter 41. Saunders Elsevier, Philadelphia, PA.

www.uptodate.com/contents/hemodialysis-anticoagulation [accessed January 20, 2014].

www.uptodate.com/Hemodynamic instability during hemodialysis: Overview [accessed January 20, 2014].

Weaver, J. (2012) Phosphate binders: new study raises questions about safety and efficacy. *Nephrology Times*, **5 (8)**, 1, 16–17.

Weigert, A.L. & Schafer, A.I. (1998) Uremic bleeding: pathogenesis and therapy. *American Journal of Medical Sciences*, **316** (2), 94–104.

Weinberg, M.A., Segelnick, S.L., Kay, L.B. *et al.* (2013) Medical and dental standardization for solid organ transplant recipients. *The New York State Dental Journal*, **79**, 35–40.

Wolfe, R.A., Ashby, V.B., & Milford, E.L. (1999) Comparison of mortality in all patients on dialysis, patients on dialysis awaiting transplantation and recipients of a first cadaveric transplant. *New England Journal of Medicine*, **341**, 1725–1730.

Yao, S.G. & Fine, J.B. (2012) A review of vitamin D as it relates to periodontal disease. *Compendium of Continuing Education in Dentistry*, **33**, 166–171.

Zhang, L., Wang, M., & Wang, H. (2005) Acute renal failure in chronic kidney disease—clinical and pathological analysis of 104 cases. *Clinical Nephrology*, **63 (5)**, 346–350.

Chapter 4

Diseases of the endocrine system

A. Diabetes	46
B. Thyroid diseases	50
C. Adrenal gland disorders	53
References	57

A. Diabetes

Clinical synopsis

Diabetes can be described as a hormonal disease with alterations in carbohydrate, protein, and lipid metabolisms resulting in elevated levels of blood glucose (Padwal *et al.* 2005). Diabetes affects virtually all organs in the body, including the macrovascular (heart) and the microvascular systems (eyes, nerves, kidney, and the periodontium in the oral cavity). Diabetics without a history of heart disease may be at a higher risk for developing cardiovascular events earlier in life than nondiabetics (Junttila *et al.* 2010).

Type 1 diabetes is caused by the destruction of pancreatic islet beta cells resulting in absolute insulin deficiency. When there is not adequate amount of insulin to allow glucose from the blood to enter the cells, the cells starve while glucose accumulates in the blood. When glucose is not available, the cells break down the available fat. As a result free fatty acids are produced and excess of fatty acids get accumulated in the blood, which may result in ketoacidosis, a potentially life-threatening condition. Type I diabetes is primarily an autoimmune process where insulin auto-antibodies produced in the body are involved in pancreatic cell destruction. Macrovascular/cardiovascular complications are not usually prevalent in type 1 diabetes (Dagogo 2004).

Type 2 diabetes is considered to be a type of insulin resistance where there is decreased insulin effectiveness with a reduced sensitivity of the cells to respond to insulin. Normally, the beta cells adjust insulin secretion levels according to the feeding or fasting cycle. If the intake of calories is greater than the expenditure of calories—nondegraded substrates are stored in the adipose tissue—the bodies' energy reservoir and the body weight increases. As the adipose mass increases, the number of insulin receptors on the adipocyte and other cell surfaces including the liver and muscle

The Dentist's Quick Guide to Medical Conditions, First Edition. Mea A. Weinberg, Stuart L. Segelnick, Joseph S. Insler, with Samuel Kramer.
© 2015 John Wiley & Sons, Inc. Published 2015 by John Wiley & Sons, Inc.

cells decreases and the tissues become resistant to the effects of insulin. Insulin must bind with these receptors and become active in bringing glucose into the cell and in stimulating glucose metabolism (Junttila *et al.* 2010). In type 2 diabetes, insulin receptors on the target tissues become insensitive or resistant to insulin. Insulin may bind to the receptor, but there is a defect in both insulin action and secretion, which makes the insulin ineffective in glucose uptake into the tissues. When insulin resistance develops, the beta cells are forced to compensate by secreting more insulin resulting in a condition known as hyperinsulinemia (Weinberg and Segelnick 2012). Over time, the beta cells of the pancreas lose their ability to produce insulin in sufficient quantities to overcome insulin resistance. This condition is referred to as impaired glucose tolerance or prediabetes. This results in high blood glucose levels, especially after meals, which is called postprandial hyperglycemia. The degree of insulin defects is influenced by many factors, including obesity, cigarette smoking, and decreased physical activity. In fact, approximately 80% of type 2 diabetics are obese or overweight (Mahler and Adler, 1999). Continued insulin resistance and insulin deficiency ultimately will result in type 2 diabetes.

Cardiovascular disease (CVD) is a major cause of mortality in diabetic patients, and the prevalence of diabetes is increasing in both developed and undeveloped countries (Berry *et al.* 2007). The prevalence of CVD is as low as 2–4% in the nondiabetic population to about 55% in adult diabetic individuals (Kahn and Flier 2000; Berry *et al.* 2007). There are several important factors that physical activity influence the development of CVD in patients with diabetes mellitus (Weinberg and Segelnick 2012):

- Central obesity (waist circumference >40 in. in men and >35 in. in women)
- Decrease in physical activity
- history of diabetes in the family
- Gender (women greater than men)
- Aging (older than 40–45 years old)
- Hyperglycemia

Metabolic syndrome

Components of the metabolic syndrome include a combination of insulin resistance obesity around the waist, abnormal lipid profile including triglyceride levels, increased LDL cholesterol, decreased HDL cholesterol, high blood pressure, and prothrombotic state (Giles and Sander 2005). Obesity, and hypertriglyceridemia may be strongly related to an increased development of diabetes (Hanson *et al.* 2002). Prothrombotic state is characterized by alterations in blood coagulation (hypercoagulation) or platelet abnormalities that may predispose the patient to intravascular clotting or arterial thrombosis (Trovasti and Anfossi 1998; Colwell and Nesto 2003). Obesity and insulin resistance are associated with increased platelet activation or clotting that can influence the development of thrombotic events in diabetics (Ajjan and Grant 2006).

Insulin resistance

Insulin resistance, which is defined as impairment in insulin-mediated glucose disposal, and a defect in insulin secretion are the primary causes of the metabolic problems seen in type 2 diabetics. Insulin resistance develops from obesity, decreased physical activity, and a genetic susceptibility (Grundy *et al.* 1999). Insulin resistance will usually develop before the onset of diabetes and often is present in prediabetic states and in conjunction with other cardiovascular risk factors such as dyslipidemia, hypertension, and prothrombotic factors (Grundy *et al.* 1999).

Diagnostic criteria and evaluation of glycemic control

The 2010 American Diabetic Association (ADA) criteria for the diagnosis of diabetes are as follows (American Diabetes Association 2011; Handelsman *et al.* 2011):

Hemoglobin A1c (HbA1c) ≥6.5%
OR
Fasting plasma glucose (FPG) ≥126 mg/dl
OR
Two-hour plasma glucose ≥200 mg/dl during an oral glucose tolerance test (OGTT)
OR
Random plasma glucose ≥200 mg/dl.

Patients with classic symptoms of hyperglycemia are diagnosed with a random plasma glucose ≥200 mg/dl (American Diabetes Association 2011; Handelsman *et al.* 2011).

The ADA recommends that either two FPG levels or HbA1c is appropriate to identify prediabetes and diabetes. Blood glucose testing can be used to screen healthy, asymptomatic individuals as well as to diagnose diabetes in individuals with symptoms of hyperglycemia such as polyuria, polydypsia, fatigue, blurred vision, and slow healing of infections.

HbA1c test is used to diagnose and monitor the diabetic patient's glycemic control over approximately 2–3 months. According to the ADA, if a patient is 40 or 50 years old, the target HbA1c is <6%, but if the person is older or is experiencing hypoglycemia, the target HbA1 would be higher (Handelsman *et al.* 2011). HBA1c levels show a relationship with the development of diabetic complications including periodontal disease (Mealey and Oates 2006).

Managing hyperglycemia

Glycemic control is primarily a determinant of diabetic microvascular complications such as retinopathy, nephropathy, neuropathy, and periodontal disease (O'Keefe *et al.* 2011). Also, it has been reported that with optimum glycemic control, in addition with better control of hypertension and atherosclerosis with cholesterol-lowering drugs, progression of diabetic-induced heart failure can be stopped or prevented (Gilbert *et al.* 2006). However, the American Heart Association has advised that even though hyperglycemia contributes to cardiovascular risk, more treatment is required besides controlling glucose in order to reverse or reduce the atherosclerotic process (Reusch 2003). It must be emphasized that although current literature has found that pursuit of very low glucose levels (HbA1$_c$ <6.0%) may not be as beneficial as once thought, failing to control hyperglycemia may considerably increase the possibility of acute metabolic events, chronic complications, and mortality (Huang *et al.* 2011). Table 4.1 summarizes glucose testing and interpretations.

Managing diabetes and hypercoagulation

Besides treating diabetic patient with antihypertensives and antihyperlipidemia drugs, antiplatelet therapy has become a major part of treatment to prevent myocardial infarction or stroke. Antiplatelet therapy in patients with type 2 diabetes has significantly reduced the cardiovascular risk. The ADA 2011 guidelines recommends low-dose aspirin therapy (75–162 mg/day) as primary prevention therapy in patients with type 1 or type 2 diabetes mellitus who are at an increased cardiovascular risk (10-year risk >10%) (Handelsman *et al.* 2011). This includes men over the age of 50 and

Table 4.1 Fasting/oral glucose tolerance test goals set by AACE and ADA (Handelsman *et al.* 2011; American Diabetes Association 2011; Weinberg and Segelnick 2012).

Test	Values	Diagnosis
Fasting plasma glucose (FPG) 8–12 h fasting (mg/dl)	≤99	Normal
	100–125	Impaired fasting glucose
	≥126	Diabetes, confirm with a second test on a different day
Oral glucose tolerance test; 2 h after ingestion of 75 g glucose load) (mg/dl)	≤139	Normal
	140–199	Impaired fasting glucose
	≥200	Diabetes, confirm with a second test on a different day

women over the age of 60 who have at least one major risk factor (e.g., family history of CVD, hypertension, smoking, dyslipidemia, or albuminuria) (ADA) The ADA does not recommend aspirin for AVD prevention for adults with diabetes at low CVD risk because of the increased risk of bleeding. This includes men <50 years old and women <60 years old with no major additional risk factors. Aspirin (75–162 mg/day) is recommended as secondary preventive treatment in diabetics with a history of CVD. An alternative to aspirin if the patient is allergic to it can be clopidogrel (75 mg/day) (Handelsman *et al.* 2011).

Oral adverse effects from diabetes

- Periodontal disease
- Xerostomia
- Glossitis

Dental management of dental patients taking oral hypoglycemic drugs and insulin dental drug interactions (www.rxlist.com)

- Regular dose aspirin and NSAIDs (e.g., ibuprofen) increase hypoglycemic effects of insulin.
- Systemic corticosteroids increase blood glucose that will interfere with diabetic medication. This effect may be dramatic and prolonged, requiring dose increases to achieve glycemic control during concomitant therapy. Consultation with the patient's physician is recommended.
- "Azole" type antifungal medications (e.g., fluconazole): concomitant therapy may cause acute hypoglycemia. Doses should be spaced about 2 h apart.
- Fluoroquinolone antibiotics (e.g., ciprofloxacin) has been associated with a possibility of glucose and insulin dysregulation by directly inhibiting insulin release. Recommend using another antibiotic or careful monitoring with the patient's physician.

Dental notes: Management of diabetic patient

- Important to take blood pressure at every visit since diabetes can lead to cardiovascular problems including hypertension.
- Patients in the dental office should be screened and monitored for periodontal disease, since diabetes mellitus is a documented risk factor for periodontal diseases. On the other hand, patients

with periodontal disease should be cognizant of the development of diabetes mellitus. Thus patient education is an integral part of treatment of the periodontal patient with diabetes.

- The American Association of Clinical Endocrinologists (AACE) and the American Diabetes Association recommend a glycemic target range from an HbA1$_c$ of <6.5 to <7.0%, respectively (Rodbard *et al.* 2007; Farmer 2010; American Diabetes Association 2011; Handelsman *et al.* 2011).
- Other oral manifestations of diabetes mellitus include xerostomia, burning tongue/mouth, and *Candida* (fungal) infections. These factors must be monitored in diabetic patient because xerostomia can lead to increased incidence of caries.
- As diabetes progresses, many organs become affected and the patient most likely will be taking many other different types of drugs such as antihypertensives and drugs to lower cholesterol (antihyperlipidemic drugs). A review of all medications a diabetic is taking is important to determine adverse side effects and drug interactions.
- Patients should be asked at the beginning of every appointment if they had taken insulin/oral agents as directed that day, since many diabetic patients (especially those taking insulin) are susceptible to hypoglycemic reactions (profuse sweating, fainting, palpitations, hunger, nervousness, or unconsciousness). The dental clinician should ask patients if they are prone to hypoglycemic reactions. If patients become hypoglycemic, sugar, orange juice, or glucose tablets can be given provided patients should be conscious. If patients become unconscious, then additional medical assistance should be called and injection of glucagon is given. Dextrose (glucose) can also be used.
- Most diabetic patients monitor their blood glucose levels at home with a glucometer. Ask patients the results of the test for that day.
- Low-dose aspirin (75–162 mg/day) is recommended as secondary prevention treatment in diabetics with a history of CVD.Epinephrine decreases the effect of insulin due to epinephrine-induced hyperglycemia via inhibition of pancreatic release of insulin and cellular uptake of glucose. Thus, dental local anesthetic solution with epinephrine is safe for use in diabetic patients except in those who have not taken their preoperative oral hypoglycemic medication. No relation has been found between the post-extraction glucose changes and the number of cartridges administered (Tily and Thomas 2007).

B.   Thyroid diseases

Clinical synopsis

The **thyroid gland**, located on the front side of the neck, produces and releases *thyroxine* (T$_4$, levothyroxine). At the target tissues, thyroxine is converted into the active form, *triiodothyronine* (T$_3$), which enters the cells and binds to receptors. About 87% of T$_3$ is derived from T$_4$ and the remaining 13% is synthesized by the thyroid gland (Weinberg *et al.* 2012). Iodine is required for the synthesis of T$_4$ and is provided by dietary intake of iodized salt. For therapeutic purposes (e.g., medications for replacement of thyroid hormone), T$_4$ is used because more constant blood levels can be achieved due to its longer duration of action with a half-life of 7 days rather than T$_3$ with a half-life of 1 day (Weinberg *et al.* 2012).

Thyroid stimulating hormone (TSH), which comes from the hypothalamus, stimulates the growth of the thyroid gland and synthesis and secretion of the thyroid hormones. The thyroid forms a *negative feedback loop* whereby secretion of TSH declines as the blood level of thyroid hormones rises, (T$_4$) and vice versa (e.g., peaks at night and lower levels during the day).

Once released into the bloodstream, thyroid hormones can exist in the bound (to a protein) or unbound form. Thyroid hormones are highly protein bound (99.9% for T$_4$ and 99.5% for T$_3$) so that only a little of the free unbound form actually binds to receptors and produces an effect in the body.

The conversion to T_3 is critical because T_3 has greater biological activity than T_4. Hypothyroidism is defined as a diminished thyroid hormone formation. Hashimoto's thyroiditis, an autoimmune disorder of the thyroid gland, is presumably the most common cause of primary hypothyroidism. Other causes may include treatment of a patient with radioactive iodine during when the thyroid gland becomes inactive (hypothyroid) and requires replacement therapy, thyroid gland failure, cretinism (congenital hypothyroidism), tumors, or drug induced (e.g., lithium, iodides, and sulfonylureas). Diagnosis is based on elevated levels of TSH. Initially, T_4 levels may be normal, but later on in the disease there are decreased levels. Symptoms of hypothyroidism in adults, also known as myxedema, include slowed body metabolism, slurred speech, depression, bradycardia, weight gain, low body temperature, and intolerance to cold environments. Treatment of hypothyroidism is with L-thyroxine.

Hyperthyroidism (thyrotoxicosis) or excessive production of thyroid hormones must be treated by reducing the levels of the thyroid hormones. The most common type of hyperthyroidism is called Graves' disease, an autoimmune disease, in which the body develops antibodies against its own thyroid gland. Other causes of hyperactivity includes multinodular goiter or Plummer's disease (enlargement of thyroid gland) and tumors. Pharmacologic treatment options include the following antithyroid drugs such as propylthiouracil and methimazole (Tapazole) or radioactive iodine. After radioactive iodine, the patient usually becomes hypothyroid and must take thyroid replacement medications.

Thyroid storm or thyroid crisis is a state of exaggerated hyperthyroidism-characterized hyperpyrexia (temporary increase in body temperature), which can be as low as 38 °C or 100.4 °F and a rapid pulse rate. Thyroid storm is due to severe stress, surgery, or infection. This is a medical emergency.

Cancer of the thyroid

The dentist may be the first clinician to detect a problem in the thyroid region. Diagnosis of thyroid cancer is initially made by palpation and observation of lump or nodule in the thyroid area. There are no laboratory blood values that will aid in the diagnosis. Any suspicious palpable thyroid nodule should be referred immediately to a physician. The majority of thyroid cancers are either the papillary or follicular type (Schlumberger 1998). Treatment of either cancer routinely includes surgery followed by radioactive iodine therapy (RAI). Surgery involves either a thyroidectomy that removes the entire thyroid gland or lobectomy that removes only the affected side of the thyroid gland) (Schlumberger 1998; Walter *et al.* 2007). Radioactive iodine is done after surgery to look for areas of thyroid tissues that absorb and concentrate the iodine and then destroy any remaining cancerous thyroid tissue (Schlumberger 1998). RAI is also the modality of choice in the treatment of hyperthyroidism of Graves' disease. Thyroid hormone supplementation is required after RAI therapy. External beam radiation is used for medullary and anaplastic thyroid cancers that are more aggressive. If the patient previously was treated for thyroid cancer, ask them what type of cancer they had and whether radiotherapy or RAI was used. This will make a difference in dental management of these patients. In patients that have had or will have RAI or radiotherapy therapy to the head and neck area, special management must be taken into consideration. Chapter 14 will address this subject.

The dentist should reinforce meticulous oral home care before, during, and after cancer treatment. Consider fluoride supplements in office/home. Radioiodine may affect oral health with the development of postradioiodine xersotomia. This adverse effect increases with increasing radioactive iodine doses (e.g., 100 millicuries) (Walter *et al.* 2007). For this reason, the lowest dose (e.g., 30 millicuries) possible is administered initially (Schlumberger *et al.* 2012).

Diagnostic/lab values (Stagnaro-Gree *et al.* 2011)

- To determine whether an individual has hyperthyroidism, or hypothyroidism, a blood test is taken that measures unbound T_4 and TSH levels.
- Tyroxine (T_4): this is a measure of bound and free thyroxine (affects tissue function) and a measure of thyroid function. Normal range: 4.5–12.5 mcg/dl.
- Triiodothyronine (T_3): reference range: 80–220 ng/dl.
- TSH: reference range: 0.3–3.
- Hypothyroidism: TSH levels elevated (primarily) and T_4 levels are low.
- Hyperthyroidism: TSH levels low; T_3 and T_4 levels are high.

Oral manifestations of thyroid disorders (Chandna and Bathla 2011)

Hypothyroidism:

- Delayed tooth eruption
- Delayed wound healing; increased chance for oral infection
- Enamel hypoplasia
- Mouth breathing
- Glossitis
- Salivary gland enlargement
- Dysgeusia (distortion of the sense of taste)
- Anterior open bite
- Macroglossia

Hyperthyroidism:

- Increased incidence of periodontal disease
- Increased incidence of dental caries
- Enlargement of thyroid gland
- Burning mouth syndrome
- Accelerated tooth eruption
- Development of connective tissue diseases such as Sjogren's syndrome or systemic lupus erythematous

Dental notes: Management of patient with thyroid disorder

- Assess the patient's clinical status. Usually no special precautions are followed when treating dental patients who are well controlled with thyroid medication.
- There may be a relative delayed wound healing in patients with hypothyroidism (Chandna and Bathla 2011).
- Patient with hypothyroidism are more susceptible to developing CVD (Chandna and Bathla 2011). Monitor the patient.
- Some patients with comorbid cardiovascular conditions (e.g., atrial fibrillation) may be taking warfarin. Avoid aspirin, NSAIDs, and acetaminophen in patients on warfarin therapy (Hughes *et al.* 2011). Consult with the patient's physician.
- There are no specific dental drug–drug interactions.
- Most patients presenting to the dental office will be controlled and under the care of a physician; however, patients may be seen with undiagnosed hypothyroidism or hyperthyroidism, where routine dental treatment may result in adverse outcomes. If there is no documentation on the

patient's medical history about thyroid disorders, but several signs and symptoms point to thyroid disease, it is prudent to get a medical consult from the patient's physician.

- Reduce stress and anxiety levels in patients with hyperthyroidism, which could trigger a thyrotoxic crisis (Chandna and Bathla 2011).
- Monitor vital signs in a hyperthyroid patient.
- Epinephrine (1:100,000) is limited to two cartridges in hyperthyroid patients; however, patients with thyroid storm will most likely not be seen in the dental office, since it is a life-threatening disorder and patients are very ill (Huber and Terezhalmy 2008).
- Monthly blood tests should be done to maintain normal thyroid hormone levels. The dentist must be cognizant in recognizing signs and symptoms of thyroid disorders especially hyperthryoid crisis and when necessary, refer to their physician (Pinto and Glick 2002).

C. Adrenal gland disorders

Clinical synopsis

Adrenal corticosteroids provide replacement therapy in adrenal insufficiency, hypopituitarism, and congenital adrenal hyperplasia and are also used for their anti-inflammatory and immuno-suppressive effects in treating such diseases as rheumatoid arthritis, asthma, and nephrotic syndrome.

The adrenal glands are located next to the kidneys and are made up of the adrenal medulla, adrenal cortex. The adrenal medulla produces and secretes epinephrine and norepinephrine that stimulate the sympathetic division of the central nervous system. Epinephrine is responsible for converting stored glycogen (carbohydrates) into glucose in the liver. This process is called glycogenolysis.

The adrenal cortex produces and releases steroid hormones into the circulation which allow the body to endure stresses put upon it such as injury, disease, and mental strain. The release of **corticosteroids** by the adrenal cortex is controlled by the hypothalamus and anterior pituitary gland via adrenocorticotropic hormone (ACTH), which stimulates corticosteroid release. All human steroids are synthesized from cholesterol found in the body. Three natural adrenal corticosteroids that the body produces and secretes are classified by their actions:

1. **Mineralocorticoids.** The primary mineralocorticoid is aldosterone. Mineralocorticoids exhibit salt-retaining activity in the body and regulate blood pressure. They conserve or maintain the body's concentration of water at a near constant level. They exert most of their effect on the kidneys via the renin–angiotensin mechanism, causing selective excretion of excess potassium in the urine and at the same time retain sodium. The medical use of mineralocorticoids is limited, primarily used for the treatment of hypoadrenalism. Examples of mineralocorticoids include aldosterone and fludrocortisone.
2. **Glucocorticoids.** Hydrocortisone (cortisol) is the primary glucocorticoid. (Hydrocortisone equivalent means that hydrocortisone is equal in potency to cortisol.) Most adrenal corticosteroids exhibit both glucocorticoid and mineralocorticoid activities, although in different potencies and ratios. **Glucocorticoids** regulate energy metabolism by breaking down proteins (e.g., muscles) and lipids (e.g., body fats) and converting them into glucose (gluconeogenesis). They also convert carbohydrates stored in the form of glycogen to glucose and make them available in the blood for tissue uptake. About 20–30 mg of cortisol (equivalent to 5–7.5 mg prednisone) is secreted in the body daily. When the body is under stress, cortisol production may increase up to 300 mg/day (equivalent to 60 mg prednisolone) (Montgomery *et al.* 1990; Gibson and Ferguson 2004). It has

been reported that in response to major surgery, cortisol levels in a patient may increase up to 75–150 mg/day, and in response to minor surgery to 50 mg/day (Kehlet and Binder 1973; Miller *et al.* 2001). When administered, corticosteroids are generally intended to reach a target level, equal to or less than the normal daily output of cortisol by the adrenal cortex, which is 20–30 mg/day (Miller *et al.* 2001). For instance, hydrocortisone or cortisol is prescribed at 20 mg/day and equivalents to this include prednisone, which is much more potent, prescribed at 5 mg/day and dexamethasone, which is most potent, is prescribed at 0.75 mg/day (Miller *et al.* 200).

Glucocorticoids also suppress inflammatory processes (anti-inflammatory) within the body (e.g., bee sting, arthritis), have anti-allergic properties, and are important to the body's immunological defense reactions. Other conditions include the following:

- Asthma
- Rheumatoid arthritis
- Bursitis
- *Pneumocystis jiroveci* pneumonia in HIV-infected patients
- Viral croup (upper airway obstruction with cough in children)
- Systemic lupus erythematous (SLE), pemphigus, erythema multiforme, lichen planus
- Ulcerative colitis
- Antirejection for organ transplant
- Inflammatory conditions of the eye and skin disorders (e.g., pemphigus vulgaris and erythema multiforme)
- Stress-induced shock syndrome
- Severe allergic reactions
- Joint diseases (given as intra-articular injections every 1–6 weeks)
- Organ transplant
- Addison's disease
- Aphthous stomatitis, burning mouth

Steroid hormones act by controlling the rate of protein synthesis inside cells. When taken systemically, glucocorticosteroids are absorbed into the circulation and enter sensitive cells, where they bind to protein receptors and regulate the levels of specific proteins and enzymes, which result in its anti-inflammatory effects. Corticosteroids also exert an anti-inflammatory effect by inhibiting the release of histamine from mast cells.

3. **Gonadocorticoids** (sex hormones). Male and female sex hormones produced by the adrenal cortex supplement those produced by the testes and ovaries. The female hormones are called estrogen and progesterone, and the male androgens include testosterone; the androgens are referred to as anabolic steroids.

Diagnostic/lab values

Physical or mental stress overrides the controlling mechanisms of ACTH secretion and leads to loss of the normal circadian variation of plasma cortisol, causing ACTH secretion which will turn on cortisol synthesis and secretion by the adrenal cortex. Adrenocortical disorders can be diagnosed by measuring the level of cortisol in the plasma or urine. There are no dental implications in these lab values. Morning values of cortisol are higher while evening values are lower.

Dental notes: Adverse effects of corticosteroids and dental management

- Steroid-induced diabetes mellitus
  - Monitor patients taking long-term oral corticosteroids for diabetes and periodontal disease.

- Dental-induced stress: under stress (e.g., dental) the amount of cortisol increases up to 300 mg/day depending on the dental procedure. Endogenous cortisol production stops when exogenous (oral) corticosteroids are ingested.
- Does a patient taking systemic corticosteroids require supplemental steroids before a dental procedure under *local anesthesia* (Table 4.2)?
  - An "older" theory concerning the need for steroid supplementation in patients taking steroids was called the "rule-of-twos" which stated that if the patient was currently on 20 mg of cortisone (equivalent to 5 mg prednisone) daily for 2 weeks or longer within the past 2 years, then it was necessary to give supplemental steroids to prevent an adrenal crisis (Sharuga 2008).
  - Adrenal crisis is associated with a stressful event that is caused by the failure of cortisol levels to meet the body's increased requirements for cortisol and is primarily a mineralocorticoid steroid deficiency, not a glucocorticoid deficiency. Adrenal crisis is a medical emergency characterized by abdominal pain, weakness, hypotension, dehydration, nausea, and vomiting. Adrenal crisis in dental patients is a rare event especially in patients with secondary adrenal insufficiency who are taking the steroid for a medical disorder; however, certain risk factors put the patient at risk for having an adrenal crisis including poor health, infection, hemorrhage, trauma, use of a barbiturate general anesthetic, and an unrecognized adrenal insufficiency (Sharuga 2008; Khalaf *et al.* 2013).
  - *Minor dental procedure under local anesthetic:* It has been concluded in clinical studies that patients taking under 7.5 mg prednisone, long-term, do not require supplemental "steroid coverage" for routine dentistry, including minor surgical procedures under profound local anesthesia with adequate postoperative pain control (Gibson and Ferguson 2004). The target steroid level is 5 mg of prednisone. The low incidence of significant adrenal insufficiency precludes the addition of supplemental steroids (Gibson and Ferguson 2004).
  - According to the most current guidelines, general dental procedures do not require patients who are taking long-term steroids to supplement with additional steroids (Gibson and Ferguson 2004).
  - Patients taking high doses of systemic steroids should double the regular dose on the day of the surgery (medical consult is needed) (Gibson and Ferguson 2004).
  - If adrenal insufficiency is suspect, refer the patient to an endocrinologist.
  - The higher the dose of systemic corticosteroid taken, the greater the risk for developing adrenal suppression.
  - Patients taking corticosteroid inhalers and alternate day dosing of systemic steroids are at a low risk for developing adrenal crisis. Patients with asthma taking chronic (>6 months) 5 mg prednisone per day do not require supplemental steroids for routine restorative procedures and simple single tooth extractions.
  - Know the dosing equivalents: 20 mg hydrocortisone (cortisol) = 5 mg prednisone = 0.75 mg dexamethasone. For example, a patient is taking 30 mg prednisone for rheumatoid arthritis for the past 5 months; 30 mg prednisone is equivalent to 120 mg cortisol, which is adequate coverage for routine minor dental procedures.
  - Take and monitor blood pressure before and after the dental procedure.
  - Remember, according to Gibson and Ferguson (2004), corticosteroid supplementation should not exceed levels of cortisol produced under stress which is up to 300 mg/day. In addition, daily doses of steroids at or <5–7 mg prednisone are thought to be under the physiological threshold for causing adrenal suppression (Gibson and Ferguson 2004).
- Does a patient taking systemic corticosteroids require supplemental steroids before a dental procedure under *general anesthesia*?
  - The need for supplemental steroids depends on the surgical procedure and the regular dose the patient is taking.

- For major oral/periodontal surgery under general anesthesia, supplemental steroids (doubling the dose) may be required depending upon the dose of steroid and the duration of treatment (Gibson and Ferguson 2004). It is important to obtain a medical consultation from the patient's physician.
  - Supplements should only be given in amounts equivalent to the normal physiological response to surgical stress.
  - Consult with the patient's endocrinologist.
- Make sure to schedule the patient in the morning and make sure the patient has taken the steroid within 2 h of the dental procedure because at this time the cortisol levels are the highest (Miller *et al.* 2001).
  - Try to make appointment as stress-free as possible. Administer profound anesthesia with long-acting anesthetic and adequate analgesic for after the procedure. In addition, utilization of adjunctive stress/pain reducing methods can be utilized including hypnosis or biofeedback.
  - Avoid NSAIDs and aspirin when patients are taking systemic corticosteroids due to increased risk for developing gastric lesions including ulcers and bleeding.
  - Epinephrine can safely be administered in patients taking systemic corticosteroids; epinephrine is synthesized in the adrenal medulla, not adrenal cortex.

Table 4.2 Guidelines for patients taking systemic corticosteroids (Sharuga 2008; Miller *et al.* 2001).

Risk category and dental procedure	Supplemental steroids
Low risk: 1. Minor nonsurgical dental procedures without local anesthetic	Minimal increase in cortisol secretion Target steroid level is about 5 mg prednisone No supplemental dose needed—regular steroid dose
Mild risk: 2. Minor periodontal and oral surgery with local anesthetic (e.g., single tooth extraction, periodontal scaling and root planning)	Target steroid level is about 5 mg prednisone Adrenal insufficiency is prevented when circulating levels of glucocorticoids are about 25 mg of hydrocortisone equivalent/day which is equivalent to a dose of about 5–6 mg of prednisone (prednisone is supplied as 1, 2.5, 5, 10, 20, 50 mg tab). This should be taken 1–2 h before treatment. This is regular dosing and no supplemental steroids are required.
Moderate to major risk: 3. Major dental surgery (multiple extractions, impacted wisdom teeth extraction, quadrant periodontal surgery, multiple implants under general anesthesia longer than 1 h (usually in the hospital)	Requires physician's consultation. Need glucocorticoid levels of 50–100 mg/day of hydrocortisone equivalent on the day of surgery and for at least 1 day after surgery. Intra-muscular injection of 100 mg hydrocortisone one hour prior to surgery or if the patient is already taking 5 mg prednisone, then double the dose to 10 mg taken 2 h before extractions/surgery, then 10 mg for 1 day following surgery and then return to normal dosing. Prescribe analgesics as needed.

Adapted from Little *et al.* (2008).
National Endocrine and Metabolic Diseases Information Service. Available at: http://endocrine.niddk.nih.gov/pubs/addison/addison.htm [accessed January 21, 2014].

References

Ajjan, R. & Grant, P.J. (2006) Coagulation and atherothrombotic disease. *Atherosclerosis*, **186**, 240–259.

American Diabetes Association (2011) Classification and diagnosis. *Diabetes Care*, **34 (Suppl. 1)**, S11–S61.

Berry, C., Tardif, J.C. &, Bourassa, M.G. (2007) Coronary heart disease in patients with diabetes. *Part I: recent advances in prevention and noninvasive management. Journal of the American College of Cardiology*, **49**, 631–642.

Chandna, S. & Bathla, M. (2011) Oral manifestations of thyroid disorders and its management. *Indian Journal of Endocrinology and Metabolism,* **15 (Suppl 2)**, S113–S116.

Colwell, J.A. & Nesto, R.W. (2003) The platelet in diabetes: focus on prevention of ischemic events. *Diabetes Care*, **26**, 2181–2188.

Dagogo, J.S. (2004) Hypoglycemia in type 1 diabetes mellitus: pathophysiology and prevention. *Treatments in Endocrinology*, **3 (2)**, 91–103.

Farmer, A.J. (2010) Chapter 25. Monitoring diabetes. In: R.I.G. Holt, C.S. Cockram, A. Flyvbjerg, & B. Goldstein (eds.) *Textbook of Diabetes*, 4th ed. Blackwell Publishing Ltd, Oxford.

Gibson, N. & Ferguson, J.W. (2004) Steroid cover for dental patients on long-term steroid medication. Proposed clinical guidelines based upon critical review of the literature. *British Dental Journal*, **197**, 681–685.

Gilbert, R.E., Connelly, K., Kelly, D.J. *et al.* (2006) Heart failure and nephropathy: catastrophic and interrelated complications of diabetes. *Clinical Journal of the American Society of Nephrology*, **1**, 193–208.

Giles, T.D. & Sander, G.E. (2005) Pathophysiologic, diagnostic, and therapeutic aspects of the metabolic syndrome. *The Journal of Clinical Hypertension*, **7**, 669–678.

Grundy, S.M., Benjamin, I.V., Burke, G.L. *et al.* (1999) Diabetes and cardiovascular disease: a state for healthcare professionals from the American Heart Association. *Circulation,* **100**, 1134–1146.

Handelsman, Y., Mechanick, J.I., Blonde, L. *et al.* (2011) American Association of Clinical Endocrinologists Medical Guidelines for Clinical Practice for Developing a Diabetes Mellitus Comprehensive Care Plan. *Endocrine Practice*, **17 (Suppl. 2)**, 1–53.

Hanson, R.L., Imperatore, G., Bennett, P.H. *et al.* (2002) *Diabetes*, **51 (10)**, 3120–3127.

Huang, E.S., Liu, J.Y., Moffet, H.H. *et al.* (2011) Glycemic control, complications, and death in older diabetic patients. *Diabetes Care*, **34 (6)**, 1329–1336.

Huber, M.A. & Terezhalmy, G.T. (2008) Risk stratification and dental management of the patient with thyroid dysfunction. *Quintessence International*, **39**, 139–150.

Hughes, G.J., Patel, P.N., & Saxena, N. (2011) Effect of acetaminophen on international normalized ratio in patients receiving warfarin therapy. *Pharmacotherapy*, **31**, 591–597.

Junttila, M.J., Barthel, P., Myerburg, R.J. *et al.* (2010) Sudden cardiac death after myocardial infarction in patients with type 2 diabetes. *Heart Rhythm*, **7 (10)**, 1396–1403.

Kahn, B.B. & Flier, J.S. (2000) Obesity and insulin resistance. *Journal of Clinical Investigation*, **106**, 473–481.

Kehlet, H. & Binder, C. (1973) Adrenocortical function and clinical course during and after surgery in unsupplemented glucocorticoid-treated patients. *British Journal of Anaesthesiology*, **45**, 1043–1048.

Khalaf, M.W., Khader, R., Cobetto, G. *et al.* (2013) Risk of adrenal crisis in dental patients. Results of a systematic search of the literature. *Journal of the American Dental Association*, **144**, 152–160.

Little, J.W., Falace, D.A., Miller, C.S. *et al.* (2008) *Dental Management of the Medically Compromised Patient*, 7th ed, pp. 236–247. Mosby, St. Louis.

Mahler, R.J. & Adler, M.L. (1999) Type 2 diabetes mellitus: update on diagnosis, pathophysiology, and treatment. *Journal Clinical Endocrinology & Metabolism*, **84 (4)**, 1165–1171.

Mealey, B.L. & Oates, T.W. (2006) Diabetes mellitus and periodontal disease. *Journal of Periodontology*, **77**, 1289–1303.

Miller, C.S., Little, F.W., & Falace, D.A. (2001) Supplemental corticosteroids for dental patients with adrenal insufficiency: reconsiderations of the problem. *Journal of the American Dental Association*, **132**, 1570–1579.

Montgomery, M.T., Hogg, J.P, Roberts, D.L. *et al.* (1990) The use of glucocorticoids to lessen the inflammatory sequelae following third molar surgery. *Journal of Oral Maxillofacial Surgery*, **48**, 179–187.

O'Keefe, J.H., Abuannadi, M., Lavie, C.J. *et al.* (2011) Strategies for optimizing glycemic control and cardiovascular prognosis in patients with type 2 diabetes mellitus. *Mayo Clinic Proceedings*, **86 (2)**, 128–138.

Padwal, R., Majumda, S.R., Johnson, J.A. *et al.* (2005) A systematic review of drug therapy to delay or prevent type 2 diabetes. *Diabetes Care*, **28**, 736–744.

Pinto, A. & Glick, M. (2008) Management of patients with thyroid disease: oral health considerations. *Journal of the American Dental Association*, **133** (7), 849–858.

Reusch, J.E.B. (2013) Diabetes, microvascular complications, and cardiovascular complications: what is it about glucose? *Journal of Clinical Investigations*, **112** (7), 986–988.

Rodbard, H.W., Blonde, L., Braithwaite, S.S. *et al.* (2007) American Association of Clinical Endocrinologists medical guidelines for clinical practice for the management of diabetes mellitus. *Endocrine Practice*, **13 (Suppl. 1)**, 1–68.

Schlumberger, M.J. (1998) Papillary and follicular thyroid carcinoma. *New England Journal of Medicine*, **338**, 297–306.

Schlumberger, M., Catargi, B., Borget, I. *et al.* (2012) Strategies of radioiodine ablation in patients with low-risk thyroid cancer. *The New England Journal of Medicine,* **366**, 1663–1673.

Sharuga, C.R. (2008) Corticosteroid supplementation. Is it still relevant? Dimensions of *Dental Hygiene*, **6**, 16–17, 19.

Stagnaro-Gree, A., Abalovich, M., Alexander, E. *et al.* (2011) Guidelines of the American Thyroid Association for the diagnosis and management of thyroid disease during pregnancy and postpartum. *Thyroid*, **21**, 1081–1126.

Taylor, J.J., Preshaw, P.M., & Lalla, E. (2013) A review of the evidence for pathogenic mechanisms that may link periodontitis and diabetes. *Journal of Clinical Periodontology/Journal of Periodontology*, **84**, S113–S134.

Tily, F.E. & Thomas, S. (2007) Glycemic effect of administration of epinephrine-containing local anaesthesia in patients undergoing dental extraction, a comparison between healthy and diabetic patients. *International Dental Journal*, **57**, 77–83.

Trovasti, M. & Anfossi, G. (1998) Insulin, insulin resistance and platelet function: similarities with insulin effects on cultured vascular smooth muscle cells. *Diabetologia*, **41**, 609–622.

Walter, M.A., Turtschi, C.P., Schindler, C. *et al.* (2007) The dental safety profile of high-dose radioiodine therapy for thyroid cancer: long-term results of a longitudinal cohort study. *The Journal of Nuclear Medicine*, **48**, 1620–1625.

Weinberg, M.A. & Segelnick, S.L. (2012) Managing heart-related complications in patients with diabetes. *US Pharmacist*, **27**, 68–76.

Weinberg, M.A., Theile, C., & Fine, J.B. (2012). *Oral Pharmacology for the Dental Hygienist,* 2nd ed. Pearson, Upper Saddle River, NJ.

Chapter 5

Disorders of the cardiovascular system

A. Hypertension	59
B. Angina Pectoris	68
C. Myocardial infarction	70
D. Heart failure	73
E. Arrhythmias	75
F. Valvular heart disease	78
G. Epinephrine in cardiac patients	79
References	80

A.   Hypertension

Clinical synopsis

Hypertension is defined as a sustained elevation in arterial pressure due to the amount of blood in the vessel being greater than the space available. In December 2013, the Joint National Committee on Prevention, Detection, Evaluation, and Treatment of High Blood Pressure released its eighth report (*JNC-VIII*) which varies from the JNC-VII from 2003 (Chobanian *et al.* 2003; James 2014). Other guidelines that have been published include ACCOMPLISH, ON-TARGET, TRANSCEND, HYVET, the Cochrane Collaboration analysis of beta-blockers, ACCORD-BP for hypertension, and JUPITER, SPARCL, ENHANCE, ARBITER 6, and ACCORD-Lipid for dyslipidemia. These trials should be considered as temporary guidelines until existing guidelines are updated. The 2013 classification of blood pressure is summarized in Table 5.1.

According to the new guidelines, emphasis is put on whether starting antihypertensive therapy at specific blood pressure thresholds in adults with hypertension improve overall health (James 2014). According to *JNC-VIII*, normal blood pressure goal in a person ≥60 years of age is <150/90 mmHg. Pharmacologic therapy is initiated if blood pressure is ≥150/90 in order to reach the goal of <150/90. If there are comorbidities such as diabetes in a person ≥18 years of age, then the new blood pressure goal is <140/90 mmHg. Pharmacologic therapy is initiated if blood pressure is <140/90 in order to reach the goal of <140/90. In people <60 years of age, a blood pressure of

The Dentist's Quick Guide to Medical Conditions, First Edition. Mea A. Weinberg, Stuart L. Segelnick, Joseph S. Insler, with Samuel Kramer.
© 2015 John Wiley & Sons, Inc. Published 2015 by John Wiley & Sons, Inc.

Table 5.1   JNC-VIII classification of blood pressure for adults (James 2014).

Category	Systolic (mmHg)	Diastolic (mmHg)
Normal		
≥60 years old	<150	<90
<60 years old	<140	<90
≥18 years old	<140	<90

Table 5.2   Major risk factors for hypertension (Dalen *et al.* 2011).

Smoking
Obesity
Sedentary lifestyle
Alcohol
Stress
Male gender
Family history of CV disease
Postmenopause
Sodium intake

<140/90 mmHg is the goal. Additionally, there is now emphasis on elevated systolic pressure (SBP) being an important risk factor for cardiovascular (CV) disease, rather than elevated diastolic blood pressure (Kannel *et al.* 1969; Fifth Report of the Joint National Committee on Detection, Evaluation, and Treatment of High Blood Pressure 1993; Chobanian *et al.* 2003). The systolic blood pressure is the important factor in controlling blood pressure (Hyman and Pavlik 2001; Basile 2002).

According to the 2013 guidelines, the selection of appropriate medication is based on race: In the non-black population, the initial drug of choice is thiazide diuretic, calcium channel blockers (CCBs), angiotension-converting enzyme inhibitors (ACEIs), or angiotensin receptor blocker (ARB). In the black population, the initial drug of choice is either a thiazide diuretic or CCB (James 2014).

Blood pressure is regulated by the sympathetic nervous system and the kidneys. Hypertension having no identifiable cause is termed primary or essential and accounts for 90% of all cases. It results in an increase in systolic and diastolic pressure due to alterations in the mechanisms regulating cardiac output and total peripheral vascular resistance. Secondary hypertension is the term given to elevated blood pressure due to a known physical abnormality.

Although the etiology of essential hypertension is relatively unknown, certain genetic and environmental risk factors are thought to cause hypertension and are listed in Table 5.2.

Risk factors for secondary hypertension include renal disease, hyperthyroidism, medication, (estrogen), Cushing's disease (glucocorticoid excess), diabetes mellitus, and pheochromocytoma (rare malignant neoplasm). Complications arising from hypertension include stroke and renal failure, which leads to heart failure.

Only about 40% of treated hypertensive patients are actually well controlled (Cutler *et al.* 2008). Most patients are not even aware that they have high blood pressure. This is interpreted that most likely a majority of dental patients coming to the dental office are not controlled.

Three factors are responsible for creating blood pressure and controlling cardiac function: cardiac output, peripheral resistance, and blood volume.

- *Cardiac output* is the volume or amount of blood pumped out per minute by the ventricle of the heart and is determined by the heart rate and stroke volume, which is the amount of blood pumped by a ventricle in one contraction.
- *Peripheral resistance* (afterload) refers to the resistance of blood vessels to blood flow.
- *Blood volume* is the total amount of blood in the circulatory system, which is approximately 5 l.

Other factors include the following:

- *Preload:* the volume of blood returned to the heart before it beats.
  Contractility: the forcefulness with which the heart contracts.

Medications

Treatment of essential hypertension is aimed at restoration of the balance between cardiac output and total peripheral vascular resistance, so that the blood pressure (cardiac output times total peripheral vascular resistance) falls to acceptable levels before irreversible damage occurs to organ systems such as the eyes, the kidneys, or the CV system. Secondary hypertension is treated by removing the causative agent, re-evaluating the CV system for damage, and initiating treatment, if necessary.

It is important to realize that treatment of hypertension not only involves pharmacotherapy, but major lifestyle modifications, including weight reduction, limiting alcohol consumption, increasing aerobic physical activity, restricting sodium intake, and smoking cessation.

There are over 100 drugs that have been approved by the US Food and Drug Administration (FDA) for the treatment of hypertension. Thus, it is important that a drug be selected that is most appropriate for the specific needs of the patient. Many patients with hypertension will have a comorbidity (another coexisting disease) which makes choosing the correct medication more challenging to prevent any drug–drug or drug–disease interactions. For instance, patients with hypertension and arthritis may be taking a nonsteroidal anti-inflammatory drug (NSAID) (e.g., ibuprofen) that could lower the effects of some antihypertensive drugs. *The desired target blood pressure goal is lower than 140/90 in patients without compelling indicators, and lower than 130/80 on patients with compelling indicators or comorbidities such as diabetes mellitus or renal disease* (James 2014).

The JNC VII hypertension guidelines recommended five classes of drugs for initial therapy with thiazide diuretics being the drug of choice for the majority of patients without evidence to prescribe another type of drug. If a patient had concurrent diabetes mellitus (type 1), an ACE inhibitor or ARB is recommended; if the patient has concurrent heart failure, an ACE inhibitor or diuretic is recommended; if the patient had a previous heart attack, a beta-blocker is recommended and; in the elderly patient, a diuretic is preferred.

With the newer JNC VIII hypertension guidelines, there is a selection of four specific medication classes including ACEI, ARB, CCB, or diuretics. Dosing is based on randomized controlled trials (RCT), and specifically is based on categories such as race, gender, smokers, coronary artery disease, previous stroke, chronic kidney disease (CKD), and diabetic subgroups (James 2014). The JNC 8 panel developed a table of drugs and doses with specific nine recommendations (James 2014).

Diagnostic/lab tests

1. Vital signs: Blood pressure, pulse rate, and breathing rate. Depending on the circumstances, record blood pressure at the start, during, and the end of the dental procedure (www.dental.pacific.edu/Documents/dental_prof/Medically_Complex.pdf).

2. If the systolic reading is >140 mmHg or diastolic reading is >90 mmHg after two readings in contralateral arms and 5 min apart, then the patient has stage 1 hypertension according to the classification in Table 5.1.

3. Even if the patient is "controlled" with antihypertensive medications, the patient is still considered to have hypertension and must be dentally managed accordingly.

4. *The desired target blood pressure goal is lower than 140/90 in patients without compelling indicators, and lower than 130/80 on patients with compelling indicators or comorbidities such as diabetes mellitus or renal disease (Basile 2002).*

Dental notes: Medication management of the hypertensive patient

Diuretics:
Diuretics were the first drugs used in the treatment of hypertension, in the 1950s. They are still considered to be the drug of choice because they produce few adverse effects and are very effective for treating mild to moderate hypertension.

There are three classes of diuretics: thiazides, loop, and potassium-sparing, which act in different parts of the kidney. Diuretics act by increasing the volume of urine production by excretion of excess fluid in the body.

Because of increased loss of fluids, common adverse effects such as electrolyte disturbance with loss of sodium, potassium, and magnesium; dehydration; orthostatic hypotension (due to reduced blood volume); and xerostomia occur.

Thiazide Diuretics: Thiazide diuretics act in the distal tubule of the kidney to inhibit sodium chloride (NaCl) reabsorption back into the blood allowing an increased level of sodium in the tubule, which holds water, resulting in increased urination and a lowering of blood pressure. Because of the increased sodium load in the tubule, excretion of potassium is usually increased, resulting in hypokalemia. Hydrochlorothiazide is the prototype thiazide.

Thiazide Diuretics:

- Chlorothiazide (Diuril)
- Hydroclorothiazide (Hydrodiuril)

Over months, the diuretic effect of thiazides decreases, with kidney function returning to normal in regard to sodium (sodium reabsorbs back into the blood and is not excreted), but the antihypertensive effect remains the same. Thiazides are effective in lowering blood pressure of 10–15 mmHg in patients with *mild essential hypertension.* Thiazides may increase total cholesterol and the loss of electrolytes, which may predispose the patient with heart disease to arrhythmias. Potassium supplements (e.g., food or drugs) may be necessary to replenish the lost potassium. Thiazides are contraindicated in diabetics because they increase blood glucose and may decrease the effectiveness of antidiabetic drugs. Monitoring of blood electrolytes including K^+, N^+, Mg^+, Cl^-, and serum lipids and cholesterol is essential.

Patients taking diuretics may develop orthostatic hypotension. Common signs include dizziness, light-headedness, pale skin, and nausea. Management of the patient is by monitoring the blood pressure. After moving the dental chair from a supine position, have the patient remain in an upright position for a few minutes before dismissing them.

Potassium-sparing diuretics:

- Amiloride (Midamor)
- Spironolactone (Aldactone)
- Triamterene (Dyrenium)

Potassium-sparing/thiazide diuretics:

- Amiloride/hydrochlorothiazide (HCTZ) (Moduretic)
- Spironolactone/HCTZ (Aldactazide)
- Triamterene/HCTZ (Dyazide)

Potassium-sparing diuretics act in the distal tubule, where inhibition of sodium reabsorption results in a corresponding *reduction* in potassium excretion, so potassium supplements are not necessary. In order to equalize the potassium effects, these drugs are usually prescribed with a potassium-wasting diuretic such as hydrochlorothiazide. Thus these diuretics work differently compared with thiazides and loop diuretics.

Angiotensin-converting enzyme inhibitors

- Captopril (Capoten)
- Lisinopril (Prinivil)
- Enalapril (Vasotec)
- ramipril (Altase)
- Benazepril (Lotensin)
- Fosinopril (Monorail)
- Quinapril (Accupril)
- Moexipril (Univasc)
- Trandolapril (Mavik)

Angiotensin II receptors blockers

- Candesartan cilexetil (Atacand)
- Eprosartan (Teveten)
- Irbesartan (Avapro)
- Losartan (Cozar)
- Telmisartan (Micardis)
- Valsartan (Diovan)

Central presynaptic α_2-adrenergic release inhibitors

- Clonidine (Catapres)
- Methyldopa (Aldomet)

Peripheral presynaptic adrenergic release inhibitors

- Reserpine (Serpasil)
- Guanethidine

α_1-Adrenergic blockers (also vasodilators)

- Doxazosin (Cardura)
- Prazosin (Minipress)
- Terazosin (Hytrin)

β-Adrenergic blockers

- Atenolol (Tenormin)
- Acebutolol (Sectral)

- Betaxolol (Kerlone)
- Bisoprolol (Zebeta)
- Carteolol (Cartrol)
- Metoprolol (Lopressor)
- Labetalol (Normodyne)
- Nadolol (Corgard)
- Propranolol (Inderal)

Calcium channel blockers

- Diltiazem (Cardizem)
- Verapamil (Calan, Isoptin)
- Amlodipine (Norvasc)
- Felodipine (Plendil)
- Isradipine (Dynacirc)
- Nicardipine (Cardene)
- Nifedipine (Adalat, Procardia)
- Nisoldipine (Sular)

Direct vasodilators

- Hydralazine (Apresoline)
- Minoxidil (Loniten)
- Nitroprusside (Nitropress)

Specific dental management guidelines should be followed for patients taking different antihypertensive medications. Attention should be focused on disease recognition and adverse effects of the medications. Table 5.3 shows the key points to review when treating these patients.

Dental notes: Management of the hypertensive patient

- The patient should be asked what medications he/she is currently taking for blood pressure and whether these medications are being taken as prescribed. Specifically ask the patient whether they have taken their medication on the day of treatment and document in the chart. These medications are usually taken in the morning or at night. If the patient has not taken their medication as prescribed, it is recommended to postpone the treatment (www.dental.pacific.edu/Documents/dental_prof/Medically_Complex.pdf).
- Remember to update medical history at every appointment.
- Have good relations with the patient's physician.
- Ask the patient about their usual blood pressure and their last visit to their physician.
- In a hypertensive patient, vital signs should be monitored multiple times during every dental visit. Since these antihypertensive drugs are used to treat different types of CV/cardiac conditions and not just hypertension, the clinician should ask the patient for what condition the drug(s) is (are) being taken.
- A patient with more severe hypertension may do better with short, morning appointments that are less stressful. Adjunctive procedures including nitrous oxide/oxygen or prescribing a benzodiazepine (anti-anxiety) drug should be considered to reduce stress levels.
- Physician consultation is highly recommended in patients with blood pressure ≥140/90 mmHg.
- It is important to avoid a hypertensive crisis where the blood pressure increases very quickly.
- A study showed that the time when blood pressure is monitored during a dental procedure may be significant. It was found that blood pressure readings were significantly higher in the beginning of the dental procedure rather than at the end (Nichols 1997).

Table 5.3 Summaries of antihypertensive medications and management of patients taking these medications in the dental office.

Drugs name	Dental notes
Diuretics	NSAIDs such as naproxen sodium and ibuprofen can decrease the effectiveness of the antihypertensive action of the diuretic, resulting in rapid elevation of blood pressure Orthostatic hypotension: Monitor blood pressure. To avoid dizziness/fainting when a patient goes from the supine position, have the patient sit in an upright position for a few minutes before dismissing them Patients may need to use the restroom facilities (increased urination from the diuretic) more frequently during the dental visit. Adjust your time accordingly Xerostomia: monitor for dental caries and candidiasis No special precautions with the use of epinephrine
ACEI	NSAIDs such as naproxen sodium and ibuprofen can decrease the effectiveness of the antihypertensive action of the ACEI inhibitor, resulting in rapid elevation of blood pressure Orthostatic hypotension: Monitor blood pressure. To avoid dizziness/fainting when a patient goes from the supine position, have the patient sit in an upright position for a few minutes before dismissing them Xerostomia: monitor for dental caries and candidiasis No special precautions with the use of epinephrine
ARBs	NSAIDs such as naproxen sodium and ibuprofen can decrease the effectiveness of the antihypertensive action of the antihypertensive resulting in rapid elevation of blood pressure. Orthostatic hypotension: Monitor blood pressure. To avoid dizziness/fainting when a patient goes from the supine position, have the patient sit in an upright position for a few minutes before dismissing them Xerostomia: monitor for dental caries and candidiasis No special precautions with the use of epinephrine
Central presynaptic α_2-adrenergic release inhibitors	Least affect by combining with NSAIDs Orthostatic hypotension: Monitor blood pressure. To avoid dizziness/fainting when a patient goes from the supine position, have the patient sit in an upright position for a few minutes before dismissing them Xerostomia: monitor for dental caries and candidiasis No special precautions with the use of epinephrine
Peripheral presynaptic adrenergic release inhibitors	NSAIDs such as naproxen sodium and ibuprofen can decrease the effectiveness of the antihypertensive action of the antihypertensive resulting in rapid elevation of blood pressure Orthostatic hypotension: Monitor blood pressure. To avoid dizziness/fainting when a patient goes from the supine position, have the patient sit in an upright position for a few minutes before dismissing them Xerostomia: monitor for dental caries and candidiasis No special precautions with the use of epinephrine

(*continued*)

Table 5.3 *(cont'd)*

Drugs name	Dental notes
β₁-Adrenergic blockers (also vasodilators)	NSAIDs such as naproxen sodium and ibuprofen can decrease the effectiveness of the antihypertensive action of the antihypertensive resulting in rapid elevation of blood pressure Orthostatic hypotension: Monitor blood pressure. To avoid dizziness/fainting when a patient goes from the supine position, have the patient sit in an upright position for a few minutes before dismissing them Xerostomia: monitor for dental caries and candidiasis No special precautions with the use of epinephrine
β-Adrenergic blockers	NSAIDs such as naproxen sodium and ibuprofen can decrease the effectiveness of the antihypertensive action of the antihypertensive resulting in rapid elevation of blood pressure Orthostatic hypotension: Monitor blood pressure. To avoid dizziness/fainting when a patient goes from the supine position, have the patient sit in an upright position for a few minutes before dismissing them Xerostomia: monitor for dental caries and candidiasis
Atenolol (Tenormin)	No special precautions regarding use of epinephrine in local anesthetic
Acebutolol (Sectral)	No special precautions regarding use of epinephrine in local anesthetic
Betaxolol (Kerlone)	No special precautions regarding use of epinephrine in local anesthetic
Bisoprolol (Zebeta)	No special precautions regarding use of epinephrine in local anesthetic
Carteolol (Cartrol)	No special precautions regarding use of epinephrine in local anesthetic
Metoprolol (Lopressor)	No special precautions regarding use of epinephrine in local anesthetic
Labetalol (Normodyne)	Use minimal amount of epinephrine (two cartridges 1:100,000)
Nadolol (Corgard)	Use minimal amount of epinephrine (two cartridges 1:100,000)
Propranolol (Inderal)	Use minimal amount of epinephrine (two cartridges 1:100,000)
CCBs	There is no drug interaction with NSAIDs Orthostatic hypotension: Monitor blood pressure. To avoid dizziness/fainting when a patient goes from the supine position, have the patient sit in an upright position for a few minutes before dismissing them Gingival enlargement occurs most frequently with nifedipine and amlodipine. Management: meticulous oral home care and maintenance care. Referral to periodontist Xerostomia: monitor for dental caries and candidiasis
Direct vasodilators	NSAIDs such as naproxen sodium and ibuprofen can decrease the effectiveness of the antihypertensive action of the antihypertensive resulting in rapid elevation of blood pressure Orthostatic hypotension: Monitor blood pressure. To avoid dizziness/fainting when a patient goes from the supine position, have the patient sit in an upright position for a few minutes before dismissing them Xerostomia: monitor for dental caries and candidiasis No special precautions with the use of epinephrine

- What is the maximum blood pressure that a patient should have for a dentist to treat? There are no specific articles addressing this; however, it is generally accepted not to perform surgery or dental procedures if the blood pressure is over 160/95. If a reading of 180/110 is obtained, after a few minutes, the blood pressure should be retaken. If the reading is still 180/110 or higher, no dental procedures should be started and emergency medical care should be initiated (www.heart.org/ HEARTORG/Conditions/HighBloodPressure/AboutHighBloodPressure/Hypertensive-Crisis-UCM-301782-Article.jsp).
- If the patient has had a mastectomy, blood pressure should be taken on the other side.
- Lymphoedema can occur if the patient has had lymph nodes removed from the arm from which blood pressure is taken. In such conditions, recommend taking blood pressure in the leg right above the knee.
- In morbidly obese patients, pressure can be taken in the popliteal artery in the ankle.
- Any hypertensive drug has the ability to cause orthostatic hypotension, a fall in blood pressure of 20/10 mmHg or more within 5 min of standing from a supine position, which can result in syncope (Bradley and Davis 2003). Care must be taken to allow the patient to remain sitting upright for a few minutes after being in a supine position to this.
  - Using vasoconstrictors in the hypertensive patient is *not* contraindicated. In the hypertensive patient, high doses (about four or more cartridges) of epinephrine may cause excessive cardiac stimulation, resulting in angina or cardiac arrhythmias which can lead to increased blood pressure and stroke. Bader *et al.* (2002) has documented that the use of epinephrine in local anesthetics in uncontrolled hypertensive patients was associated with small, nonsignificant increases in systolic and diastolic blood pressure. They found that the heart rate was higher but the diastolic pressure was lower for both hypertensive and nonhypertensive patients.
  - Patients taking a nonselective β-blocker such as propranolol (Inderal), nadolol (Corgard), or timolol (Blocarden) may have an increased vasopressor response to epinephrine. Blood pressure should be monitored before and during dental treatment for any changes. The initial dose should be minimal (1/2 cartridge), injected slowly using aspiration to avoid intravascular injection. After waiting and monitoring for toxicity for a few minutes, more of the anesthetic may be injected (Lifshey 2004). Do not use more than two cartridges of epinephrine 100,000 (equivalent to <0.034 mg).
  - Always aspirate to avoid intravascular injection.
  - If necessary blood pressure can be taken after an injection.
  - The maximum dose of epinephrine to be used in a patient with controlled hypertension or cardiovascular disease is 0.04 mg which is equivalent to two cartridges (0.017 mg EPI (epinephrine) per cartridge 1:100,000; note that the volume in a cartridge is now 1.7 with a range from 1.7 to 1.8 ml). The benefits for maintaining adequate anesthesia outweigh the risks for toxicity. Careful monitoring for toxicity (e.g., increased blood pressure, cardiac arrhythmias including tachycardia) is important.
  - Epinephrine 1:50,000 should be avoided, as well as retraction cord containing epinephrine (Perusse *et al.* 1992; Hersh and Moore 2008).
  - Levonordefrin, a vasoconstrictor contained in mepivacaine, primarily stimulates α-adrenergic receptors. Since this will increase blood pressure, levonordefrin should not be used in the hypertensive patient. Either mepivacaine plain without vasoconstrictor or lidocaine with 1:100,000 epinephrine (minimum two cartridges) is appropriate.
  - Xerostomia including a dry, sore mouth caused by diuretics and central-acting adrenergic inhibitors are dealt with by educating the patient to increase fluid intake, avoid alcohol and alcohol-containing mouthrinses, and use artificial salivary drugs. Monitor for signs of demineralization and treat with topical fluorides or remineralizing pastes.
  - Gingival enlargement is a common adverse effect of CCBs (e.g., nifedipine). Discontinuation of the drug usually results in a disappearance of the enlargement. Treatment involves meticulous

oral home care and possible surgical removal of excess gingiva. Consultation with the patient's physician is recommended.

○ ACEIs cause angioedema characterized by swelling of the lips and tongue. Notify the patient's physician.

○ ACEIs and thiazide diuretics can cause an oral lichenoid reaction or lichen planus–like lesions. Be aware and treat accordingly.

○ The kidney plays a major role in controlling blood pressure by regulating blood volume. When blood pressure increases in the blood vessels, the kidney can excrete more sodium, which will lower blood volume, resulting in a decrease in cardiac output and the blood pressure returning to normal. An important drug–drug interaction occurs when an NSAID such as naproxen sodium or ibuprofen is taken with all antihypertensive medications except CCBs. This combination of drugs reduces the antihypertensive effect of the antihypertensive drug, which may result in elevated blood pressure. Patients taking antihypertensive medications (except for CCBs) should not take any NSAIDs for more than 5 days.

○ Smoking cessation should be part of the treatment plan in the hypertensive patient.

B. Angina Pectoris

Clinical synopsis

Clinic

Angina pectoris (AP) occurs when the metabolic demands of the heart exceed the ability of the coronary arteries to supply adequate blood flow and oxygen to the heart. Although the typical symptom of angina is severe chest pain upon exertion, angina may develop unexpectedly with minimal or no exertion.

The majority of myocardial ischemia or reduced blood flow represents a manifestation of atherosclerosis. Other risk factors for AP include smoking, elevated serum lipids, family history, obesity, male gender, sedentary lifestyle, hypertension, and a type A personality.

Stable angina occurs when chest pain is intermittent on exertion but relieved by rest. Each attack generally resembles the previous attack, to such an extent that the patient can predict the attack and change his way of life to avoid the precipitating cause. The classical symptoms are squeezing chest pain that radiates to the left arm, right arm, or both, and to the jaw. There may be shortness of breath, nausea, vomiting, and sweating. Acute coronary syndromes (ACS) or myocardial ischemia include unstable angina and myocardial infarction (MI). *Unstable angina* occurs when oxygen demand exceeds oxygen supply at rest and the frequency and severity of attacks increases. *Variant angina* (Prinzmetal's angina) is due to a heart vasospasm, often occurring during sleep. About 90% of patients present with stable angina and 10% have unstable angina that progresses to myocardial infarction and requires antiplatelet drugs and/or surgery (American Academy of Periodontology 1996).

Dental notes: Medications for angina

The goals of treatment are to reduce morbidity and mortality and to control angina. Risk factors must be controlled, including smoking and alcohol cessation.

The goal of drug therapy is to reduce angina by restoring a balance between the supply and demand of the oxygen supply to the heart, either by increasing oxygen supply or decreasing oxygen demand.

Table 5.4 lists the drugs used in the treatment of angina (Table 5.4).

Beta-blockers have been proven to reduce mortality and are used in patients with stable angina who require long-term treatment or in patients who also have hypertension. These drugs decrease

Table 5.4 Dental management of patients on antianginal drugs.

Drugs	Mechanism of action	Dental management
Nitrates		
Nitroglycerin (NitroBid, Nitrostat, Nitro-Dur)	Dilates and relaxes coronary blood vessels	Headache, dizziness and/or flushing, orthostatic hypotension. Monitor blood pressure. Allow patient to sit in an upright position in dental chair for a few minutes before dismissing them
Isosorbidedinitrate (Isordil)		No special precautions with epinephrine
Calcium channel blockers		
Amlodipine (Norvasc) Bedpridil (Vasocor) Diltiazem (Cardizem) Nifedipine (Procardia, Adalat) Verapamil (Calan, Isoptin)	Slows heart rate and dilates coronary arteries	Orthostatic hypotension: Allow patient to sit in an upright position in dental chair for a few minutes before dismissing them gingival enlargement (especially with nifedipine) No special precautions with epinephrine
Cardioselective beta-blockers		
Atenolol (Tenormin): β_1 Metoprolol (Lopressor): β_1	Reduces cardiac load and thus oxygen demand	NSAIDs such as naproxen sodium and ibuprofen can decrease the effectiveness of the antihypertensive action of the antihypertensive resulting in rapid elevation of blood pressure
Non-cardioselective beta-blockers		
Nadolol (Corgard)		Orthostatic hypotension: Monitor blood pressure. To avoid dizziness/fainting when a patient goes from the supine position, have the patient sit in an upright position for a few minutes before dismissing them
Propranolol (Inderal)		No special precautions with epinephrine EXCEPT with non-cardiac selective beta-blockers

myocardial oxygen demand by decreasing heart rate, contractility, and tension. Cardioselective β-blockers are preferred so that only the β_1-receptors are stimulated. These drugs are *cardioselective* because they do not cause bronchoconstriction and the hypoglycemic effects of nonselective beta-blockers. The non-cardioselective beta-blockers will block both β_1 and β_2 receptors, so these drugs should be used with extreme caution in patients with asthma and diabetes. Since non-cardioselective beta-blockers block both the β_1 and β_2 receptors, allowing only alpha-1 receptors to be stimulated, there is an increased vasoconstriction. Thus, the amount of epinephrine 1:100,000 is limited to two cartridges.

Dental notes: Management of the patient with angina

- It is important to determine the severity and stability of the angina. Upon review of the patient's medical history, the patient's last attack, the precipitating factor, and the factor that relieved the attack should be determined.
- Ask the patient what triggers an attack and what relieves the attack.
- Must determine the severity and stability of the angina.
- If patient is taking nitroglycerin, have their bottle within reach.
- If chest pains develop while the patient is in the dental chair, stop all procedures, tell the patient to catch their breath and take nitroglycerin. Then wait a few minutes, take blood pressure and heart rate. Give them oxygen.
- Patients taking any form of nitrates must be careful when sitting up and getting out of the dental chair. Orthostatic hypotension may develop whereby the patient will get dizzy. Have the patient remain in an upright position in the chair for a few minutes before attempting to get out. Otherwise, there are no contraindications or complications to dental treatment. No special precautions are needed with epinephrine.
- It is usually not necessary to discontinue aspirin for routine periodontal debridement.
- The use of vasoconstrictors in local anesthetics in stable angina patients is recommended to obtain profound anesthesia and reduce stress; however, it is suggested to use a maximum of two cartridges containing 1:100,000 epinephrine. A local anesthetic with 1:200,000 epinephrine can also be used (e.g., articaine 4%). In a 1.7 ml cartridge, 1:200,000 dilution concentration contains 0.0085 mg of epinephrine versus 0.017 mg in 1:100,000 concentration. Short appointments are recommended. Mild or moderate (conscious) sedation may be indicated.
- Elective dentistry should be postponed in patients with unstable angina.

C. Myocardial infarction

Clinical synopsis

An MI or heart attack occurs when the blood flow through the coronary arteries is blocked and the muscle cells supplied by the blocked vessels die. The area of dead tissue is called an infarct. Different invasive surgical interventions are used after the initial MI attack including percutaneous coronary interventions, laser angioplasty, stents, or coronary artery bypass graft (CABG). These procedures attempt to improve blood flow (http://emedicine.medscape.com/article/155919-treatment).

Diagnostic/lab tests

Electrocardiogram (EKG) readings, enzyme assays (e.g., SGOT, LDH, and CK/CPK), stress test, international normalized ratio (INR) for patients on warfarin.

Dental notes: Medication management of the MI dental patient

In order to reduce the chance of another MI, a patient may take:

- Triple oral antithrombotic therapy that includes (Schömig *et al.* 2009) the following:
  - low-dose aspirin for its antiplatelet actions
  - platelet $P2Y_{12}$ receptor blocker: clopidogrel (Plavix), aspirin/dipyridamole (Aggrenox), prasugrel (Effient) (Cattaneo 2010)

- ◦ anticoagulant: warfarin (Coumadin)
- ◦ to prevent recurrent ischemic events
- In the past there has been much controversy whether it is safe to take a patient off of an anticoagulant or antiplatelet drug to avoid excessive bleeding during an invasive dental procedure. As far back as 1998, Wahl reported that the incidence of thromboembolic events is increased by 0.2% in patients in whom oral anticoagulation is stopped before a surgical procedure. If an oral anticoagulant is discontinued, a "rebound hypercoagulable state" occurs, during which period an increase in clotting factors and thrombin activity is observed. Warfarin inhibits the synthesis of "new" clotting factors II, VII, IX, and X but does not interfere with the already synthesized and circulating factors in the blood. These factors are still able to function until their half-lives are over so that until the remaining coagulation factors disappear there will always be a risk of abnormal coagulation. This results in a transient hypercoagulation. The half-life of factor II is 60 h; factor VII is 4–6 h; factor IX is 24 h; and factor X is about 3 days (http://emedicine.medscape.com/article/821038-overview#a0104).

Currently, the clinical significance of a hypercoagulable state is unclear (Jeske and Suchko 2003). There is no doubt that keeping patients on an anticoagulant/antiplatelet during dental surgery will most likely result in excessive bleeding; in most cases, it has been reported that it is more easily handled than if the anticoagulant/antiplatelet drugs were discontinued which could result in a medical emergency such as a stroke (Ardekian *et al.* 2000).

- The activity of warfarin is expressed using the INR. In patients taking warfarin, an INR reading should be measured within 24 h, but not more than 72 h, before the dental procedure. For a patient not taking warfarin, a normal coagulation profile is an INR of 1.0.
- In 1992, the American College of Chest Physicians recommended that the therapeutic range of continuous anticoagulant is an INR between 2.0 and 3.0 for all conditions except artificial heart valves, for which the recommended INR is between 2.5 and 3.5. Minor surgical procedures such as a single tooth extraction can be safely performed without altering the warfarin dose with an INR 3. Anticoagulation alterations are required if INR is >4. The target INR differs based on the indication for taking warfarin. For example, if the patient is taking warfarin for atrial fibrillation (AF), deep vein thrombosis or pulmonary embolus, the INR should be 2.5 (range 2.0–3.0). If the patient is taking warfarin for mechanical prosthetic heart valves, stents, or recurrence of embolism, then the INR should be 3.5 (range 2.5–3.5).
- The following are common dental drug–drug interactions:
  - ◦ Erythromycin and clarithromycin (Biaxin) are inhibitors of P450 cytochrome enzymes, which will decrease the metabolism of warfarin, thus increasing warfarin blood levels and causing hypoprothrombinemia.

Box 5.1   International Normalized Ratio (INR) Guidelines for Dental Treatment (Goldhaber 2006).

- All patients should have an INR below 4
- Acceptable range INR 2.0–3.0 in patients with:
  - ◦ Pulmonary embolus
  - ◦ Deep vein thrombosis (DVT)
  - ◦ AF
  - ◦ Bileaflet mitral value
- Acceptable range INR 3.0–4.0 in patients with:
  - ◦ Mechanical heart valves
  - ◦ Recurrence of embolism while on warfarin

- ◦ Azithromycin inhibits warfarin clearance and cause hypoprothrombinemia; monitor prothrombin times (Horn and Hansten 2009).
- ◦ Fluconazole (Diflucan) increases warfarin blood levels by inhibiting CYP2C9 enzymes.
- ◦ Metronidazole inhibits enzymes that metabolize warfarin. These two drugs should be avoided.
- ◦ There is an increased risk for bleeding with concomitant administration of aspirin and other NSAIDs such as ibuprofen.
- ◦ Acetaminophen and warfarin significantly elevate INR, which puts the patient at an increased risk for hemorragic complications (Hughes *et al.* 2011). If it is necessary to recommend/prescribe acetaminophen alone or in combination with a narcotic, then it is necessary to adequately monitor and/or adjust the dosages. A consultation with the patient's physician is recommended. Avoid "prn" dosage.
- • In addition, patients may take:
  - ◦ beta-blocker to reduce the workload of the heart by blocking the β_1-receptors on heart muscle cells
    - • the beta-blocker binds to the beta-receptors on the heart muscle cell and prevents them from being stimulated
    - • watch for orthostatic hypotension
  - ◦ ACEI
    - • blocks angiotensin in the blood allowing vasodilation and lowering of blood pressure and thus has a direct action on the heart which has a protective effect
    - • watch for orthostatic hypotension
  - ◦ CCB: monitor for gingival enlargement
  - ◦ Cholesterol lowering "statin" drugs: avoid prescribing clarithromycin and erythromycin and "azole" antifungal agents (e.g., fluconazole).
    - • Adverse effect of statins is myopathy or rhabdomyolysis. Ask patient if they have either condition. It is advised to have the patient walk around every so often to offset muscle aches.

Dental notes: Management of the MI patient

- • Always get a medical consult.
- • During the first month post-MI, there is an increased risk for developing a second episode (Skaar *et al.* 2012). Therefore, no dental treatment should be performed for the first 30 days. As a general rule, treatment should not be started for 6 months post-MI; however, a recent study documented that it can be earlier, at least 3 months (Skaar *et al.* 2012).
- • Generally, dental treatment should be delayed 3 months post-CABG surgery (Lifshey 2004; Skaar *et al.* 2012). The reason for waiting this long is to prevent a secondary CV episode. Monitor blood pressure and heart rate at every appointment.
- • Epinephrine 1:100,000 should be limited to a maximum of two cartridges.
- • Have short and stress reduction appointment.
- • According to the most current AHA Guidelines, no antibiotic prophylaxis is required for a patient with coronary stents (Wilson *et al.* 2007).
- • Aspirin and NSAIDs such as ibuprofen or naproxen sodium are contraindicated in patients who take warfarin because of an increased risk for bleeding. Any morphine analogues including hydrocodone (Vicodin) can be used but only for a few days. Extra-strength Tylenol taken with warfarin may cause a substantial increase in INR. So, the recommended analgesic is Regular-strength Tylenol.
- • Both prescription and Over-the-counter (OTC) NSAIDs have a black box warning emphasizing the potential for increased risk of CV events. NSAID use among patients with first-time MI was

associated with persistently increased risk of all-cause mortality (e.g., the number of deaths in a given age group per the population in that age group in contrast to the total number of deaths relative to the total population which is the crude death rate) and of a composite of coronary death or nonfatal recurrent MI, respectively, for at least 5 years thereafter. NSAIDs have no apparent safe treatment window among patients with MI (Olsen *et al.* 2012).

- If a patient is suspected to have an MI on a dental visit, then the emergency medical system should be activated. Have the patient lie down on the floor and assess the airway, breathing, and circulation (ABCs) and monitor vital signs.

D. Heart failure

Clinical synopsis

Heart failure occurs when decreases in contractility prevent the heart from pumping forcefully enough to deliver blood to meet the body's demands. Decreases in cardiac output activate reflex responses in the sympathetic nervous system which attempt to compensate for the reduced cardiac output. These reflex responses include increase in heart rate, increased preload, which causes edema, and increased afterload. Ultimately, the heart fails.

Heart failure is classified into systolic dysfunction (left ventricular) and diastolic dysfunction (right ventricular). Causes of left ventricular heart failure (decreased emptying of the left ventricle) include hypertension, coronary artery disease, mitral regurgitation, anemia, and Paget's disease. These conditions impair the ability of the heart muscle to contract. Symptoms of left heart failure include cough, dyspnea during exercise or when lying flat and pulmonary edema. Right ventricular heart failure occurs with a decreased emptying of the right ventricle. Symptoms include pitting edema (fluid accumulation in the interstitial spaces is especially seen in the ankles), liver enlargement, nausea, vomiting, anorexia, and abdominal distention.

Diagnostic/lab tests

No specific tests are required for dental treatment.

Dental notes: Dental management of patient with heart failure

- See Table 5.5 for dental notes on dental management of medications for patient with heart failure.
- Patients with heart failure may take similar drugs (e.g., duiretics, ACEIs, and beta-blockers) as a hypertensive patient. Thus, when recording the type of medication, it is also important to record the indication for usage.
- Administration of a vasoconstrictor (1:100,000 epinephrine) in a local anesthetic should be limited to two cartridges. Excessive doses of epinephrine can lead to dysrhythmic activity (Moreno-Gomez *et al.* 2009)
- Some patients may not be able to tolerate a supine position.
- Avoid NSAIDs in patient with heart failure; recommend acetaminophen but be cautious while prescribing the maximum dose.
- Nitrous oxide sedation is contraindicated in patients with heart failure.
- Digoxin increases the gag reflex; difficulty when taking impressions.
- In patients with refractory heart failure, dental treatment should be conducted only after close consultation with the physician/cardiologist (Findler *et al.* 2013).

Table 5.5 Drugs in the treatment of heart failure.

Drugs	Dental management
Diuretics *Loop diuretics* Furosemide (Lasix)	NSAIDs such as naproxen sodium (Aleve) and ibuprofen (Advil, Motrin) can decrease the effectiveness of the antihypertensive action of the thiazide diuretic, resulting in rapid elevation of blood pressure. Monitor blood pressure Orthostatic hypotension: Monitor blood pressure. To avoid dizziness/fainting when a patient goes from the supine position, have the patient sit in an upright position for a few minutes before dismissing them. Monitor blood pressure Patients may need to use the restroom facilities (increased urination from the diuretic) more frequently during the dental visit. Adjust your time accordingly Xerostomia: monitor for dental caries and candidiasis. Monitor salivary consistency No special precautions with the use of epinephrine
Positive inotropics ***Cardiac glycosides*** Digoxin (Lanoxin)	No interactions with NSAIDs No xerostomia Avoid epinephrine Interaction with tetracycline including doxycycline and minocycline; space doses apart about 2 h Interaction with "azole" antifungal drugs; space doses apart about 2 h Interaction with clarithromycin and erythromycin; prescribe azithromycin instead
Adrenergic receptor agonist Dobutamine (Dobutrex) dopamine	Orthostatic hypotension: Monitor blood pressure. To avoid dizziness/fainting when a patient goes from the supine position, have the patient sit in an upright position for a few minutes before dismissing them. Monitor blood pressure Xerostomia: monitor for dental caries and candidiasis. Monitor salivary consistency No special precautions with the use of epinephrine
Vasodilators Hydralazine (Apresoline)	NSAIDs such as naproxen sodium (Aleve) and ibuprofen (Advil, Motrin) can decrease the effectiveness of the antihypertensive action of the ACE inhibitor resulting in rapid elevation of blood pressure. Monitor blood pressure Orthostatic hypotension: Monitor blood pressure. To avoid dizziness/fainting when a patient goes from the supine position, have the patient sit in an upright position for a few minutes before dismissing them. Monitor blood pressure. Xerostomia: monitor for dental caries and candidiasis. Monitor salivary consistency No special precautions with the use of epinephrine.
ACEI Captopril (Capoten) Enalapril (Vasotec)	NSAIDs such as naproxen sodium (Aleve) and ibuprofen (Advil, Motrin) can decrease the effectiveness of the antihypertensive action of the ACE inhibitor resulting in rapid elevation of blood pressure. Monitor blood pressure

(continued)

Table 5.5   (*cont'd*)

Drugs	Dental management
Lisinopril (Prinivil, Zestril)	Monitor for angioedema of lips and tongue
Quinapril (Accupril) Fosinopril (Monopril)	Orthostatic hypotension: Monitor blood pressure. To avoid dizziness/fainting when a patient goes from the supine position, have the patient sit in an upright position for a few minutes before dismissing them. Monitor blood pressure Xerostomia: monitor for dental caries and candidiasis. Monitor salivary consistency No special precautions with the use of epinephrine
Calcium channel blockers Diltiazem (Cardizem) Verapamil (Calan, Isoptin) Amlodipine (Norvasc)	Orthostatic hypotension: Monitor blood pressure. To avoid dizziness/fainting when a patient goes from the supine position, have the patient sit in an upright position for a few minutes before dismissing them. Monitor blood pressure Xerostomia: monitor for dental caries and candidiasis. Monitor salivary consistency
Felodipine (Plendil) Isradipine (Dynacirc) Nicardipine (Cardene) Nifedipine (Adalat, Procardia) Nisoldipine (Sular)	No special precautions with the use of epinephrine

E.   Arrhythmias

In an unstimulated neuron, potassium ions (K^+) are present in higher concentration inside the cell than outside, and sodium ions (Na^+) are found in higher concentration outside the cell than inside. In this situation, the neuron is polarized. If the cell membrane becomes depolarized, allowing the rapid movement of K^+ ions outside the cell and Na^+ inside the cell, a stimulation or action potential results, which causes the cell to contract. This action potential is the stimulus that normally initiates the contraction of the heart. During the depolarization phase, the cell cannot be reactivated by an electrical impulse and is considered refractory to further stimulation. For the cell to return to a resting state, Na^+ ions must be pumped out of the cell and K^+ ions back into the cell, known as repolarization. This action potential process is spontaneous or automatic.

In the normal heart, an electrical impulse or contraction originates from the sinoatrial (SA) node, a small mass of tissue in the right atria, and travels through the internodal tracts in the atrium to the atrioventricular (AV) node. At the AV node, a momentary delay of the impulse allows for atrial contraction and ventricular filling. The electrical impulse then travels through the bundle of His (collection of heart muscle), bundle branches, and Purkinje fibers to stimulate the ventricles to contract and pump blood into the systemic circulation.

An arrhythmia occurs when either the impulse rhythm does not start in the SA node or the rate of heartbeats is abnormal (normally the heart beats about 70–80 times per minute), or it is not under automatic control.

Classification of arrhythmias is based on the anatomical site of the abnormal rhythm:

Atrial (atrium)
Ventricular (ventricle) or
Supraventricular (atrium or above the ventricles)

When the heart beats too slowly but at a regular rate, it is called sinus bradycardia. There is an increased parasympathetic stimulation that causes the heart to beat slowly. If the heart beats too fast, it is called sinus or ventricular tachycardia or atrial flutter. Of the different arrhythmias seen in clinical practice, the most common is AF, where the heart beats without regard for impulses originating from the SA node. Other types of arrhythmias are ventricular tachycardia, ventricular fibrillation, and premature ventricular contractions.

Long QT syndrome is diagnosed by a prolonged QT interval of the electrocardiogram (ECG). Risk factors for developing include cardiac and noncardiac drugs and genetics. Many drugs that the dentist prescribes have the potential for triggering episodes of polymorphic ventricular dysrhythmias, called torsades de pointes, which occasionally terminate in sudden death (Cavero *et al.* 2000; De Ponti *et al.* 2002). Accurate measurement of the QT interval requires an ECG.

The nonarrhythmic dental drugs that have a great potential to cause prolonged QT interval (or long QT syndrome), specifically torsades de pointes, include erythromycin, clarithromycin, levofloxacin (less likely), "azole" antifungals (e.g., fluconazole, clotrimazole), chloral hydrate, epinephrine, and amitriptyline in otherwise healthy individuals (Karp and Moss 2006). These individuals, if they develop drug-induced long QT syndrome, may have an underlying genetic cardiac defect making them more susceptible to disruptions in heart rhythm from drugs. This interaction may be more common than has been documented and is considered to be a sometimes fatal adverse event that is reportable to the FDA Adverse Event Reporting System (AERS) (De Ponti *et al.* 2002; Poluzzi *et al.* 2010). Certain patients are more susceptible to the cardiac toxic effects of these QT-prolonging drugs (Owens 2004). Preventive measures should be taken to avoid a torsades de pointes episode. Dental management is geared toward the removal of the physical activity and psychological stressors (Karp and Moss 2006). It is recommended that dentists prescribing these antibiotics and "azole" antifungal agents consult with a cardiologist to assure the status of their ECG. Patients with long QT syndrome may be better treated in an outpatient hospital setting where a potential cardiac event can be appropriately managed (Karp and Moss 2006).

Medications: Anti-arrhythmic agents

- Anti-arrhythmic agents suppress arrhythmia by blocking either autonomic function or calcium, potassium, or sodium channels, which slows the conduction of the cardiac impulse. Anti-arrhythmics should only be used to treat symptomatic arrhythmias. Based upon these mechanisms, there are four Vaughan Williams classifications of antiarrhythmics:
- Class I drugs, the largest group of antiarrhythmics, have a mechanism of action similar to local anesthetics. These drugs block sodium entry into the cell, thus preventing the transmission of the nerve impulse and reducing the rate of depolarization. Table 5.6 lists the anti-arrhythmic drugs.
- Most patients with heart arrhythmias take anticoagulants too.
- Three newer oral anticoagulants (dabigatran (Pradaxa), rivaroxaban (Xarelto), and apixaban (Eliquis)) have been approved as alternatives to warfarin for patients with AF. There is a trend toward lower mortality with these novel drugs. Other advantages of the new agents include convenience (no INR testing), lack of dietary or drug–drug interaction, and rapid anticoagulation after an oral dose (rather than days for warfarin). A major disadvantage is that it is expensive. (http://medcitynews.com/2013/05/update-on-anticoagulation-for-atrial-fibrillation-encouraging-news-for-rivaroxaban-xarelto/#ixzz2bfi1XOCg).
- Avoid excessive amount of epinephrine. Limit to two cartridges of 1:100,000.
- Avoid intraligamentary injection of epinephrine.

Table 5.6 Anti-arrhythmic drugs.

Drug
Class I: Sodium Channel Blockers
Class I-A Quinidine (Quinidine) Procainamide (Pronestyl) Disopyramide (Norpace)
Class I-B Lidocaine (Xylocaine) Tocainide (Tonocard) Mexiletine (Mexitil)
Class I-C Flecainide (Tambocor) Propafenone (Rythmol)
Class II β-Adrenergic Blockers Esmolol (Brevibloc) Metoprolol (Lopressor) Propranolol (Inderal)
Class III Potassium Channel Blockers Amiodarone (Cordarone) Bretylium (injectable) Sotalol (Betapace)
Class IV Calcium Channel Blockers Diltiazem (Cardizem) Nifedipine (Adalat, Procardia) Verapamil (Calan)

Dental notes: Dental management of patient with heart arrhythmias

- A medical consult is recommended to know what kind of arrhythmia is present and how controlled the patient is.
- Determine the type of drugs the patient is taking for a specific CV condition. There are no special precautions when treating a patient with controlled arrhythmias. The patient's pulse should be taken to determine normal rate and rhythm.
- The most common arrhythmia is AF and they have a high risk for a stroke.
- In patients taking warfarin, an INR reading should be measured within 24h, but not more than 72h, before the dental procedure.
- Pacemakers are implanted in patients with arrhythmias to keep heart at a normal rate and rhythm. Today almost all pacemakers have an internal shield that allows ultrasonic scalers, pulp testers, instrument cleaning systems, and any other electronic units to be used without problems; however, it is still controversial because although all pacemakers today have shields, they have not been fully tested and approved for ultrasonic use and could interfere with electrical impulse (Roedig *et al.* 2010). In such cases, it is recommended to contact the manufacturer. The patient will most likely be carrying a card with information on it.
- Do not take blood pressure on left arm of a patient with a pacemaker inserted on left side.
- Antibiotic prophylaxis is not required.
- Monitor blood pressure and pulse at every appointment and make short less stressful appointment.

F.   Valvular heart disease

Clinical synopsis

Cardiovalvular disorders encompass patients with heart valve defects. The major concern is patients that have a heart valve replacement. There are essentially three types of valves: mechanical or prosthetic valves, donor valve, and bioprosthetic or tissue valves that are from animal donors, usually porcine in origin. Tissue valves last much longer, up to 10–20 years (Schmelzeisen *et al.* 2009).

Patients who have had prosthetic cardiac valve replacement usually begin anticoagulation immediately after surgery to reduce the risk of thromboembolism. Heparin is administered first to minimize the delay in achieving therapeutic anticoagulation. This is called "bridging" (Goldhaber

Table 5.7   Prophylactic antibiotic regimens for oral and dental procedures (Wilson *et al.* 1997).

Situation	Drug	Regimen (to be taken 30–60 min before dental procedure)
Oral	Amoxicillin	Adults: 2.0 g; children: 50 mg/kg
Unable to take oral medications	Ampicillin or Cefazolin or ceftriaxone*	Adults: 2.0 g IM or IV; children: 50 mg/kg IM or IV Adults: 1 g IM or IV; children: 50 mg/kg
Allergic to penicillins or ampicillin, oral	Cephalexin* or Clindamycin or Azithromycin or clarithromycin	Adults: 2 g; children: 50 mg/kg Adults: 600 mg; children: 20 mg/kg Adults: 500 mg; children: 15 mg/kg
Allergic to pencillins or ampicillin and unable to take oral medications	Cefazolin or ceftriaxone* or Clindamycin	Adults: 1 g IM or IV; children: 50 mg/kg IM or IV

*If emergency treatment is necessary before the allotted time, the patient should be premedicated with antibiotics.

Table 5.8   Antibiotic prophylaxis recommendations for dental procedures (Wilson *et al.* 1997).

Higher incidence	Lower incidence
Dental extractions	Restorative dentistry (operative and prosthodontic)
Periodontal procedures: surgery, scaling and root planing, probing and recall maintenance	Local anesthetic injections (all except intraligamentary)
Implant placement and reimplantation of avulsed teeth	Placement of rubber dams
Root canal instrumentation when beyond apex (endodontics)	Postoperative suture removal
Subgingival placement of antibiotic fibers or strips	Placement of removable prosthodontic/orthodontic appliances
Placement of orthodontic bands (not brackets)	Taking oral impressions or radiographs
Intraligamentary local anesthesia injection Prophylactic cleaning of teeth and implants	Fluoride treatment

2006). Low-molecular-weight heparin has also been used in place of heparin. The anticoagulation regimen depends on the valve type. For mechanical valves, the patient may take warfarin and aspirin. For mitral bioprosthetic valve replacement, warfarin is initiated and if the patient has AF or previous thromboembolism, warfarin is used indefinitely. For aortic valve and sinus rhythm, anticoagulation is optional.

Dental notes: Dental management of patients with heart valve replacement

- Medical consultation recommended
- All patients require AHA antibiotic prophylaxis (Tables 5.7 and 5.8)
- Functional heart murmurs do not require antibiotic prophylaxis
- Patients will take an antiplatelet such as aspirin and/or warfarin. An INR reading is required before dental procedures if they are taking warfarin. For most mechanical heart valves, the target INR ranges between 2.0 and 3.5 (see Box 5.1).

G. Epinephrine in cardiac patients

Although epinephrine stimulates both α- and β-receptors, at low doses (1–2 cartridges: 0.18 mg) when used in dental anesthesia, epinephrine does not stimulate α-receptors very much but does stimulate the β_2-receptors by binding to them because these receptors have a higher affinity for epinephrine. Thus, epinephrine selectively stimulates β_2-receptors, resulting in vasodilation of blood vessels in skeletal muscle. This vasodilation reduces diastolic blood pressure. With an increase in systolic blood pressure and a decrease in diastolic blood pressure, there is no real change in mean blood pressure. Therefore, it is important to inject slowly and aspirate. The primary effect at high doses (e.g., used in emergency anaphylaxis and cardiac arrest: 0.5–1 mg) is vascular smooth muscle contraction through stimulation of α-receptors followed by a β_1-adrenergic effect, resulting in increased systolic and diastolic blood pressure.

Summary: Dental notes on the cardiac patient

Table 5.9 lists the time interval after a cardiac procedure that a patient should commence with dental procedures. The reason for delaying dental treatment after cardiac surgery or procedures is to prevent a second CV event or procedure resulting from vascular inflammation (Skaar *et al.* 2012). Dentist must use clinical judgment regarding the risk versus benefits for performing elective dental procedures on a recent cardiac patient.

Table 5.9 Recommendations when to start dental treatment after cardiac surgery (www.colgate.com/app/CP/US/EN/OC/information/Articles/Oral-and-Dental-Health-Basics/Medical-Conditions/Heart-Disease-and-Oral-Health/article/Cardiovascular.cvsp; Skaar *et al.* 2012).

Cardiac procedure	How soon after to initiate dental treatment
Coronary artery bypass graft (CABG)	6 months: no antibiotic premedication
Pacemaker	At least within the first few weeks; no antibiotic premedication
Cardiac stent	3 months; generally no antibiotic premedication
Angioplasty or catherization	No need to postpone treatment; no antibiotic premedication
Artificial valves or shunts	Minimum 3 months; antibiotic prophylaxis required
Myocardial infarction	Minimum 6 months; no antibiotic premedication

References

American Academy of Periodontology (1996) Periodontal management of patients with cardiovascular diseases. *Journal of Periodontology*, **67**, 627–635.

Ardekian, L., Gaspar, R., Peled, M., *et al.* (2000) Does low-dose aspirin therapy complicate oral surgical procedures? *The Journal of the American Dental Association*, **131**, 331–335.

Bader, J.D., Bonito, A.U., & Shugars, D.A. (2002) A systematic review of cardiovascular effects of epinephrine on hypertensive dental patients. *Oral Surgery Oral Medicine Oral Pathology Oral Radiology Endodontics*, **93**, 647–653.

Basile, J.N. (2002) Systolic blood pressure. It is time to focus on systolic hypertension—especially in older people. *British Journal of Medicine,* **325 (7370)**, 917–918.

Bradley, J.G. & Davis, K.A. (2003) Orthostatic hypotension. *American Family Physician* **68**, 2398–2398.

Cattaneo, M. (2010) Update on antithrombotic therapy. New P2Y12 inhibitors. *Circulation*, **121**, 171–179.

Cavero, I., Mestre, M., & Guillon, J.M. (2000) Drugs that prolong QT interval as an unwanted effect: assessing their likelihood of inducing hazardous cardiac dysrhythmias. *Expert Opinion in Pharmacotherapy*, **1 (5)**, 947–973.

Chobanian, A.V., Black, H.R., Cushman, W.C. *et al.* (2003). The seventh report of the Joint National Committee on Prevention, Detection, Evaluation, and Treatment of High Blood Pressure. *Journal of the American Medical Association,* **289**, 2560–2571.

Cutler, J.A., Sorlie, P.D., Wolz, M. *et al.* (2008) Trends in hypertension prevalence, awareness, treatment, and control rates in United States adults between 1988–1994 and 1999–2004. *Hypertension*, **52**, 618–827.

Dalen, H., Thorstensen, A., Romundstad, P.R. *et al.* (2011) Cardiovascular risk factors and systolic and diastolic cardiac function: a tissue Doppler and speckle tracking echocardiographic study. *Journal of the American Society of Echocardiography*, **24**, 322–332.

De Ponti, F., Poluzzi, E., Cavalli, A. *et al.* (2002) Safety of non-antiarrhythmic drugs that prolong the QT interval or induce torsade de pointes: an overview. *Drug Safety*, **25**, 263–286.

Fifth Report of the Joint National Committee on Detection, Evaluation, and Treatment of High Blood Pressure. (JNC V)(1993) *Archives of Internal Medicine*, **153**, 154–183.

Findler, M., Elad, S., Kaufman, E. *et al.* (2013) Dental treatment for high-risk patients with refractory heart failure: a retrospective observational comparison study. *Oral Medicine,* **44**, 61–70.

Goldhaber, S.Z. (2006) "Bridging" and mechanical heart valves. Perils, promises, and predictions. *Circulation*, **113**, 470–472.

Hersh, E.V. & Moore, P.A. (2008) Adverse drug interactions in dentistry. *Periodontology* **2000**, 46, 109–142.

Horn, J.R. & Hansten, P.D. (2009) More evidence of a warfarin-antibiotic interaction. *Pharmacy Times*, June 27. Published online Monday, June 15, 2009.

Hughes, G.J., Patel, P.N., & Saxena, N. (2011) Effect of acetaminophen on international normalized ratio in patients receiving warfarin therapy. *Pharmacotherapy*, **31**, 591–597.

Hyman, D.J. & Pavlik, V.N. (2001) Characteristics of untreated hypertension in the United States. *New England Journal of Medicine*, **345**, 479–486.

James, P. (2014) Evidence-based guideline for the management of high blood pressure in adults. Report from the Panel Members Appointed to the Eight Joint National Committee (JNC 8). *Journal of the American Medical Association*, published online December 18, 2013, E1–E14.

Jeske, A.H. & Suchko, G.D. (2003) Lack of a scientific basis for routine discontinuation of oral anticoagulation therapy before dental treatment. *The Journal of the American Dental Association*, **134**, 1492–1497.

Kannel, W.N., Schwartz, M.J., & Mcnamara, P.M. (1969) Blood pressure and risk of coronary heart disease. *The Framingham study. Disease of the Chest*, **56**, 43–52.

Karp, J.M. & Moss, A.J. (2006) Dental treatment of patients with long QT syndrome. *Journal of the American Dental Association*, **137**, 630–637.

Lifshey, F.M. (2004) Evaluation of and treatment considerations for the dental patient with cardiac disease. *New York State Dental Journal*, **70**, 16–19.

Moreno-Gomez, G., Guardia, J., Cutando, A., *et al.* (2009) Pharmacological interactions of vasoconstrictors. *Medicina Oral Patologia Oral Y Cirugia Bucal*, **14**, E20–E27.

Nichols, C. (1997) Dentistry and hypertension. *Journal of the American Dental Association*, **128**, 1557–1562.

Olsen, A.M.S., Fosbøl, E.L., & Lindhardsen, J. (2012) Long-term cardiovascular risk of NSAID use according to time passed after first-time myocardial infarction: a Nationwide Cohort Study. *Circulation*, **126 (16)**, 1955–1963.

Owens, R.C. Jr. (2004) QT prolongation with antimicrobial agents: understanding the significance. *Drugs*, **64**, 1091–1124.

Perusse, R., Goulet J.-P., & Turcotte, J.-Y. (1992) Contraindications to vasoconstrictors in dentistry. Part I. *Oral Surgery Oral Medicine Oral Pathology*, **74**, 679–786.

Poluzzi, E., Raschi, E., Motola, D., *et al.* (2010) Antimicrobials and the risk of torsades de pointes: the contribution from data mining of the US FDA Adverse Event Reporting System. *Drug Safety*, **33**, 303–314.

Roedig, J.J., Shah, J., Elayi, C.S. *et al.* (2010) Interference of cardiac pacemaker and implantable cardioverter-defibrillator activity during electronic dental device use. *Journal of the American Dental Association*, **141**, 521–526.

Schmelzeisen, R., Yabroudi, F., & Dannan, A. (2009) Pre-and post-operative dental focus of patients with prosthetic heart valves. *The Internet Journal of Cardiovascular Research*, **6 (1)**, 2–3. DOI:10.5580/1fe0.

Schömig, A., Sarafoff, N., & Seyfarth, M. (2009) Triple antithrombotic management after stent implantation: when and how? *Heart*, **95**, 1280.

Skaar, D., O'Connor, H., Lunos, S., *et al.* (2012) Dental procedures and risk of experiencing a second vascular event in a Medicare population. *Journal of the American Medical Association*, **143**, 1190–1198.

Wahl, M.J. (1998) Dental surgery in anticoagulated patients. *Archives of Internal Medicine*, **158**, 1610–1616.

Weinberg, M.A., Westphal Theile, C., & Fine, J.B. (2012) Cardiovascular pharmacology. *Oral Pharmacology*, 2nd edn. In: M. A. Weinberg, C. Westphal Theile, & J. B. Fine. Pearson Publications, Upper Saddle River, NJ.

Wilson, W., Taubert, A., & Gewitz, M. (2007) Prevention of infective endocarditis guidelines from the American Heart Association: a guideline from the American Heart Association rheumatic fever, endocarditis, and Kawasaki disease committee, council on cardiovascular disease in the young, and the council on clinical cardiology, council on cardiovascular surgery and anesthesia, and the quality of care and outcomes Research Interdisciplinary Working Group. *Circulation*, **116**, 1736–1754.

Chapter 6

Pregnancy, lactation, and oral contraceptives

A. Pregnancy and lactation	82
B. Oral contraceptives	89
References	90

A. Pregnancy and lactation

Clinical synopsis

Preventive dental care should be provided to pregnant patients as early as possible. The first trimester is from week 1 to week 12, second trimester is from week 13 to week 28, and third trimester is from week 29 to week 40, which includes delivery.

Many dentists refuse dental care to pregnant patients because of misconceptions regarding the safety of treatment. In 2012, the Health Resources and Services Administration in cooperation with the American College of Obstetricians and Gynecologists and the ADA (American Dental Association), which was coordinated by the National Maternal and Child Oral Health Resource Center, created a consensus statement stressing that dental care is safe and important throughout pregnancy (Fox 2013). It is advisable to do preventive, emergency, and routine restorative and periodontal therapy throughout the pregnancy period to help reduce the risk of developing oral infections that could happen during the last trimester (American Academy of Pediatric Dentistry 2012); however, the patient's obstetrician should be consulted if there are any concerns.

Dental management: Drug safety and drug interactions in pregnant patients

- Avoid prescribing drugs, including antibiotics, sedatives, and analgesics in the first trimester.
- The Food and Drug Administration (FDA) requires that all prescription drugs absorbed systemically or that are known to be potentially harmful to the fetus be given a pregnancy category of A, B, C, D, or X. Table 6.1 lists all categories (Lynch *et al.* 1991). Before prescribing any mediation to a pregnant patient, know to what FDA pregnancy category the drug belongs to.

The Dentist's Quick Guide to Medical Conditions, First Edition. Mea A. Weinberg, Stuart L. Segelnick, Joseph S. Insler, with Samuel Kramer.
© 2015 John Wiley & Sons, Inc. Published 2015 by John Wiley & Sons, Inc.

Table 6.1 FDA pregnancy categories.

Drug category	Description	Breastfeeding
A	Controlled studies in women fail to show a risk to the fetus	Yes
B	Animal or human studies have not shown a significant risk to the fetus. No controlled studies in pregnant women. Drugs that have been found to have adverse effects in animals but no well-controlled studies of humans	Yes
C	Drugs for which there are no adequate studies, either animal or humans, or drugs shown to have adverse fetal effects in animals but for which no human data are available	Yes
D	Fetal risk in humans is evident	No
X	Studies in animals or humans have shown definitive fetal risk. These drugs are contraindicated in women who are or may become pregnant.	No

- The question of nitrous oxide use in pregnant patients is still controversial based on concerns about adverse effects associated with chronic exposure (Becker and Rosenberg 2008). Nitrous oxide/oxygen, which has no FDA pregnancy *category*, can be administered safely to a pregnant patient if topical and/or local anesthesia is not adequate, but do not administer more than 30% nitrous oxide and consult with the patient's obstetrician (New York State Department of Health 2006). Nitrous oxide is *contraindicated* in the first trimester of pregnancy due to increased incidence of spontaneous abortion (Rowland *et al.* 1995). Consult with the patient's obstetrician for using intravenous sedation or general anesthesia. Local anesthetics are safe to administer to pregnant women as long as it is given in the correct dose and administered properly avoiding intravascular injection (Giglio *et al.* 2009).

- Epinephrine is a natural hormone produced in the body. Epinephrine acting as a vasoconstrictor in local anesthetics actually reduces the toxicity of the local anesthetic without harming the fetus; however, intravascular injection should be avoided. According to Michalowicz *et al.* (2008), dental treatment (e.g., scaling and root planing, temporary or permanent restorations, endodontic therapy, or extraction) with the administration of topical anesthetics and local anesthetics containing 1:100,000 epinephrine is safe and does not significantly increase the risk of any adverse events in pregnant women at week 13–21 of gestation. In this clinical study, different anesthetics were used including topical 5% lidocaine and 1% dyclonine and injectable local anesthetics such as 2% lidocaine with 1:100,000 epinephrine, 4% prilocaine with epinephrine, and prilocaine without a vasoconstrictor. *It cannot be over-emphasized to avoid intravascular injection.* The authors concluded that data from larger clinical studies are needed to confirm the safety of dental care in pregnant women. It must be emphasized that since epinephrine stimulates cardiac function, when administering epinephrine, careful technique (e.g., aspirate to avoid intravascular injection) and proper dosing are demanded (Fayans *et al.* 2010).

- Lidocaine, an amide, is associated with the least medical/dental complications. Lidocaine with 1:100,000 epinephrine (0.017 mg of epinephrine in a 1.7 ml cartridge of lidocaine) is a pregnancy category B drug in contrast to mepivacaine 3% (without a vasoconstrictor), articaine, and bupivacaine which are a category C drug. The concern about epinephrine is its effect on uterine muscle, but there are no studies to confirm this effect on pregnant women (New York State Department of Health 2006). Lidocaine with epinephrine in a ratio of 1:100,000 and lidocaine plain without epinephrine can be administered throughout pregnancy.

- Mepivacaine has been shown to cause fetal bradycardia and should be avoided during pregnancy (Shnider *et al.* 1968).
- The highest concentration in fetal circulation occurs with prilocaine and the lowest concentration is with bupivacaine and lidocaine is in between (Singh 2012).
- Long-acting local anesthetics are not necessary or recommended.

Drug dosing

Pregnancy and the first weeks of life represent two physiologic situations in which there is a continual and significant change in the levels of plasma proteins, and it may therefore be necessary to adjust the doses of medication during these times (Moore 1998).

The majority of systemic drugs passes into *human* milk by passive diffusion and appear in minute amounts, usually <1% of the maternal dose. The higher the dosage, the more the drug transfers into milk. Different features of the drug including molecular weight, fat solubility, and the half-life will affect the amount of drug that is transferred into the milk. The pH of milk is 7, which is slightly lower than plasma (pH 7.4) so that drugs that are weak bases (e.g., erythromycins, tetracycline, diazepam, and codeine) will achieve high concentrations in breast milk and should be avoided. There is usually no need to reduce the dose of an antibiotic prescribed to a pregnant patient.

Table 6.2 lists the drugs used in dentistry that are considered safe during pregnancy and breastfeeding (Turner *et al.* 2006).

Antibiotics prescribed during pregnancy and nursing

- Some antibiotics have adverse effects on the developing fetus. Choosing the appropriate antibiotic requires consideration of the effects on both the mother and the fetus. The first trimester starts at conception and continues through the eleventh week. During this period, there is an increase in blood volume and hepatic and renal blood flow which can alter the serum antibiotic concentrations. Thus, the safety of many antibiotics varies with the period of gestation and the maturity of the fetus. The time when the embryo is most vulnerable to a teratogenic agent occurs between days 18 and 60 (Lynch *et al.* 1991; Moore 1998; Lomaestro 2009).
- Penicillin VK and amoxicillin are thought to be safe to prescribe during pregnancy. If the patient is allergic to penicillin, clindamycin is recommended. Also, erythromycin (except estolate form) and metronidazole can be prescribed which have been reported to have minimal fetal risk. Tetracyclines including tetracycline HCl, doxycycline hyclate, and minocycline HCl are category D drugs and are contraindicated and should be avoided (Moore 1998). Also, clarithromycin, which is a category C drug, should be avoided; however, azithromycin, a category B drug, is safe to prescribe.

Analgesics prescribed during pregnancy and nursing

- Aspirin should be avoided especially late in pregnancy due to delivery complications and postpartum bleeding in the mother.
- Nonsteroidal anti-inflammatory drugs (NSAIDs) including ibuprofen and naproxen (Aleve) may prolong pregnancy and should be avoided especially during the first trimester and in late pregnancy (third trimester); however, if used after the first trimester then they should be used only for 24–72 h.

Table 6.2 List of drugs used in pregnancy and lactating women.

Drugs	FDA category	Can this be used during pregnancy?	Can this be used during nursing?
Antibiotics			
Amoxicillin	B	Yes	Yes
Penicillin VK	B	Yes	Yes
Erythromycin base or ethylsuccinate	B	Yes (except for esolate form)	Yes
Clarithromycin	C	No	No data is available. Manufacturer cautions its use to nursing mothers
Azithromycin	B	Yes; no human studies; give when benefits outweigh risk	Not enough information. Manufacturer advises caution
Fluroquinolones (e.g., ciprofloxacin, levaquin)	C	No	Discontinue breastfeeding or do not use ciprofloxacin
Clindamycin	B	Yes; when benefit outweighs risk	Excreted in mother's milk. Decision to either discontinue nursing or choose another antibiotic
Metronidazole	B	Yes; but not in first trimester	Discontinue breast-feeding for 12–24 h. Best to prescribe another antibiotic
Tetracyclines	D	No	No
Analgesics			
Acetaminophen	B	Yes	Yes
Aspirin	C/D (risk for use during third trimester)	No. Aspirin use in pregnancy has been associated with alterations in both maternal and fetal hemostasis. Avoid in first and third trimester	No
Ibuprofen (and all NSAIDs including naprosyn and naproxen)	B/D (D in third trimester; do not recommend during the third trimester)	After first trimester for 24–72 h only. Best to avoid in third trimester due to effects on the fetal cardiovascular system (closure of the ductus arteriosus). Not in third trimester	No data is available. Effects on nursing baby are not known

(continued)

Table 6.2   *(cont'd)*

Drugs	FDA category	Can this be used during pregnancy?	Can this be used during nursing?
Codeine (e.g., acetaminophen with codeine)	C/D (in third trimester)	Only give if benefit outweighs the risks. Codeine is the only narcotic analgesic that has shown a statistically significant association with teratogenicity (involving respiratory tract malformations; depression)	Codeine is metabolized to morphine which can result in morphine overdose in the baby especially if mothers are ultra-rapid metabolizers of codeine. Signs of morphine overdose in a nursing baby include limpness, increased sleepiness, or difficulty in breathing
Hydrocodone (e.g., Vicodin)	C/D (in third trimester)	Neonatal respiratory depression	No. Codeine is metabolized to morphine which can result in morphine overdose in the baby especially if mothers are ultra-rapid metabolizers of codeine. Signs of morphine overdose in a nursing baby include limpness, increased sleepiness, or difficulty in breathing
Antifungal agents			
Nystatin	B	Yes	Yes
Clotrimazole (topical)	B	Yes	Yes
Local Anesthetics			
Lidocaine (with epinephrine)	C (epinephrine)	Yes	Yes
Mepivacaine	C	No (causes fetal bradycardia)	Caution
Bupivacaine	C	No	Yes
Etidocaine	B	Yes	Yes
Prilocaine	B	Yes	Yes
Articaine	C	No	Caution
Marcaine	C	No	Caution
Benzocaine (topical)	C	No	No data
Anesthesia			
Nitrous oxide	Not classified	Controversial: consult with obstetrician; use lower levels of nitrous oxide (30%)	Controversial; consult with patient's prenatal care provider

(continued)

Table 6.2 *(cont'd)*

Drugs	FDA category	Can this be used during pregnancy?	Can this be used during nursing?
Antianxiety/sedation drugs			
Benzodiazepines (e.g., diazepam, alprazolam)	D	No	No
Triazolam and Temazepam	X	No	No
Barbituates	D	No	No
Oral rinses			
Chlorhexidine gluconate 0.12%	B	Yes	Yes
Nystatin oral suspention, topical	B	Yes	Yes
Periodontal local drug delivery			
PerioChip (chlorhexidine)	C (but mouth rinse is B)	No	No
Arestin (minocycline)	D	No	No
Atridox (doxycycline)	D	No	No
Antifungal/antiviral drugs			
Ketoconazole	C	No	No
Fluconazole	C	No	No
Acyclovir, systemic	C	No	No
Valacyclovir, systemic	B	Yes	Yes

Adapted from New York State Department of Health. Oral Health Care during Pregnancy and Early Childhood. Practice Guidelines. August 2006; Moore, 1998; Turner et al. 2006; www.drugs.com/pregnancy.

Use of NSAIDs during pregnancy has been associated with oligohydramnios, premature closure of the fetal ductus arteriosus with subsequent persistent pulmonary hypertension of the newborn, fetal nephrotoxicity, and periventricular hemorrhage (Collins 1981; Macones *et al.* 2001; Black and Hill 2003). Probably, it is best to avoid all NSAIDs during pregnancy.
- Acetaminophen alone but not in combination with codeine is the safest analgesic for pregnant patients and nursing mothers. Acetaminophen is hepatotoxic; caution with maximum dose.
- On August 17, 2007, the FDA warned breastfeeding mothers who take codeine, either in combination with another analgesic or in any form of cough syrup, that babies are at increased risk for morphine overdose. Newborn babies are especially sensitive to the effects of the smallest dosages of narcotics. Codeine is metabolized to morphine, and in women who are "ultra-rapid" metabolizers of codeine, adverse effects of morphine can be seen very quickly versus women who normally slowly metabolize codeine into morphine. The FDA warns nursing mothers to observe for morphine overdose in their babies. Being an ultra-rapid metabolizer of codeine is due to a mutation in the gene coding for cytochrome P450 enzyme (CYP2D6) in the liver. It is relatively uncommon but could occur.

(http://www.fda.gov/Safety/MedWatch/SafetyInformation/SafetyAlertsforHumanMedicalProducts/ucm152107.htm)

Sedative/hypnotics and anti-anxiety medications

- Benzodiazepines including alprazolam and diazepam are pregnancy category D drugs and can cause fetal cleft lip and palate; avoid the use of benzodiazepines (Dolovich *et al.* 1998).
- Barbiturates are category D drugs and should not be used in pregnancy or during breastfeeding.

Antifungal/antiviral agents

- Although the use of azoles as topical agents for superficial infections is both efficacious and well tolerated in the pregnant patient, especially when used for short periods, systemic azole therapy is not recommended in pregnancy (Sobel 2000; Colemen *et al.* 1998).
- Since nystatin is not absorbed if taken orally, it is only available in topical or oral rinse formulations. Systemic absorption after topical use is negligible.
- Systemic valacyclovir (Valtrex) is safe during pregnancy and breastfeeding.
- Systemic acyclovir is not safe to prescribe during pregnancy or breastfeeding; topical acyclovir is a pregnancy category B drug and is safe to prescribe (Ratanajamit *et al.* 2003).

Oral adverse effects of pregnancy

- Pregnancy-associated gingivitis: Gingival inflammation may occur in the majority of pregnant women primarily during the second month as a result of an exaggerated response to the increased production of estrogen and progesterone. The patient's periodontal condition (e.g., bleeding, redness) should be closely monitored during pregnancy. The gingivitis usually resolves postpartum. There is also an increased levels of some bacteria including *Prevotella intermedia, Bacteriodes,* and *Porphromonas gingivalis* (Tarsitano and Rollings 1993; Amar and Chung 1994; Armitage 1999).
- Pregnancy-associated pyogenic granuloma: Pyogenic granuloma can develop due to Flucuations in hormones and will usually disappear postpartum or can be surgically excised.
- Frequent vomiting and gastric reflux can cause erosion of the lingual surface of the maxillary anterior teeth. Studies have shown that is is not advisable to brush immediately after vomiting or acid reflux. It is recommended to wait for about 15 min before rinsing or brushing teeth.
- Xerostomia can occur in some patients.
- In the past few years, the relationship between poor periodontal health and delivering preterm low-weight babies has been controversial. The most recent literature from the European Federation of Periodontology and American Academy of Periodontology report that scaling and root planing do not improve birth outcomes in pregnant patients with periodontal disease (Michalowicz *et al.* 2013).

Dental notes: The pregnant patient

- The greatest risk for spontaneous miscarriage is in the first trimester. As it is believed that most of the fetal development takes place in the first trimester, elective dental care should be postponed until the second trimester (fourteenth week), during which period only minimal harm occurs to the fetus. A clinical study in 2008 examined the safety of dental treatment in pregnant patients and reported that elective dental treatment (e.g., treatment of moderate-to-severe caries or fractured or abscessed teeth) was safe at 13–21 weeks' gestation (Michalowicz *et al.* 2008). Emergency care (e.g., active infection or abscess) during the first trimester may outweigh the risks than if treatment was not done.
- Epinephrine 100,000 is safe to administer to pregnant women as long as intravascular injection is avoided (Little et al. 2008; Michalowicz *et al.* 2008; Giglio *et al.* 2009).

- The second trimester is the most ideal time for routine dental treatment; however, scaling can be performed at any time (Giglio *et al.* 2009).
- In early third trimester, routine dental treatment can be performed, but later in the trimester, the patient may be uncomfortable and patient positioning becomes important.
- If the patient has comorbid conditions, it is recommended to obtain a consult from the obstetrician.
- Radiographs are safe to take on pregnant patients as needed following universal precautions taking care to protect the patient's thyroid and pelvic area with a lead apron and thyroid collar. Some obstetricians have recommended wearing two aprons. In addition, the pregnant dental assistant as well the pregnant dentist should also wear a lead apron (Hilgers *et al.* 2003). Only necessary radiographs should be taken using E speed film or digital, rectangular collimation and long cone (Langlais and Langland 1995; Hilgers *et al.* 2003; American Dental Association 2012). If there are any reservations concerning the treatment of the pregnant patient, consider a consultation with the patient's obstetrician (American Academy of Periodontology 2004).
- Oral prophylaxis and polishing can be performed during the entire pregnancy.
- Positioning the pregnant patient is important for medical reasons. During the second and third trimester, the patient should be positioned in the dental chair on her left side to avoid or relieve supine hypotensive syndrome whereby the uterus partially obstructs the inferior vena cava; avoid supine position in late pregnancy. Careful patient positioning with the right hip elevated will shift the uterus to the left which is off the vena cava. Monitor vital signs during treatment. The head should also be kept above the feet. Have oxygen available if needed.
- Hypertension during pregnancy is of concern. Blood pressure should also be monitored. Hypertension in the pregnant women is classified as being mild if ≥140/90 mm Hg and severe if ≥160/110 mm Hg (New York State Department of Health 2006).
- Gestational diabetes can occur in some pregnant women (Hilger *et al.* 2003). If the patient is being treated for gestational diabetes, they should be asked about their HbA1c and fasting glucose levels. This usually reverses after delivery.
- Do not place the pregnant patient in a supine position due to breathing changes (increased rate of respiration and dyspnea) that can occur during pregnancy.
- It is important to educate the patient on good oral hygiene and nutrition during pregnancy.
- Monitor pregnant patient for signs of gingivitis as a result of elevated levels of progesterone/estrogen. Frequently a pyogenic granuloma is seen at the labial interdental papilla.
- If community water is not fluoridated, pregnant women can be prescribed 1 mg/day (tablet or drops) of sodium fluoride from the third to ninth month until dental formation is completed and during breastfeeding for caries prevention in the child (Maturo *et al.* 2011). Remember fluoride is pregnancy category C drug so application should follow evidence-based guidelines (Giglio *et al.* 2009).

B.   Oral contraceptives

- The prescribing of antibiotics is still a controversial issue.
- All women of child-bearing age should be asked if she is taking an oral contraceptive before prescribing an antibiotic. Even though there are limited case reports regarding this interaction, it is still considered to be a potential drug interaction.
- Essentially, interactions between oral contraceptive and antibiotic are rare but still it can occur (DeRossi and Hersh 2002). The concentration of estrogen today has drastically decreased in women than years ago; however, a small decrease in efficacy especially in the "low-dose" (<35 µg

of estrogen) combination oral contraceptives when taken with an antibiotic has been documented (Burroughs and Chambliss 2000).

- ○ Ethinyl estradiol, an estrogen present in oral contraceptives, is absorbed only at about 40–50% systemically in an inactive form. The remainder undergoes extensive first-pass metabolism. In the gut, inactive ethinyl estradiol becomes active by the action of bacterial gut flora. The active ethinyl estradiol is then reabsorbed in the small intestine. Thus, there is a concern when taking antibiotics, especially broad-spectrum, because bacteria that are needed to activate ethinyl estradiol for the oral contraceptive to be effective are destroyed by antibiotics (Gibson and McGowan 1994). This activation by bacterial gut flora does not occur with progestins, the other component of oral contraceptives.
- ○ There is conflicting reports on which antibiotics are the offending agents. Additionally, drug interactions may be more common with the low-dose estrogen oral contraceptives (Gibson and McGowan 1994). The first report, published in 1971, established the link between oral contraceptives and antibiotics, that is with rifampin, an antituberculosis drug (Gibson and McGowan 1994).
- ○ The American College of Obstetricians and Gynecologists concluded that clarithromycin, tetracycline, doxycycline, ampicillin, quinolones, and metronidazole do not affect oral contraceptive levels as do the broad-spectrum antibiotics such as amoxicillin that may reduce estrogen levels (Archer and Archer 2002; Horn and Hansten 2003; Lomaestro 2009). Since it cannot be predicted which women will be at greater risk for this drug interaction, it has been suggested that women use an additional contraceptive method while taking antibiotics and for at least 1 week after completing the antibiotics (Osborne 2004). It is plausible that some women may have low levels of ethinyl estradiol due to differences in the pharmacokinetics of the drug which would result in oral contraceptive failure when taking antibiotics (Bauer and Wolf 2005).
- ○ In 2004, The World Health Organization (WHO) reported that there have been uncertainties that broad-spectrum antibiotics may lower oral contraceptive effectiveness; however, pregnancy rates are similar in women taking oral contraceptives concurrently with or without antibiotics (WHO 2004).
- The ADA Council on Scientific Affairs recommends advising patients of the potential risk of antibiotics reducing the effectiveness of the oral contraceptive and advising the patient to discuss with her physician the use of an additional nonhormonal type of contraception and to continue adherence with oral contraceptives while on antibiotics (ADA Council on Scientific Affairs 2002). In any case, it is best to advise the female patient taking oral contraceptives to select a nonhormonal back-up birth control for the next 7 days weeks after discontinuation of the antibiotic or through the end of the current cycle, whichever is longer, switch the patient to an OC with a higher dose of estrogen and progestin for one cycle or to abstain from sexual activity (Osborne 2002; Horn and Hansten 2003).

References

Amar, S. & Chung, K.M. (1994) Influence of hormonal variation on the periodontium in women. *Periodontology 2000*, **6**, 79–87.

American Academy of Pediatric Dentistry (2012). Guideline oral health care for the pregnant adolescent. **35 (6)**, 150–156.

American Academy of Periodontology (2004) Task Force on Periodontal Treatment of Pregnant Women. *Journal of Periodontology*.

American Dental Association (2012) Dental Radiographic Examinations: Recommendations for Patient Selection and Limiting Radiation Exposure. www.ada.org/sections/professionalResources/pdfs/Dental_Radiographic_Examinations_2012_pdf [accessed on January 2, 2014].

American Dental Association Council on Scientific Affairs (2002) Antibiotic interference with oral contraceptives. *Journal of the American Dental Association*, **133**, 880.

Archer, J.S. & Archer D.F. (2002) Oral contraceptive efficacy and antibiotic interaction: a myth debunked. *Journal of the American Academy of Dermatology*, **46**, 917–923.

Armitage, G.C. (1999) Development of a classification system for periodontal diseases and conditions. *Annuals of Periodontology*, **84**, 1–6.

Bauer, K.L. & Wolf, D. (2005) Do antibiotics interfere with the efficacy of oral contraceptives? *The Journal of Family Practice*, **54**, 1079–1080.

Becker, D.E. & Rosenberg, M. (2008) Nitrous oxide and the inhalation anesthetics. *Anesthesia Progress*, **55**, 124–131.

Black, R.A. & Hill, D.A. (2003) Over-the-counter medications in pregnancy. *American Family Physicians*, **67**, 2517–2524.

Burroughs, K.E. & Chambliss, M.L. (2000) Antibiotics and oral contraceptive failure. *Arch Fam Med*, **9 (1)**, 81–82.

Colemen, T.K., Rogers, P.D., Cleary, J.D. *et al.* (1998) Antifungal therapy during pregnancy. *Clinical Infectious Disease*, **27**, 1151–1160.

Collins, E. (1981) Maternal and fetal effects of acetaminophen and salicylates in pregnancy. *Obstetrics & Gynecology*, **58 (5 Suppl.)**, 57S–62S.

DeRossi, S.S. & Hersh, E.V. (2002) Antibiotics and oral contraceptives. *Dental Clinics of North America*, **46**, 653–654.

Dolovich, L.R., Addis, A., & Vaillancourt, J.M.R. (1998) Benzodiazepine use in pregnancy and major malformations or oral cleft: meta-analysis of cohort and case-control studies. *British Medical Journal*, **317**, 839–843.

Fayans, E.P., Stuart, H.R., Carsten, D. *et al.* (2010). Local anesthetic use in the pregnant and postpartum patient. *Dental Clinics of North America*, **54**, 697–713.

Fox, F. (2013) Pregnant dental patients. Health groups spread word that dental care is safe, necessary. *American Dental Association News*, May 20.

Gibson, J. & McGowan, D.A. (1994) Oral contraceptives and antibiotics: important considerations for dental practices. *British Dental Journal*, **177**, 419–422.

Giglio, J.A., Lanni, S.M., Laskin, D.M. *et al.* (2009) Oral health for the pregnant patient. *The Journal of the Canadian Dental Association*, **75**, 43–48.

Hilgers, K.K., Douglass, J., & Mathieu, G.P. (2003) Adolescent pregnancy: a review of dental treatment guidelines. *Pediatric Dentistry*, **25**, 459–467.

Horn, J.R. & Hansten, P.D. (2003) Antibiotics and oral contraceptive failure. *Pharmacy Times*, November, pp. 64–65.

Langlais, R.P. & Landland, O.E. (1995) Risk from dental radiographs. *California Dental Journal*, **23 (5)**, 33–34, 36–39.

Little, J.W., Falace, D.A., Miller, C.S. *et al.* (2008) *Dental Management of the Medically Compromised Patient*, 7th ed., pp. 268–278, 456. CV Mosby, St. Louis.

Lomaestro, B.M. (2009) Do antibiotics interact with combination oral contraceptives? *Medscape*. www.medscape.com/viewarticle/707926 [accessed on December 10, 2011].

Lynch, C., Sinnott, IV J., Holt, D.A., *et al.* (1991) Use of antibiotics during pregnancy. *American Family Physician*, **43**, 1365–1368.

Macones, G.A., Marder, S.J., Clothier, B. *et al.* (2001) The controversy surrounding indomethacin for tocolysis. *American Journal of Obstetrics and Gynecology*, **184**, 264–272.

Maturo, P., Costacurta, M., Perugia, C. *et al.* (2011) Fluoride supplements in pregnancy, effectiveness in the prevention of dental caries in a group of children. *Oral Implantology*, **4**, 23–27.

Michalowicz, B.S., DiAngelis, A.J., Novak, M.J. *et al.* (2008) Examining the safety of dental treatment in pregnant women. *Journal of the American Dental Association*, **139**, 686–695.

Michalowicz, B.S., Gustafsson, A., Thumbigere-Math, V. *et al.* (2013) The effects of periodontal treatment on pregnancy outcomes. *Journal of Periodontology,* **84**, S195–S207.

Moore, P.A. (1998) Selecting drugs for the pregnant dental patient. *Journal of the American Dental Association*, **129**, 1281–1286.

New York State Department of Health (2006) Oral Health Care during Pregnancy and Early Childhood. Practice Guidelines. August 2006.

Osborne, N.G. (2004) Antibiotics and oral contraceptives: potential interactions. *Journal of Gynecologic Surgery*, **18**, 171–172.

Ratanajamit, C., Vinther, S.M., Jepsen, P. *et al.* (2003) Adverse pregnancy outcome in women exposed to acyclovir during pregnancy: a population-based observational study. *Scandinavian Journal of Infectious Diseases*, **35**, 255–259.

Rowland, A.S., Baird, D.D., Shore, D.L. *et al.* (1995) Nitrous oxide and spontaneous abortion in female dental assistants. *American Journal of Epidemiology*, **141**, 531–538.

Shnider, M., Asling, J.H., Margolis, A.J. *et al.* (1968) High fetal blood levels of mepivacaine and fetal bradycardia. *New England Journal of Medicine*, **279 (17)**, 947–948.

Singh, P. (2012) An emphasis on the wide usage and important role of local anesthesia in dentistry: a strategic review. *Journal of Dental Research*, **9**, 127–132.

Sobel, J.D. (2000) Use of antifungal drugs in pregnancy: a focus on safety. *Drug Safety*, **23**, 77–85.

Tarsitano, B.F. & Rollings, R.E. (1993) The pregnant dental patient: evaluation and management. *General Dentistry*, **41**, 226–231.

Turner, M.D., Singh, F., & Glickman, R.S. (2006) Dental management of the gravid patient. *New York State Dental Journal*, **72**, 22–27.

World Health Organization (2004) *Medical Eligibility Criteria for Contraceptive Use*. 3rd ed. Reproductive Health and Research, WHO, Geneva.

Chapter 7

Disorders of the liver and gallbladder

A. Liver disease   93
    a. Alcoholic liver disease and cirrhosis   98
    b. Hepatitis   99
    c. Liver transplant   103
B. Gallstones   105
References   106

A. Liver disease

Diagnostic/lab values

Liver is an important organ because it metabolizes majority of the drugs; it regulates the metabolism of nutrients such as glucose, glycogen, lipids, cholesterol, and amino acids. When there is liver disease (e.g., impaired liver function), liver function tests (LFTs) including the levels of serum aminotransferase, bilirubin, and albumin must be known before prescribing any medication. In patients with abnormal LFTs who do not have cirrhosis, drug metabolism is unlikely to be significantly affected; however, LFTs should be monitored (Denk 2002; Smith and Desmond 2013).

Liver disease is classified as acute or chronic (e.g., cirrhosis and alcohol liver disease); infectious (e.g., hepatitis A, B, C, D, and E viruses, infectious mononucleosis, or secondary syphilis and tuberculosis) or non-infectious (e.g., substance abuse such as alcohol); and diseased condition due to medications (e.g., ketoconazole, methyldopa, methotrexate, and acetaminophen) (Pamplona *et al.* 2011).

Liver panel (Pincus and Abraham 2011; Pincus *et al.* 2011; http://www.webmd.com/digestive-disorders/tc/liver-function-panel-topic-overview)

The following enzymes and substances actually do not evaluate the actual function of the liver; the enzymes just tell us there is liver damage.

Alanine aminotransferase (ALT): normal range is 3.4–5.4 grams per deciliter (g/dl); a protein that gets released into the blood when liver cells are damaged; look for elevated levels in liver disease.
Aspartate aminotransferase (AST): a protein released into the blood after liver cell damage; normal range is 10–34 IU/l (international units per liter); elevated levels in liver disease.

The Dentist's Quick Guide to Medical Conditions, First Edition. Mea A. Weinberg, Stuart L. Segelnick, Joseph S. Insler, with Samuel Kramer.
© 2015 John Wiley & Sons, Inc. Published 2015 by John Wiley & Sons, Inc.

Alkaline phosphatase (ALP): a protein whose normal range is 44–147 IU/l; look for elevated levels in liver disease.

Serum bilirubin: Old red blood cells are broken down in the spleen into globin and heme; heme is then converted into bilirubin after the removal of iron, and the iron is then reused. Bilirubin is transported, bound to plasma albumin, to the liver where it is metabolized.

Normal range of total bilirubin is 0.3–1.9 mg/dl; liver disease can cause jaundice or elevated bilirubin levels.

Serum albumin: a protein synthesized by the liver; normal range is 3.4–5.4 g/dl; levels of albumin, a water-soluble, coagulable protein, may decrease in liver disease, which will lead to a decrease in clotting ability.

Coagulation defects

In addition, the liver produces vitamin K dependent coagulation factors I (fibrinogen), II (prothrombin), V, VII, IX, X, and XI. Since there will be hemostatic defects with bleeding problems, an evaluation of the patient's platelet count, partial prothrombin time (PPT), and international normalized ratio (INR) must be obtained before starting any dental procedures.

Portal hypertension can scavenge platelets formed in the spleen, resulting in thrombocytopenia. This results in increased bleeding tendencies when performing invasive dental procedures (Pamplona *et al.* 2011). Patients with liver disease also have comorbidities including diabetes, kidney disease, weight loss, malnutrition, and protein deficiency.

Platelet count: Platelets are synthesized in the bone marrow. A normal platelet count is 150,000–400,000/mm^3. For invasive dental procedures (e.g., extractions), the platelets must not be <50,000/mm^3; otherwise they require a platelet transfusion the morning of the dental procedure (Williford *et al.* 1989). Noninvasive dental procedures may be performed in patients with platelet counts ≥50,000/mm^3 (Afdhal *et al.* 2008). There is a redistribution of circulating platelets into the enlarged spleen resulting in thrombocytopenia (Peck-Radosavljevic 2000; Qamar and Grace 2009). Thrombocytopenia is defined as platelets <100,000/mm^3 and is one of the most common causes of abnormal bleeding. Levels <80,000 can be associated with bleeding problems (Little *et al.* 2008).

In summary, platelet counts >50,000/mm^3 will not cause significant bleeding problems. Platelet transfusion are required with counts <50,000/mm^3 (Radmand *et al.* 2013). The majority of patients with liver disease also have platelet destruction by the spleen.

PPT: PPT is done to check the intrinsic system of coagulation of the blood inside the vessels. Normal PTT range is 25–35 seconds; values >35 seconds indicate abnormal or prolonged bleeding.

Prothrombin time (PT): PT is done to check the extrinsic system (Factor VII) which shows the ability of the blood that leaves the vessels in the injured area to clot. Normal range is 11–15 seconds; values >15 seconds is abnormal.

• Any abnormal serum values require a medical consultation.

INR: INR allows for PT values to be standardized throughout the world. INR values in patients with liver disease vary largely among different laboratories (Tripodi *et al.* 2007). Ideally, the INR should be measured within 24 h of the dental procedure, but not more than 72 h. The INR can be taken at a laboratory with results sent to the dentist or at the dentist's office, or some patients have machines at home which take INR with the results being sent to the company, which then gets sent to the physician.

Other blood abnormalities

- Anemia: This is due to either chronic gastrointestinal bleeding, and hypersplenism secondary to portal hypertension and it may be exacerbated by folic acid or vitamin B_{12} deficiency secondary to inadequate intake or malabsorption (Casas *et al.* 2009)
- Leukopenia (abnormal decrease circulating WBCs <4000/mm³): This is due to portal hypertension-induced sequestration or bone marrow suppression from excessive alcohol (Qamar and Grace 2009)
- An impairment of macrophage, neutrophil, and T-cell function increase risk for infection (Qamar and Grace 2009).

Oral adverse effects: Liver cirrhosis (Pamplona *et al.* 2011)

- Gingival bleeding
- Glossitis
- Xerostomia
- Petechiae
- Angular chelitis
- Bruxism
- Periodontal disease
- Alcohol breath
- Sialadenosis (bilateral enlargement of the parotid glands) (Guggenheimer *et al.* 2009)

Prognosis of chronic liver disease

Child–Pugh classification is a prognostic scoring model that calculates the mortality of patients with chronic liver disease, mainly cirrhosis (Boursier *et al.* 2009). This score can be used at bedside. It uses five lab values that are added together: ascites (presence/controlled or not), encephalopathy (presence/controlled or not), serum bilirubin, serum albumin, and PT (Durand and Valla 2008). Table 7.1 shows the Child–Pugh classification (Pugh *et al.* 1973; Sloss 2009).

Table 7.1 Child-Pugh classification of risk assessment for chronic liver disease.

Parameter	1 point	2 points	3 points
Ascites	None	Mild	Moderate
Serum bilirubin	<2.0 mg/dl	2.0–3.0	>3.0
Serum albumin	>3.5 mg/dl	2.8–3.5	<2.8
Prothrombin time or	<4 s	4–6	>6
INR	<1.7	1.7–2.3	>2.3
Encephalopathy	None	Mild 1–2	Severe 3–4

Grade A: total score of 5–6; mild disease and well compensated.
Grade B: total score of 7–9; moderate disease with significant function compromise.
Grade C: total score of 10–15; severe disease or decompensated liver disease—low survival.
If a patient has a Grade B or C, either there needs to be a dosage modification or avoid prescribing the drug. Consult with the patient's physician.

Drug metabolism by the liver

Drugs that are primarily cleared by the liver *may* require dosage adjustment in patients with hepatic impairment; however, liver disease has to be advanced/severe before changes in drug metabolism/pharmacokinetics occur. Drugs are primarily metabolized by cytochrome P450 enzymes and an impaired liver cannot synthesize adequate amounts of these microsomal enzymes. There are many factors involved in assessing the effects of liver disease on drug metabolism. Beside the half-life of the drug, enzyme activity, hepatic blood flow, functional liver cell mass, and previous drug therapy are important. Consultation with the patient's physician is necessary before drug prescribing.

Unlike in renal disease whereby creatinine clearance and glomerular filtration rate can be used as a reliable indicator for adjustments in drug dosage, it is more difficult to determine indicators of liver function. The liver enzymes such as AST, ALT, gamma GT (GGT), and (ALP only indicate if there is liver cell damage but does not relate to the ability of the liver to metabolize drugs. If the drug dose has to be modified, either the dosage has to be decreased or the dosing interval is increased. Consult with the patients' physician for any dosage adjustments (Golla *et al.* 2004).

Since all drugs have to be eliminated from the body they have to be broken down into a water-soluble metabolite in the liver or eliminated unchanged (not metabolized). Most drugs are metabolized and excreted primarily by the kidneys in the urine. Other drugs that are not metabolized go through the liver intact or unchanged and are excreted in the bile (fluid secreted by the liver and stored in the gallbladder). From there, the bile with the drug enters the gastrointestinal tract and then is either eliminated in feces or reabsorbed back to the liver by enterohepatic recirculation (or enterohepatic cycling) and eventually metabolized by the liver and excreted via the kidneys in the urine. Some drugs can also change into metabolites in the liver and then excreted in the bile, which are eliminated in the feces and reabsorbed back into the blood. For example, tetracycline is not metabolized (unchanged) and undergoes enterohepatic recirculation and is excreted in both the urine and bile and recovered in the feces. Doxycycline is also not metabolized in the liver but is partially deactivated in the intestines and primarily recovered in the feces.

Local anesthetics including lidocaine, mepivacaine, bupivacaine, and prilocaine are metabolized in the liver. These agents are still well tolerated by patients with mild to moderate liver disease; however, in severe disease, changes may be necessary (Pamplona *et al.* 2011). According to Little *et al.* (2008), three cartridges of 2% lidocaine is considered to be adequate for these patients. Consultation with the patient's hepatologist is recommended (Pamplona *et al.* 2011) (Table 7.2).

Dental notes: Patient with liver disease

- **Medial consultation is required to determine:**
  ○ the patient's severity of liver impairment
  ○ bleeding tendency
  ○ drug dosage modification
  ○ complete blood count (CBC) with differential (includes the platelet count)

Antibiotic prophylaxis and infection control:
- Although there is no evidence-based literature to support antibiotic prophylaxis, it may be recommended depending on the patient's medical status, presence of oral infection, decrease in white blood cell count, and immunosuppression (Douglas *et al.* 1998). It is recommended to obtain a physician's consult. The risk of infection in patients with liver disease is up to 30% (Bernard *et al.* 1999).
- Universal protection to avoid cross-infection.

Table 7.2 Dental drugs metabolized in the liver (Pamplona *et al.* 2011).

Dental drug	Liver impairment
Acetaminophen (Tylenol)	NOT contraindicated in liver disease; limited, low-dose therapy is tolerated in hepatic disease. Maximum dose should be <2 g/day) (Douglas *et al.* 1998; Hughes *et al.* 2011)
Amoxicillin (Trimox, Amoxil)	Safe to use with usual dosage
Amoxicillin/calvulante (Augmentin) (immediate-release form)	If history of amoxicillin/clavulante-associated hepatic damage then it is contraindicated
Aspirin	Avoid due to increased risk of bleeding
Azithromycin (Zithromax)	Avoid
Clarithromycin (Biaxin)	No adjustment
Clindamycin (Cleocin)	No adjustment with hepatitis; decrease dose by 50% in cirrhosis
Codeine (with acetaminophen)	Consider to decrease dose in moderate to severe disease or avoid
Diflunisal (Dolobid)	Avoid
Doxycycline (Vibramycin, Doryx)	Administered cautiously in patients with preexisting liver disease or biliary obstruction. Reduced dosages may be appropriate, since doxycycline undergoes enterohepatic recycling. Best to give alternative antibiotic
Erythromycin (Eryc, E.E.S.)	Avoid with the estolate may cause hepatotoxicity
Hydrocodone and acetaminophen (Vicodin, Lorcet, Lortab)	Consider decreasing dose and using for 2–3 days or avoid. Avoid chronic use (Johnson 2007)
Ibuprofen (Advil, Motrin, Nuprin)	Avoid in severe hepatic disease (hepatitis and cirrhosis)
Fluconazole (Diflucan)	No adjustment in mild to moderate hepatic impairment
Metronidazole (Flagyl)	Reduce dose or avoid in severe liver disease because drug can accumulate. No dose adjustment needed with mild liver disease
Naproxen (Naprosyn) Naproxen sodium (Aleve)	Not recommended
Penicillin VK (Pen-V, V-Cillin K, Veetids)	Safe to use usual dosage
Tetracycline (Sumycin)	Avoid
Local anesthetics	Lidocaine, mepivacaine, bupivacaine, and prilocaine are metabolized in the liver. These agents are still well tolerated by patients with mild to moderate liver disease; however, in severe disease changes may be necessary
General anesthetics	Avoid: halothane, thiopentone
	Acceptable: isoflurane, nitrous oxide
Benzodiazepine: diazepam, midazolam, alprazolam	Acceptable and recommended

Platelets and bleeding tendency:

- Platelets <50,000/mm^3: bleeding tendency. While some studies report that platelet transfusions are not mandatory, most references state that when platelets are <50,000/mm^3, a platelet transfusion is necessary to get a level >50,000 (Douglas *et al.* 1998; Givol *et al.* 2012).
    - Platelet transfusion results in an immediate increase in platelet count reaching a maximum at about 1 h. Thus, patients will usually have the transfusion in the morning and dental treatment immediately following.
- INR should be ≤3.5 to perform invasive dental procedures.
- It is important to recognize the increased incidence of hypercoagulability in patients with liver disease. These patients are more prone to develop clots (deep vein thrombosis) and present as a medical emergency in the dental chair (Shah *et al.* 2013).

Drug prescribing and administration:

- Determine the degree of liver impairment by using the Child–Pugh classification. Possible drug toxicity due to altered liver metabolism; in some cases, the dosage may have to be modified.
- Local anesthetics are generally safe if total dose is kept below 7 mg/kg when combined with epinephrine (Douglas *et al.* 1998).

Other information:

- Question the patient regarding alcohol intake—type of alcohol and frequency.
- Be aware of signs and symptoms for acute or chronic liver disease: poor dental health, xerostomia, jaundice of the oral mucosa, malnutrition, spider angiomas (on face, neck, and arms), palmer erythema, ascites, and splenomegaly (Grossman *et al.* 2009; Pamplona *et al.* 2011).

a.   *Alcoholic liver disease and cirrhosis*

Clinical synopsis

Alcoholic liver disease occurs after chronic, excessive alcohol intake, which kills the hepatic cells. It is reversible unless alcohol intake continues and then it becomes a fatty liver, followed by alcoholic hepatitis and finally irreversible liver cirrhosis (Pamplona *et al.* 2011). Up to 35% of heavy drinkers develop alcoholic hepatitis and between 10 and 20% develop cirrhosis (www.Liverfoundation.org/abouttheliver/info/alcohol/).

Liver cirrhosis is a chronic condition defined as a widespread hepatic fibrosis with nodule formation resulting in death of liver cells. Essentially, damaged liver tissue is replaced by dense fibrous connective tissue, similar to tissue scaring. Hepatocellular damage causes the release of intracellular enzymes such as transaminases into the extracellular fluid. Altered pharmacokinetics occurs as a result of multiple physiological changes including reduced liver cell mass, and a reduction in the concentration of drug protein binding (Smith and Desmond 2013). In addition, the fibrous tissue contracts which may reduce the circulation of blood through the liver, causing congestion in the portal vein system (portal hypertension), which affects the function of the liver and causes increased venous pressure resulting in varices or enlarged veins in the gastrointestinal tract, esophagus, and rectum which are susceptible to rupturing (Smith and Desmond 2013).

The majority of cirrhosis is caused by excessive, chronic alcohol intake or possibly malnutrition or a combination of the two, hepatitis B, hepatitis C, or fatty liver disease (Golla *et al.* 2004). Cirrhosis usually occurs as a comorbid disease (e.g., chronic hepatitis). Cirrhosis is the final stage of alcoholic liver disease. Complications of liver cirrhosis are portal hypertension (hypertension in the portal vein system), hepatocellular carcinoma, and loss of function (Ryder and Williams

1994; Golla *et al.* 2004; Blonski *et al.* 2010). At the end-stage of cirrhosis, liver transplantation is the only definitive treatment (Golla *et al.* 2004).

Patients with alcoholic cirrhosis show an increased tolerance to anesthetics, hypnotics, and sedatives and may require dose increases to obtain a desired effect (Pamplona *et al.* 2011). Invasive dental surgery may be contraindicated in patients with alcoholic cirrhosis (Pamplona *et al.* 2011).

b. Hepatitis

Hepatitis literally means inflammation of the liver and is classified as being infectious and non-infectious (e.g., caused by drugs such as acetaminophen, ketoconazole, or alcohol).

Infectious hepatitis

Examples of infectious hepatitis are viral hepatitis, mononucleosis, tuberculosis, or secondary to syphilis. The incubation period of the virus of serum hepatitis may be as long as 6 months. Symptoms may not appear until 6 weeks after infection (Pamplona *et al.* 2011). Viral hepatitis may be caused by hepatitis A virus (HAV), hepatitis B virus (HBV), or hepatitis C virus (HCV), the latter two transmitted by blood and saliva. Hepatitis B is diagnosed by quantifying the levels of HBV DNA, HBsAg, and the antigen/antibody ratio (Pamplona *et al.* 2011).

Specific lab values: Viral hepatitis

The following are serologic tests and interpretation for viral hepatitis (Table 7.3) (Chizzali-Bonfadin *et al.* 1997; www.cdc.gov/hepatitis/hbv/pdfs/serologicchartv8.pdf).

Medications: Treatment of hepatitis B infection

Patients with active signs of liver disease (HBV infection with hepatitis B antigen present) and who would most likely develop liver damage such as cirrhosis will most likely be on medication; however,

Table 7.3   Serologic tests and interpretation for viral hepatitis.

Hepatitis B		
HBsAg	Hepatitis B surface antigen	(+): Patient currently is infectious with HBV or is a chronic carrier
Anti-HBs	Hepatitis B surface antibodies	If (−) to HBsAg and (+) to anti-HBc and (+) anti-HBs, patient is immune due to natural infection If (−) to HBsAg and (−) to anti-HBc and (+) to anti-HBs, patient is immune due to hepatitis B vaccination
HBeAg	Hepatitis B e antigen	(+) virus is replicating and patient is highly infected with HBV
IgM anti-HBc	IgM antibody to hepatitis B core antigen	(+) recent infection ≤6 months; acute infection
Anti-HBc	Total hepatitis B core antibody	(+) onset of symptoms in acute infection and remains for lifetime. Indicated previous or ongoing infection

Table 7.4   Dental drug–hepatitis B drug interactions (www.drugs.com).

Dental drug	Hepatitis B drug	Management
NSAIDs: Ibuprofen/ ibuprofen-hydrocodone/ naproxen/naproxen sodium	Telbivudine	NSAIDs affect kidney function and may increase levels of telbivudine. Consult with physician; may need dose adjustment and frequent monitoring
Aspirin/aspirin, oxycodone	Telbivudine	Consult with physician
Metronidazole	Telbivudine, interferon alfa-2b	Increase risk of nerve damage; dose adjustment; consult with physician
Corticosteroids (e.g., prednisone, hydrocortisone)	Telbivudine	Increase risk of muscle disorder; consult with physician
Tramadol, tramadol/ acetaminophen	Interferon alpha-2B, pegylated Interferon	May cause seizures if taken together; consult with physician

chronically infected patients with severe liver damage usually are not started on medication (Fung and Lok 2004). The goals of treatment are to endure viral suppression, normalization of ALT, and improvement in liver histology (Fung and Lok 2004). Currently, there are seven FDA approved drugs in the USA to treat chronic HBV: interferon alpha-2b (Intron A), pegylated interferon (Pegasys), lamivudine (Epivir HBV), Adefovir (Hepsera), entecavir (Baraclude), telbivudine (Tyzeka), and tenofovir (Viread). Most patients will probably take interferon alpha-2b or pegylated interferon. Dental drug interactions are listed in Table 7.4.

Dental notes: Patients with active hepatitis B infection

- Even though the dental professional has been vaccinated against HCB, the seroconversion (development of detectable antibodies) risk is 30% (Smith *et al.* 2001).
- Use universal infection control methods.

Hepatitis C

Hepatitis C (HCV-RNA) is the primary cause of chronic liver disease with about 8,000–10,000 deaths per year and the reason for liver transplantation; however, some patients with chronic hepatitis C may never show progression to cirrhosis (DePaola 2003; Golla *et al.* 2004; Grossman *et al.* 2009; Pamplona *et al.* 2011). Acute hepatitis C infection may present with nonspecific flu-like symptoms including fatigue, nausea, anorexia, myalgias, arthralgias, weakness, and weight loss, while the clinical features of chronic hepatitis C may show no or few symptoms (Golla *et al.* 2004; Wilkins *et al.* 2010). HCV is not efficiently transmitted, and the average rate of seroconversion after an occupational exposure to HCV-positive blood through accidental needle stick is 1.8% (US Public Health Service 2011).

Diagnostic/lab values

Direct and indirect virological tests are involved in the diagnosis of hepatitis C infection, treatment planning, and the assessment of the virological response to therapy (Pawlotsky 2002). Indirect testing utilizes serologic assays to detect specific antibody to HCV (anti-HCV), and direct assays will detect, quantify, or characterize the HCV viral particles, such as HCV RNA and core antigen

Table 7.5 Serological and virological tests and interpretation for hepatitis C.

Initial testing: ELISA (hepatitis C antibodies anti-HCV)	Recombinant immunoblot assay (detects antibodies to individual HCV antigens)	HCV RNA polymerase chain reaction	Interpretation
–			No infection
+	+	+	Current infection
+	+	–	Past infection
+	–	–	False positive

Adapted from Wilkins *et al.* (2010).

(Pawlotsky 2002). Abnormal laboratory findings or signs of cirrhosis should prompt HCV antibody testing (Wilkins *et al.* 2010). The most commonly used initial assay for detecting HCV antibodies is the enzyme immunoassay (ELISA) for anti-HCV and RT-PCR (polymerase chain reaction), which detect antibodies to HCV antigens and indicates if the patient is actively replicating HCV (Golla *et al.* 2004; Wilkins *et al.* 2010; Chevaliez and Pawlotsky 2006). If the enzyme immunoassay is positive, a confirmatory test should be performed using recombinant immunoblot assay and HCV RNA PCR. The recombinant immunoblot assay and viral load tests are used to distinguish between a resolved infection and a false-positive enzyme immunoassay (Wilkins *et al.* 2010). Table 7.5 reviews the serological tests and interpretation for hepatitis C.

Medications

Hepatitis C: There is no vaccine to prevent HCV as there is for HBV. The standard drug treatment for actively infected patients with HCV is combination medications including ribarvirin (taken orally), pegylated interferon (injectable), and protease inhibitors (orally). New research on the development of drug combinations, interferon free, has been ongoing (Table 8.6). Indications for the correct drug therapy include genetic genotype, severity of liver function, previously untreated, and previously failed therapy. Oral ribavirin by itself is not effective for inducing sustained virologic response (SVR) (Brok *et al.* 2009).

Drug treatment guidelines (http://www.hepmag.com/articles/2512_18756.shtml; Jacobson *et al.* 2013; Zein 2000)

The goal of treatment is to achieve a SVR with the absence of HCV RNA by polymerase chain reaction 6 months after discontinuing treatment (Swain *et al.* 2010). In 1994, the original proposal for the nomenclature of hepatitis C viral genotypes was published which included six different genotypes (Simmonds *et al.* 1994). Since then, there have been other proposed systems (Kuiken and Simmonds 2009). On June 20, 2013, the FDA approved the first genotyping test, Abbott RealTime HCV Genotype II, for patients with HCV(http://www.FDA.gov/NewsEvents/Newsroom/PressAnnouncements/ucm357982.htm). This is an important breakthrough because the various genotypes respond differently to the available drugs therapies (Table 7.6).

Hepatitis C genotype 1, the most common strain, is usually treated with three drugs: pegylated interferon, ribavirin, and a protease inhibitor. Treatment can last for as long 48 weeks and will result in an SVR in up to 70% of people who have never been treated for HCV (Fried *et al.* 2002; Zuezem 2004).

Table 7.6   Drug therapy for hepatitis C.

Generic name	Brand name
Telaprevir	Incivek
Boceprevir	Victrelis
Pegylated interferon	Pegasys
Ribavirin	CoPegus
Pegylated interferon alpha-2b	Pegintron
Ribavirin	Rebetol
Interferon alpha-2a	Roferon
Interferon aphacon-1	Infergen
Boceprevir	Victrelis

Genotypes 2 and 3 are treated with pegylated interferon and ribavirin. Duration of treatment ranges from 3 to 12 months, depending on hepatitis C viral load, liver damage, insulin resistance, and early response to treatment. The average time is about 6 months to prevent relapse. Sustained viral response among first-time patients taking pegylated interferon and ribavirin can be over 90% for genotype 2 and are 65% or more in HCV genotype 3 (Fried *et al.* 2002; Zuezem 2004).

Genotype 4 is treated with 48 weeks of pegylated interferon and weight-based ribavirin; SVR rates in people living with HCV being treated for the first time are as high as 70% (Fried *et al.* 2002; Zuezem 2004).

Adverse drug reactions

Adherence is a problem with patients taking combination drug therapies. Ribavirin and interferon may contribute to hemolytic anemia by inducing bone marrow suppression resulting in a decline in hemoglobin (Oze *et al.* 2006). The anemic patient may present with fatigue. Ribavirin-induced hemolytic anemia is one of the reasons patients stop taking the medication or require dose reduction (Ong and Younossi 2004). In addition, interferon therapy may cause neutropenia (decrease in peripheral white blood cell counts—neutrophils and lymphocytes) which increases the risk of infection (Ong and Younossi 2004). For this reason, antibiotic prophylaxis is recommended before dental procedures. In addition, interferon may cause *thrombocytopenia* (decrease in platelet count), due to bone marrow suppression, which increases the risk of bleeding. Other adverse reactions include cardiovascular (myocardial infarction, angina, heart failure), neurologic (neuropathy, confusion, stroke, seizures, tinnitus, and vision loss), and psychiatric (Strader *et al.* 2004; Wilkins *et al.* 2010). The majority of patients taking interferon will exhibit flu-like symptoms (Chou *et al.* 2004).

Dental notes: Patients with hepatitis C

- Consult from physician: obtain current CBC with differential and platelet counts
- Hepatitis C has been associated with lichen planus independent of medication use (Mistry *et al.* 2009)
- Some adverse drug reaction of interferon in combination with ribarvirin include lichen planus, hyperpigmentation of the tongue and the skin, systemic lupus erythematosus, and aphthous ulcers (Lindahl *et al.* 2005; Nagao *et al.* 2005; Ho *et al.* 2008; Mistry *et al.* 2009). These drug reactions may be clinically seen immediately within about 3 days or later after three or more days after first taking the medication (Vervloet and Durham 1998; Mistry *et al.* 2009).

c. Liver transplant

Patients with end-stage liver disease who have no other options are candidates for orthotopic liver transplantation. These patients may be on a "list" for liver donors for an extended time period. Before and after the liver transplantation, inflammation and infection becomes an important feature that may limit the survival of the graft. Obtaining and maintaining oral health of the pre- and post-liver transplant patient is pivotal during this process. Communication between the organ transplant team and dentist is important in formulating individualized care plans to reduce the incidence of pre- and post-transplant complications. Periodontal diseases and other oral infections may present serious risks that may compromise the success of a solid organ transplant.

Model for end-stage liver disease (MELD) score is another classification other than Child-Pugh score, which is able to accurately predict 3-month mortality among patients with chronic liver disease on the liver transplant waiting list and can be applied for allocation of donor livers (Wiesner *et al.* 2003). MELD is a chronic liver severity scoring system that utilizes the patient's laboratory values for serum bilirubin, serum creatinine, and INR or prothrombin time. This model will predict short-term survival in patients with end-stage liver disease and prioritize patients waiting for liver transplant (Freeman *et al.* 2002; Malinchoc *et al.* 2000). This model is used for patients with more severe disease.

  $40\geq$: 71.3% mortality
  30–39: 52.6% mortality
  20–29: 19.6% mortality
  10–19: 6.0% mortality
  <9: 1.9% mortality

If the donor is 18 or older, the liver would be offered first to local and regional Status 1 (medically urgent) candidates. If the liver is not accepted, it is then offered to candidates with a MELD score of 15 or higher, first locally and then regionally (United Network for Organ Sharing 2008).

Medications prescribed

Patients who undergo a major organ transplant most likely take a cocktail of immunosuppressant drugs such as azathioprine (Imuran), cyclosporine, tacrolimus (Prograf, FK506), sirolimus (Rapamune), mycophenolate, and prednisone.

Azathioprine is an antimetabolite indicated as an adjunct for the prevention of rejection in hepatic transplantation. It has a mechanism of action to reduce inflammation and interfere with the growth of rapidly dividing cells. There is a warning about chronic immunosuppression with an increased risk of malignancy. It functions to prevent organ rejection by inhibiting the production of blood cells in the bone marrow. Serious infections are a constant concern for patients receiving azathioprine and any other immunosuppressive drug. The medical consultation from the patient's physician should address the potential for severe infections occurring while the patient is taking azathioprine. The dentist should have the most recent results of the CBC before starting dental treatment. Also, there could be bleeding, oral sores, or swelling of the face, lips, tongue, or throat. There are no drug interactions that would be of concern in dentistry.

Tacrolimus is an immunosuppressive drug used to prevent rejection of liver and kidney organ transplant. There is a warning about *increased susceptibility to infection* and the possible development of lymphoma. The medical consultation from the patient's physician should address the potential for severe infections occurring while the patient is taking tacrolimus. Since hypertension is a common adverse effect, patients may be taking a calcium channel blocker that could cause gingival enlargement.

Cyclosporine is a potent immunosuppressive agent that prolongs survival of many transplants such as kidney, liver, and heart. Patients taking cyclosporine usually have hypertension and may take a calcium channel blocker such as nifedipine (Adalat, Procardia) which causes gingival enlargement. Meticulous oral home care is important with these patients and maintenance/recare appointments should be made every 3 months. Cyclosporine can cause nephrotoxicity (including structural kidney damage) and hepatotoxicity.

Table 7.7 lists the drugs prescribed by the dentist, which may have an interaction with immunosuppressant drugs taken by the organ transplant patient.

Table 7.7 Dental drug–drug interactions in the liver transplant patient (http://www.medscape.com/viewarticle/726344_6; www.rxlist.com; www.epocrates.com; Saad *et al.* 2006).

Dental drug	Liver drug	Management
Clarithromycin/ erythromycin	Cyclosporine, tacrolimus	AVOID. Increase levels of immunosuppressant drugs and possible toxicity. May increase risk of QT prolongation and cardiac arrhythmias. Best to prescribe azithromycin or clindamycin instead
Ciprofloxacin (Cipro)	Cyclosporine	AVOID. Increase cyclosporine levels with risk of nephrotoxicity
Clindamycin	Mycophenolate	Caution advised; may decrease mycophenolate levels
"Azole" antifungals (e.g., clortrimazole, fluconazole, and ketoconazole)	Cyclosporine, tracrolimus, sirolimus	Increased blood concentrations of the immunosuppressants resulting in increased potential for adverse events because of excessive immunosuppression and toxicity (e.g., nephrotoxicity, neurotoxicity). Consult with patient's nephrologist; may require a dosage reduction of the immunosuppressant
"Azole" antifungals (e.g., clortrimazole, fluconazole, and ketoconazole)	Statins	Azoles can increase plasma concentrations of statins that are CYP3A4 substrates (e.g., atorvastatin, lovastatin, and simvastatin). AVOID
Systemic corticosteroids	Cyclosporine, tracrolimus, sirolimus	All azole antifungal agents have been associated with development of adrenal insufficiency. This may be potentiated by coadministration with high-dose corticosteroids. Consult with patient's nephrologist
Metronidazole	Mycophenolate	Caution advised; may increase mycophenolate levels
Tetracycline	Mycophenolate	Caution advised; may decrease mycophenolate levels
Azithromycin, clarithromycin, erythromycin	Mycophenolate	Caution advised; may decrease mycophenolate levels
Acyclovir, valacyclovir	Mycophenolate	Caution advised; may increase levels and risk of toxicity with both drugs
Corticosteroids	Mycophenolate	Combination may increase risk of immunosuppression and infections. Caution advised

Table 7.8   Oral adverse reactions of drugs taken by liver transplant candidates.

Medication	Oral adverse reaction
Cyclosporine	Bleeding, poor wound healing, gingival enlargement
Calcium channel blockers	Gingival enlargement, xerostomia
Tacrolimus	Gingival enlargement, oral ulcers, perioral numbness or tingling
Azathioprine	Stomatitis, opportunistic infections, bleeding
Corticosteroids	Diabetes, poor wound healing, depression, adrenal suppression

Many drugs taken by the pre- and postoperative transplant patient can have oral adverse effects. Table 7.8 lists some common oral adverse effects of these medications.

Dental notes: Liver transplant patient (Guggenheimer *et al.* 2003; Byron and Osborne 2005)

- Antibiotic prophylaxis: consult with the patient's physician.
- Active oral infections: dental treatment is recommended to eliminate dental caries, abscesses, and periodontal disease. Nonrestorable teeth should be extracted. Antibiotics may be necessary after dental treatment to avoid systemic infection.
- Review oral hygiene home care pre- and postoperative transplantation.
- Have patient bring in a written list of all medications at every visit.
- Patients may be taking immunosuppressive drugs.
- Post-transplantation infection is the most common cause of organ rejection in the immunosuppressed patient.
- Bleeding tendencies: A consultation from the patient's physician is required. Obtain a recent platelet count; many patients may have a decreased platelet count ($<50,000/mm^3$) and require a platelet transfusion that should be done the morning of the same day of the dental extraction. Many patients may be taking an anticoagulant (e.g., warfarin) and require an INR reading within 24 h (but not more than 72 h) of the dental procedure.
- Current CBC differential

B. Gallstones

Clinical synopsis

Bile is formed in the liver and stored in the gallbladder. Gallstones (biliary calculi or cholelithiasis) are formed as concretions in the gallbladder consisting of a core of a mixture of cholesterol, bilirubin (bile pigment formed by the breakdown of red blood cells), and protein. In most cases, there are no symptoms; the stones remain silent until an attack occurs when the gallbladder empties vigorously stirring up the stones. Once the stones move, they become wedged in the neck of the gallbladder. Laparoscopic surgery is required only if there are symptoms.

Dental notes: Management of the patient with gallstones

- There are no specific dental management problems with patients with gallstones.
- Some risk factors that can be monitored in the dental office include smoking, heavy drinking, diabetes, and imbalanced diet.

References

Afdhal, N., McHutchison, J., Brown, R., *et al.* (2008) Thrombocytopenia associated with chronic liver disease. *Journal Hepatology*, **48**, 1000–1007.

Bernard, B., Grange, J.D., Khac, E.N., *et al.* (1999) Antibiotic prophylaxis for the prevention of bacterial infections in cirrhotic patients with gastrointestinal bleeding: a meta-analysis. *Hepatology*, **29**, 1655–1661.

Blonski, W., Kotlyar, D.S., & Forde, K.A. (2010) Non-viral causes of hepatocellular carcinoma. *World Journal of Gastroenterology*, **16**, 3603–3615.

Boursier, J., Cesbron, E., Tropet, A.L., *et al.* (2009) Comparison and improvement of MELD and Child-Pugh score accuracies for the prediction of 6-month mortality in cirrhotic patients. *Journal of Clinical Gastroenterology*, **43**, 580–585.

Brok, J., Gluud, L.L., & Gluud, C. (2009) Ribavirin monotherapy for chronic hepatitis C. *Cochrane Database of Systematic Reviews*, (**4**), CD005527.

Byron, R.J. Jr. & Osborne, P.D. (2005) Dental management of liver transplant patients. *General Dentistry*, **53**, 66–69.

Casas R.G., Jones E.A., & Otero, R.M. (2009) Spectrum of anemia associated with chronic liver disease. *World Journal of Gastroenterology*, **15**, 4653–4658.

Chizzali-Bonfadin, C., Adlassnig, K.P., Kreihsl, M., *et al.* (1997) Knowledge-based interpretation of serologic tests for hepatitis on the World Wide Web. *Clinical Performance and Quality HealthCare* **5**, 61.

Chevaliez, S. & Pawlotsky, J.M. (2006) Hepatitis C virus serologic and virologic tests and clinical diagnosis of HCV-related liver disease. *International Journal of Medical Sciences*, **3 (2)**, 35–40.

Chou, R., Clark, E.C., & Helfand, M. (2004) U. S. Preventive Services Task Force. Screening for hepatitis C virus infection: a review of the evidence for the U.S. Preventive Services Task Force. *Annals of Internal Medicine*, **140 (6)**, 465–479.

Denk, H. (2002) Drug induced liver injury. *Verhandlungen der Deutschen Gesellschaft für Pathologie*, **86**, 120–125.

DePaola, L.G. (2003) Managing the care of patients infected with blood-borne disease. *Journal of the American Dental Association*, **134**, 350–358.

Douglas, L.R., Douglass, J.B., Sieck, J.O., *et al.* (1998) Oral management of the patient with end-stage liver disease and the liver transplant patient. *Oral Surgery Oral Medicine Oral Pathology Oral Radiology, and Endodontology*, **86**, 55–64.

Durand, F. & Valla, D. (2008) Assessment of prognosis of cirrhosis. *Seminars in Liver Disease*, **28**, 110–122.

Freeman, R.B. Jr., Wiesner, R.H., Harper, A. *et al.* (2002) The new liver allocation system: moving toward evidence-based transplantation policy. *Liver Transplantation Journal*, **8**, 851–858.

Fried, M.W., Shiffman, M.L., Reddy, K.R. *et al.* (2002) Peginterferon alfa-2a plus ribavirin for chronic hepatitis C virus infection. *New England Journal of Medicine*, **347**, 975–982.

Fung, S.K. & Lok, A.S. (2004) Treatment of chronic hepatitis B: who to treat, what to use, and for how long? *Clinical Gastroenterology and Hepatology*, **2**, 839–848.

Givol, N., Goldstein, G, Peleg, O. *et al.* (2012) Thrombocytopenia and bleeding in dental procedures of patients with Gaucher disease. *Haemophilia*, **18**, 117–121.

Golla, K., Epstein, J.B., & Cabay, R.J. (2004) Liver disease: current perspectives on medical and dental management. *Oral Surgery Oral Medicine Oral Pathology Oral Radiology, and Endodontology*, **98**, 516–521.

Grossman S. M., Teixeira, R., de Aguiar, M.C., *et al.* (2009) Oral mucosal conditions in chronic hepatitis C in Brazilian patients: a cross-sectional study. *Journal of Public Health in Dentistry*, **69**, 168–175.

Guggenheimer, J., Close, J.M., & Eghtesad, B. (2009) Sialadenosis in patients with advanced liver disease. *Head and Neck Pathology*, **3**, 100–105.

Guggenheimer, J., Eghtesad, B., & Stock, D.J. (2003) Dental management of the (solid) organ transplant patient. *Oral Surgery Oral Medicine Oral Pathology Oral Radiology and Endodontology*, **95**, 383–389.

Ho, V., Mclean, A., & Terry, S. (2008) Severe systemic lupus erythematosus induced by antiviral treatment for hepatitis C. *Journal Clinical Rheumatology*, **14**, 166–168.

Hughes, G.J., Patel, P., & Saxena, N. (2011) Effect of acetaminophen on International Normalized Ratio: clinician awareness and patient education. *Pharmacotherapy*, **31 (6)**, 591–597.

Jacobson, I.M., Gordon, S.C., Kowdley, K.V., *et al.* (2013) Sofosbuvir for hepatitis C genotype 2 or 3 in patients without treatment options. *New England Journal of Medicine*, **368**, 1867–1877.

Johnson, S.J. (2007) Opioid safety in patients with renal or hepatic dysfunction. Pain Treatment Topics. November 30, 2007. http://paincommunity.org/blog/wp-content/uploads/Opioids-Renal-Hepatic-Dysfunction.pdf [accessed on August 24, 2013].

Kuiken, C. & Simmonds, P. (2009) Nomenclature and numbering of the hepatitis C virus. *Methods in Molecular Biology*, **510**, 33–53.

Lindahl, K., Stahle, L., Bruchfeld, A. *et al.* (2005) High-dose ribavirin in combination with standard dose peginterferon for treatment of patients with chronic hepatitis C. *Hepatology*, **41**, 275–279.

Little, J.W., Falace, D.A., Miller, C.S. *et al.* (2008) Liver disease. In: J.W. Little, D.A. Falace, C.S. Miller, et al. (eds), *Dental Management of the Medically Compromised Patient*, 7th edn, pp. 140–161. Mosby Elsevier, St. Louis, MO.

Malinchoc, M., Kamath, P.S., Gordon, F.D. *et al.* (2000) A model to predict poor survival in patients undergoing transjugular intrahepatic portosystemic shunts. *Hepatology*, **31**, 864–871.

Mistry, N., Shapero, J., & Crawford, R.I. (2009) A review of adverse cutaneous drug reactions resulting from the use of interferon and ribavirin. *Canadian Journal of Gastroenterology*, **23**, 677–683.

Nagao, Y., Kawaguchi, T., Ide, T., *et al.* (2005) Exacerbation of oral erosive lichen planus by combination of interferon and ribavirin therapy for chronic hepatitis C. *International Journal of Molecular Medicine*, **15**, 237–241.

Ong, J.P. & Younossi, Z.M. (2004) Managing the hematologic side effects of antiviral therapy for chronic hepatitis C: anemia, neutropenia, and thrombocytopenia. *Cleveland Clinic Journal of Medicine*, **71 (3 Suppl.)**, S17–S21.

Oze, T., Hiramatsu, N., Kurashige, N., *et al.* (2006) Early decline of hemoglobin correlates with progression of ribavirin-induced hemolytic anemia during interferon plus ribavirin combination therapy in patients with chronic hepatitis C. *Journal of Gastroenterology*, **41**, 862–872.

Pamplona, M.C., Muñoz, M.M., & Pérez, M.C.S. (2011) Dental considerations in patients with liver disease. *Journal Clinical Experimental Dentistry*, **3 (2)**, e127–e134.

Pawlotsky, G.M. (2002) Use and interpretation of virological tests for hepatitis C. *Hepatology*, **36**, S65–S73.

Peck-Radosavljevic, M. (2000) Thrombocytopenia in liver disease. *Canadian Journal of Gastroenterology*, **13 (Suppl. D)**, 60D–66D.

Pincus, M.R. & Abraham, N.Z (2011). Interpreting laboratory results. In: R.A. McPherson & M.R. Pincus (eds). *Henry's Clinical Diagnosis and Management by Laboratory Methods*, 22nd ed, Chapter 8. Saunders Elsevier, Philadelphia, PA.

Pincus, M.R., Tierno, P., Fenelus, M., *et al.* (2011) Evaluation of liver function. In: R.A. McPherson & M.R. Pincus (eds). *Henry's Clinical Diagnosis and Management by Laboratory Methods*, 22nd ed, Chapter 21. Saunders Elsevier, Philadelphia, PA.

Pugh, R.N., Murray-Lyon, I.M., & Dawson, J.L. (1973) Transection of the oesophagus for bleeding oesophageal varices. *British Journal of Surgery*, **60**, 646–649.

Qamar, A.A. & Grace, N.D. (2009) Abnormal hematological indices in cirrhosis. *Canadian Journal of Gasteroenterology*, **23**, 441–445.

Radmand, R., Schilsky, M., Jakab, S. *et al.* (2013) Pre-liver transplant protocols in dentistry. *Oral Surgery, Oral Medicine, Oral Pathology, Oral Radiology*, **115**, 426–430.

Ryder, S.D. & Williams, R. (1994) Liver disease. *Postgraduate Medical Journal*, **70**, 162–184.

Shah, N.L., Northup, P.G., & Caldwell, S.H. (2013) Coagulation abnormalities in patients with liver disease. *UpToDate,* Topic 13932. Version 21.0.

Simmonds, P., Alberti, A., & Alter, H.J. (1994) A proposed system for the nomenclature of hepatitis C viral genotypes. *Hepatology*, **19**, 1321–1324.

Sloss, A. (2009) Prescribing in liver disease. *Australian Prescriber*, **32**, 32–35.

Smith, A.J., Cameron, S.O., Bagg, J., *et al.* (2001) Management of needlestick injuries in general dental practice. *British Dental Journal*, **190**, 645–650.

Smith, E. & Desmond, P. (2013) Prescribing in patients with abnormal liver function tests. *Australian Family Physician*, **42**, 30–33.

Strader, D.B., Wright, T., Thomas, D.L., *et al.* (2004) American Association for the Study of Liver Diseases. Diagnosis, management, and treatment of hepatitis C. *Hepatology*, **39 (4)**, 1147–1171.

Swain, M.G., Lai, M.Y., Shiffman, M.L. *et al.* (2010) A sustained virologic response is durable in patients with chronic hepatitis C treated with peginterferon alfa-2a and ribavirin. *Gastroenterology*, **139**, 1593–1601.

Tripodi, A., Chantarangkul, V., Primiganani, M. *et al.* (2007) The international normalized ratio calibrated for cirrhosis (INR(liver)) normalizes prothrombin time results for model for end-stage liver disease calculation. *Hepatology*, **46**, 520–527.

U.S. Public Health Service (2001) Updated U.S. Public Health Service guidelines for the management of occupational exposures to HBV, HCV, and HIV and recommendations for postexposure prophylaxis. *MMWR Recommendations and Reports*, **50 (RR-11)**, 1–52.

United Network for Organ Sharing (March, 2008) Questions and Answers for Transplant Candidates about MELD and PELD. www.unos.org/docs/MELD_PELD.pdf [accessed on July 16, 2014].

Vervloet, D. & Durham, S. (1998) ABC of allergies: adverse reactions to drugs. *British Medical Journal*, **316**, 1511–1514.

Wiesner, R., Edwards, E., Freeman, R., *et al.* (2003) Model for end-stage liver disease (MELD) and allocation of donor livers. *Gastroenterology*, **124 (1)**, 91–96.

Wilkins, T., Malcolm, J.K., Raina, D. *et al.* (2010) Hepatitis C: diagnosis and treatment. *American Family Physician*, **81**, 1351–1357.

Williford, S.K., Salisbury, P.L., Peacock, J.E. *et al.* (1989) The safety of dental extractions in patients with hematologic malignancies. *Journal of Clinical Oncology*, **7**, 798–802.

Zein, N.N. (2000) Clinical significance of hepatitis C virus genotypes. *Clinical Microbiological Reviews*, **13**, 223–235.

Zeuzem, S. (2004) Heterogeneous virologic response rates to interferon-based therapy in patients with chronic hepatitis C: who responds less well? *Annals of Internal Medicine*, **140**, 370–381.

Chapter 8

Diseases of the neurological system

A. Parkinson's disease	109
B. Multiple sclerosis	113
C. Seizures	116
References	123

A. Parkinson's disease

Clinical synopsis

Parkinson's disease (PD) is a chronic degenerative disease of the nervous system with loss of cells in the substantia nigra and the degeneration of the dopaminergic pathway (neurons that synthesize dopamine) resulting in decreased dopamine in the brain (Jenner et al. 2013). The usual age of onset is 50–70 years but rapidly increases over the age of 60 and only 4% of cases are under the age of 50. In addition, the incidence of PD varies by race and ethnicity (Van Den Eeden *et al.* 2003). Although the cause of PD is relatively unknown, there are most likely some environmental and genetic risk factors involved (Klein and Westenberger 2012). Early PD is diagnosed as a disease that is present less than 5 years or an individual who has not yet developed motor complications from levodopa. (Clarke and Moore 2003; Dickerson 2005).

The most common pathologic brain changes and the histological hallmark of PD is the presence of Lewy's bodies in the substantia nigra (Wakabayashi *et al.* 2007). Lewy's bodies are essentially abnormal aggregates of protein (alpha-synuclein) that develops inside nerve cells and are associated with nerve cell loss and serve as a marker for neuronal degeneration (Takahashi and Wakabayashi 2001; Wakabayashi *et al.* 2007). The four classic motor symptoms of Parkinsonism are resting tremor, muscle rigidity, bradykinesia, and postural instability (Jankovic 2008). A resting, nonessential tremor may be the first detectable sign/symptoms of PD; however, a majority of patients do not display a tremor until later in the disease process. The resting tremor presents as a fine "pill-rolling" movement of the hands. With movement, the tremor usually disappears. Muscle rigidity presents as stiffness with increased muscle tone making it difficult to move. Bradykinesia, the most noticeable of all symptoms, is a difficulty and slowness in initiating movement. Patient may have difficulty in chewing, swallowing, and speaking. They show an expressionless (stare) face. Postural instability presents as poor posture and imbalance, which may result in falls. Non-motors symptoms, some of which have

The Dentist's Quick Guide to Medical Conditions, First Edition. Mea A. Weinberg, Stuart L. Segelnick, Joseph S. Insler, with Samuel Kramer.
© 2015 John Wiley & Sons, Inc. Published 2015 by John Wiley & Sons, Inc.

implications in dentistry, include loss of smell, pain, sialorrhea, mood changes, sleep disturbances, excessive salivation, cognitive issues (e.g., memory loss, slow thinking, confusion, and speech impairment), bladder problems, pain, and orthostatic hypotension. Approximately 90% of individuals with PD will also develop dysphagia or swallowing disorders (Sapir *et al.* 2007). Dysphagia symptoms in PD include difficulty with lingual motility, reduced initiation of swallow, difficulty with bolus formation, delayed pharyngeal response, and decreased pharyngeal contraction.

Diagnostic lab values

PD is diagnosed strictly based on clinical features; there are no blood or other tests to diagnose PD.

Medications

Treatment for PD is currently focused on restoring (neuro-restorative) or preventing (neuroprotection) progressive nerve cell degeneration (Goetz 2013). Since the key feature in PD is loss of dopamine in the brain, replacement of the neurotransmitter dopamine is needed to treat the motor symptoms of PD. Dopamine cannot cross the blood–brain barrier; however, levodopa, the metabolic precursor of dopamine as well as epinephrine, can cross the blood–brain barrier and thus is the cornerstone medication of symptomatic therapy for early PD (Factor 2007). Since levodopa may be metabolized before it gets through the blood–brain barrier, it is combined with carbidopa (Sinemet), a decarboxylase inhibitor, which reduces the peripheral conversion of levodopa to dopamine allowing more levodopa to get through the blood–brain barrier. Carbidopa does not cross the blood–brain barrier (Salat and Tolosa 2013).

The addition of a catechol-*O*-methyltransferase inhibitor such as entacapone to the levodopa/carbidopa combination (Stalevo) will improve the bioavailability of levodopa and increase its transportation across the blood–brain barrier (Salat and Tolosa 2013).

While levodopa is used to improve motor symptoms, there are motor complications or dyskinesia resulting from its use. Dopamine agonists (e.g., Requip), which stimulate dopamine receptors, reduce dyskinesia and motor complications from L-dopa (Street and Stacy 2007).

In chronic, long-term use, plasma levels of levodopa are usually erratic with highs and lows due to its short half-life of 90 min or less. The concept of "wearing-off" occurs when symptoms appear again before the next dose of levopoda is given. This time may be difficult for the dentist to deal with dyskinesias. During "OFF" period dyskinesias, levodopa occurs in low concentrations. The key to treatment is to maintain levodopa concentrations during the "OFF" period (Giron and Koller 1996).

Dental drug–drug interactions

Table 8.1 lists the commonly encountered drug–drug interactions with PD.

Table 8.1 Dental drug–drug interactions.

Dental drugs	Management
Epinephrine + levodopa	Concurrent administration may increase the cardiac adverse effects (e.g., cardiac arrhythmias) of levodopa. Levodopa is actually a precursor to epinephrine
Erythromycin + levodopa/carbidopa/entacapone	Entacapone levels may increase due to biliary excretion altered. Use alternative antibiotic
General anesthetics (halothane) + levodopa	Cardiac arrhythmias

Dental notes

A medical consultation is recommended to acquire the stage of PD, the frequency of wearing-off and OFF periods the patient experiences, and if the patient has diminished cognitive ability. If the patient has a caregiver, dental care must be discussed with them. This information will help to schedule the best time of the day for a dental visit. Maintenance of oral health may be compromised due to tremors, muscle rigidity, and cognitive disorder. Recommend to schedule short appointments of about 1–2 h after the patient has taken their medication when their medication has reached peak blood levels (Friedlander *et al.* 2009). Schedule more frequent recare appointments. An electric toothbrush is a good recommendation. Some patients may be able to successfully use only one hand. Oral rinses are not recommended because of an increased chance for choking (Noble 2009).

The dentist should be aware of both motor and non-motor symptoms that may interfere with dental treatment. Most common obstacles when treating a patient with PD is difficulty in keeping their mouth open, involuntary head and tongue movements, and difficulties in wearing dentures due to either xerostomia or retention (www.toolkit.parkinson.org/content/dental-encounter). Table 9.2 reviews more dental implications of PD (Ford 2004–2005; Friedlander *et al.* 2009; Noble 2009). Table 8.2 lists the management of dentally related adverse effects of PD.

Table 8.2 Dental adverse effects of Parkinson's disease.

Dental-related effects of Parkinson's disease	Dental notes
Dyskinesia: difficulty and reduced muscle movement due to long-term use of levodopa. Jaw involvement and lips and mouth are also affected	Orobuccal dyskinesias and bruxism can hinder dental treatment. Bruxism is also an adverse effect of levodopa. Assist the patient on and off the dental chair. Interferes with oral home care procedures. The lower jaw moves up and down repetitively as they try to keep their mouth open.
Bradykinesia: difficulty and slowness in initiating movement. Expressionless "poker" face. Poor coordination of muscles of the tongue and throat	Makes dental treatment difficult. Cheek and lip control is problematic
Essential tremor: Pill-rolling movement of fingers	Pill-rolling tremor occurs as a circular movement with the index finger is in contact with the thumb. Oral hygiene practices may be difficult. Work with the patient's caregiver
Dystonia: dystonic spasms are painful sustained twisting movements and postures. Affects arms, legs, neck, face, tongue, jaw, and swallowing muscles	Later in the day appointments may be preferred when the dystonia occurs early in the morning which is relieved by physical activity and/or medication. Difficulty in restricting head and tongue movement. Some patients have lip and cheek muscles that are very strong and is difficult to work on these patients; consider local anesthesia to "turn of the muscles" when doing dental procedures. Inquire from the patient if they do have dystonia and when does it usually occur. Otherwise, early in the day appointments may be preferred

(continued)

Table 8.2 *(cont'd)*

Dental-related effects of Parkinson's disease	Dental notes
Akathisia: restlessness	Patient is unable to sit still which most likely will interfere with dental treatment. Make sure the patient is securely in the chair and will not fall off
Neck pain	This neck pain is mainly persistent. Ask the patient if they feel better while in the dental chair
Akinesia: unable to initiate muscle movement	Difficulty in retracting and gaining access into the oral cavity
Dysphagia: difficulty with tongue movement and reduced initiation of swallow. Impaired gag reflex	Use of bite block will help to keep mouth open. Should be cautious with aspiration because of slow swallowing. Aspiration or inhalation of oral bacteria may be a consequence. Having the dental chair at no more than a 45° angle will help the patient better in swallowing. May have difficulty with rubber dam placement
Sialorrhea: Excessive saliva resulting in drooling may be due to slowing of the involuntary swallowing movements	If severe, anticholinergics can be prescribed: benzatropinemesilate or trihexphenidyl hydrochloride However, these drugs also have many adverse and annoying adverse effects. Botulinum toxin has also been suggested (Merello 2008). Essentially, management of sialorrhea is difficult with no positive therapies
Xerostomia: from PD or medication	Increase water intake, fluoride application. Avoid alcohol-containing rinses (rinsing may be difficult for the patient). Monitor for dental caries, periodontal disease, and for problems with dentures
Orthostatic hypotension: levodopa lowers blood pressure	Supine position in dental chair is not recommended. Rather have the patient sit in a 45° angle (Friedlander *et al.* 2009). This position is also important for airway protection
Loss of balance (postural instability)	Hold the patient's arm when walking to the dental chair and when procedures are finished
Musculoskeletal pain	Pain in the hip, back, and neck will make dental treatment difficult
Hand contractures	Immobility of hands for an extended amount of time causes the development of band-like tendons, called contractures, to develop resulting in prolonged flexion of the hand. This makes oral home care difficult. Talk with the patient's care giver
Non-motor symptoms: depression and forgetfulness	Patients must be reminded to maintain oral hygiene care. Talk with their caregiver
Pain: can come from anywhere in the body including the teeth	Obtain physicians consult to determine the extent of pain
Loss of bladder control: from PD or medication	Have patient go to the restroom before dental treatment

Dental care (Ford 2004–2005)

- Use of electric tooth brush
- Topical stannous fluoride gel (at home and dental office)
- Oral rinses are NOT recommended since the patient may experience choking

B. Multiple sclerosis

Clinical synopsis

Multiple sclerosis (MS), myasthenia gravis, muscular dystrophy amyotrophic lateral sclerosis, and Huntington's disease are progressive degenerative neuromuscular diseases that can affect or alter dental treatment.

MS is a chronic, inflammatory, immune-mediated condition that results in generalized destruction of the myelin sheaths of the neurons in the spinal cord and the brain. The destroyed myelin sheaths are replaced by hardened, white plaques that interfere with normal transmission of nerve impulses. The etiology of the destruction is relatively unknown; however, genetic, autoimmunity, and possibly a virus may play a role. Symptoms of MS involve both motor and sensory tracts, depending on the area in the central nervous system (CNS) affected. These symptoms include irregular twitching of facial muscles (facial myokymia), abnormal sensations, spastic paralysis, muscle weakness in limbs (arms, hands, feet, legs), pain, fatigue, tremor, depression, speech disturbance, exaggerated reflexes, and visual disturbances (e.g., nystagmus and double vision), which are the most common early symptoms (Fiske *et al.* 2002). Trigeminal neuralgia is commonly presented as pulsating pain radiating along the trigeminal nerve presenting as facial pain. MS usually affects females more than males and usually in the 20–30 year age range. Patients can have MS for many years with few symptoms, while others have primary progressive MS and become disabled quickly; however, in the majority of cases, the disease follows a relapsing–remitting pattern, with short-term episodes of neurologic deficits that resolve completely or almost completely (Luzzio 2014). Table 8.3 lists dentally related effects of MS and its management (Chemaly *et al.* 2000).

MS is classified into different categories (Goldenberg 2012):

- Relapsing–remitting where the patient has flare-up and then periods of remission. After each flare-up, there is usually a new neurologic deficit. Most patients are in this category.
- Primary-progressive where the patient is continuously progressing without any periods of remission.
- Secondary-progressive where the patient gradually gets worse.
- Progressive–relapsing where there is disease progression with relapses that worsen from the beginning.

Diagnostic/lab values

The diagnosis of MS is based upon patient interview, clinical examination, radiographic and supplementary laboratory tests such as an magnetic resonance imaging (MRI) and lumbar puncture (Fischer *et al.* 2009).

Medications

The goal of therapy is to reduce relapse rate, prolong remission, reduce the onset of new MS lesions, and delay the progression of long-term disability (Tullman 2013). In progressive disease,

Table 8.3 Denta related effects of multiple sclerosis.

Orally related effects	Dental notes
Trigeminal neuralgia	Review history of neurological problems with the patient. Pain in trigeminal neuralgia may last anywhere from minutes to hours and is usually bilateral. Trigeminal neuralgia can be triggered by toothbrushing, chewing, or touching. Patient should be referred to physician (Scully and Schotts 2001; Reich and Campbell 2010)
Facial palsy (Bell's palsy, seen later on in disease) or facial myokymia (irregular twitching of facial muscles)	Difficulty in performing oral home care
Paresthesia of face or limbs	Difficulty in performing oral home care
Neuropathy of the mental nerve resulting in numbness of the lower lip and chin, with or without accompanying pain	Refer to physician
Clenching, bruxism/attrition due to muscle spasticity	Night guard
Xerostomia due to medications	Over-the-counter (OTC) salivary substitutes and dry mouth relief products (Reich and Campbell 2010)

it is the slow progression that drives most of the disability (http://www.medscape.com/viewarti cle/812373_2). High-dose intravenous corticosteroids are used to hasten acute MS exacerbations but they do not change the extent of recovery. Most patients have daily symptoms, and a combination of pharmacotherapy and nonpharmacologic therapies is used in the symptomatic treatment of MS. There are disease-modifying drugs that are FDA approved to reduce the relapse rate and delay disability (Tullman 2013). Table 8.4 lists the common medications used in MS with corresponding dental implications (Fox 2010; Tullman 2013). Medications are used to treat acute relapse and aggressive phases.

Dental notes

Table 8.5 reviews how to modify dental treatment for the patient with MS (Elemek and Almas 2013). Treatment alterations depend on the level of impairment and fatigue. It is preferred to have short and early morning appointments after the patient has taken the prescribed medications. Many patients may be wheel-chair bound. It is ideal to place patient in a semi-supine position due to problems with airway and gag flexes. Frequent suctioning is necessary. If the disease is stable and not progressing, routine dental treatment is provided; however, if the patient has more advanced and progressing disease, additional aids may be necessary such as a mouth prop or rubber bite block which can assist in keeping the patient's mouth open. Contending with tongue movements and swallowing problems can be difficult. Using a dental assistant can help with this. In-office fluoride application and antimicrobial rinsing (e.g., chlorhexidine) should be considered in the high caries risk patient.

Table 8.4   Medications for multiple sclerosis.

Drugs	Indications	Dental notes
Steroids Oral/IV methylprednisone (Solu-Medrol)	Accelerates recovery from an acute exacerbation	Adrenal atrophy, more prone to bacterial infections, diabetes, ulcers (avoid prescribing/ recommending NSAIDs). Consult with rheumatologist regarding dosing of steroid for long, invasive dental procedures
Wakefulness-promoting agents Modafinil (Provigil) Amantadine (Symmetrel)	Fatigue	Modafinil: serious rash, ulcers in mouth, difficulty swallowing and breathing Amantadine: xerostomia
Potassium channel blocker Dalfampridine (Ampyra)	Improve walking	Dizziness, upset stomach
Muscle relaxants Baclofen (Lioresal) Tizanidine (Zanaflex) Diazepam (Valium)	Spasticity (involuntary movements and contractions; muscle relaxant)	Dizziness, hypotension, fatigue
Immunosuppressants Azathioprine (Imuran) Methotrexate	Suppress T-lymphocytes	Anemia, neutropenia (more susceptible to bacterial infections), thrombocytopenia (increase incidence of bleeding). Obtain medical consultation and CBC values. Avoid NSAIDs. Oral effects include stomatitis, ulcers, gingivitis, candidiasis, herpes simplex infections, and parotid gland enlargement
Disease modifying drugs (DMDs) Beta interferons (IM, SC) Avonex, Rebif, Betaseron, and Extavia Glatiramer acetate (SC) Natalizumab (IV) Fingolimod (oral) Mitoxantrone (IV) Teriflunomide (oral) Dimethyl fumarate (oral)	Relapsing–remitting MS	Angular cheilitis, stomatitis, xerostomia, candidiasis, flu-like symptoms (interferon) and dysgeusia. Anemia, neutropenia and thrombocytopenia. Obtain CBC values

(continued)

Table 8.4   *(cont'd)*

Drugs	Indications	Dental notes
Pain relief drugs Gabapentin (Neurotin) Pregabalin (Lyrica) Carbamazepine (Tegretol) Phenytoin	Relief of pain due to trigeminal neuralgia	Phenytoin: Gingival enlargement Carbamazepine: neutropenia, thrombocytopenia. Avoid chronic use of acetaminophen with carbamazepine
Anticholinergics Oxybutynin (Ditropan)	Control of bladder function; bladder dysfunction occurs in more than 90% of MS patients (Goldenberg 2012)	Xerostomia: increased caries and periodontal risk

Table 8.5   Dental treatment modifications in the MS patient.

Dental procedure	Dental notes	Dental management
Periodontal/home care	Patient may have problems in performing adequate home care because of difficulties in swallowing, xerostomia, muscle spasticity (including tongue movements). This puts the MS patient in a high caries and periodontal risk category	May require a care giver at home to help. Electric devices may assist. Schedule frequent recare appointments (McGrother *et al.* 1999; Elemek and Almas 2013)
Prosthodontics	Due to muscle spasticity the patient may have trouble holding a full or partial denture in their mouth or in the worst case scenario even swallow the denture	When possible treatment plan for fixed prosthesis
Cariology	A significant relationship has been found between MS and the development of dental caries with a reported 21% increased incidence	Have patient placed on routine recare appointments

C.   Seizures

Clinical synopsis

Epilepsy is a relatively common CNS disorder characterized by the repeated occurrence of **seizures,** or the abnormal, excessive discharges of brain neurons and changes in the electrical activity in the brain. Convulsions or violent, involuntary contractions of the voluntary muscles may or may not occur with a seizure. If a seizure occurs, it is often intermittent and brief. Drooling and tongue biting are common symptoms.

Seizures may result from hypoxia (lack of oxygen), birth injury to the brain, fever, alcohol intoxication/ withdrawal, brain tumors, head trauma, or stroke. In some patients, epilepsy may be genetic.

The Commission of Classification and Terminology of the International League Against Epilepsy classifies seizures as (Commission on Classification and Terminology of the International League Against Epilepsy 1989) follows:

Partial (focal) seizures
- Simple partial seizure (no loss of consciousness)
- Complex partial seizure (impairment of consciousness)
- Secondarily generalized seizure

Generalized seizures
- Tonic–clonic seizures (most common type; formerly called grand mal; an aura or symptoms may appear before the seizure occurs; jerking of the extremities with loss of consciousness)
- Absence seizures (formerly called petit mal; occurs in young children and adolescents aged 2–12 years; many seizures a day with a momentary loss of consciousness with eye blinking and muscle jerks)
- Myoclonic seizures (sudden, short jerks or muscle contractions of the extremities that can occur at any age; associated with hereditary disorders)
- Clonic seizures (contraction and relaxation of muscles of the entire body)
- Tonic seizures (increased muscle tone; loss of bladder and bowel control)
- Atonic seizures (sudden loss of muscle tone similar to slumping to the ground)
- Febrile seizures (occurs in children and lasts for just a few minutes; the child has a fever)

Unclassified epileptic seizures
Status epilepticus (emergency situation characterized by continuous, prolonged seizures longer than 20 min)

Diagnostic tests/lab values (National Institute for Health and Clinical Excellence 2012)

- Electroencephalogram (EEG)
- Neuroimaging (MRI and computed tomography [CT])
- Neuropsychological assessment
- Other tests
  - Adults: blood tests (e.g., plasma electrolytes, glucose, and calcium)
  - Children: blood and urine biochemistry
  - 12 lead electrocardiogram (ECG)

Medications

Table 8.6 lists the drugs prescribed for epileptic seizures and Table 8.7 lists the common oral adverse effects of anti-epileptic drugs (AEDs).

Table 8.8 lists the potential dental drug interactions with AEDs (www.rxlist.com; www.epocrates.com)

During the intraoral examination, there are specific findings that should be noted in an epileptic patient. Box 8.1 reviews the common oral features and their management.

Dental notes

If the patient is poorly controlled, it is recommended to obtain a medical consultation. It has been documented that patients with poorly controlled epilepsy with frequent generalized tonic–clonic seizures exhibit poor oral health in comparison to patients that are well controlled and/or have seizures that do not involve the masticatory apparatus and in patients that do not have epilepsy

Table 8.6   Anti-epileptic drugs.

Type of seizure	Drug of choice	Alternative drug
Complex/partial seizures	Carbamazepine (Tegretol) Valproic acid (Depakene, Depakote) Phenytoin (Dilantin)	Phenobarbital (Luminal) Primidone (Mysoline) Gabapentin (Neurontin) Lamotrigine (Lamictal)
Generalized tonic–clonic (grand mal) seizures (most common form of seizure)	Carbamazepine (Tegretol) Phenytoin (Dilatin) Topiramate (Topamax) Levetiracetam (Keppa)	Phenobarbital (Luminal) Gabapentin (Neurontin) Lamotrigine (Lamictal)
Absence (petitmal) seizures	Ethosuximide (Zarontin)	Clonazepam (Clonopin) Valproic acid (Depakene, Depakote)
Febrile seizures in children	Phenobarbital (Luminal)	
Myoclonic seizures	Clonazepam (Klonopin)	
Status epilepticus	Lorazepam (Ativan) (IV)	

Table 8.7   Common oral adverse effects of AEDs (Aragon and Burneo 2007; Gurbuz 2011).

Anti-epileptic drugs	Common oral adverse effects
Phenytoin (Dilantin)	Gingival enlargement, delayed healing, gingival bleeding
Valproic acid (Depakote, Depakene)	Bone marrow suppression that can impair wound healing and increase postoperative bleeding (thrombocytopenia; decrease platelet aggregation) and infections, gingival enlargement, petechiae, xerostomia
Carbamazepine (Tegretol)	Agranulocytosis (severe low neutrophil count; delayed healing), aplastic anemia, xerostomia, gingival bleeding (thrombocytopenia), caries
Phenobarbital	Drowsiness. Xerostomia, stomatitis
Gabapentin (Neurontin)	Xerostomia, stomatitis (ulcerations in mouth), gingivitis, glossitis, orofacial edema, dysgeusia
Lamotrigine (Lamictal)	Stevens–Johnson syndrome (severe form of erythrema multiforme), cleft lip, and palate
Levetiracetam (Keppra)	Gingivitis, xerostomia, stomatitis, orofacial edema

(Karolyhazy *et al.* 2003). Involvement of the masticatory apparatus due to powerful contraction of the masticatory muscles includes attrition, abrasion, fractured teeth. In addition, there may be oral soft tissue injury including tongue and cheek biting (Karolyhazy *et al.* 2003). In addition, it has been reported that epileptic patients have more missing teeth and become edentulous earlier (Gurbuz 2011).

Table 8.8 Dental drug–antiepileptic drug interactions.

Drug	Dental drug	Management of interaction
Valproic acid/ valproate sodium	Aspirin, NSAIDs	Especially with high doses of aspirin or NSAIDs, increased bleeding due to antiplatelet effects; may increase valproic acid levels. Monitor effects
Valproic acid/ valproate sodium	Erythromycin	Combination may increase valproic acid levels. Use alternative drug such as azithromycin
Valproic acid/ valproate sodium	Clarithromycin (Zithromax)	Combination may increase valproic acid levels; avoid concurrent use. Use alternative drug such as azithromycin
Valproic acid/ valproate sodium	Lorazepam	Combination may increase lorazepam (a benzodiazepine) with risk of CNS depression. Avoid concurrent use
Valproic acid/ valproate sodium	Tricyclic antidepressants (sometimes prescribed for bruxism)	Combination may increase levels of antidepressant. Avoid concurrent use
Valproic acid/ valproate sodium	Alprazolam (Xanax)/ diazepam (Valium)	Combination may increase CNS depression due to additive effect; caution should be used
Valproic acid/ valproate sodium	Hydrocodone/ibuprofen	Combination with ibuprofen may increase risk of bleeding due to antiplatelet effect. May increase CNS depression. Caution with combination use
Valproic acid/ valproate sodium	Any opiates (codeine, hydrocodone, oxycodone)	May increase CNS depression due to additive effects; caution should be used
Carbamazepine	Azole antifungals (e.g., fluconazole)	Contraindicated. Do not use these two drugs concurrently. Combination may increase carbamazepine levels and decrease antifungal levels
Carbamazepine	Acetaminophen (alone or in combination with a narcotic including codeine, oxycodone, hydrocodone)	Combination may increase risk of acetaminophen liver toxicity; avoid using together
Carbamazepine	Ciprofloxacin (Cipro)	Combination may increase carbamazepine levels. Avoid using together
Carbamazepine	Erythromycin/ clarithromycin (Zithromax)	Combination may increase carbamazepine levels. Avoid using together. Use azithromycin
Carbamazepine	Tramadol (Ultram)	Combination may decrease tramadol levels and may alter seizure control. May increase CNS depression. Avoid using together
Carbamazepine	Diflunisal (Dolobid)	Combination may increase risk of syndrome of inappropriate antidiuretic hormone (SIADH); continued secretion of ADH causing hyponatremia; monitor for adverse effects or use alternative drug

(continued)

Table 8.8   *(cont'd)*

Drug	Dental drug	Management of interaction
Carbamazepine	NSAIDs (e.g., ibuprofen, naproxen, and naproxen sodium)	Combination may increase risk for SIADH; continued secretion of ADH resulting in hyponatremia. Monitor for adverse effects or use alternative drug
Gabapentin (Neurontin)	Acetaminophen/codeine and any narcotic combination including hydrocodone and oxycodone. Meperidine (Demerol)	Combination may increase CNS depression; caution is advised
Gabapentin (Neurontin)	Barbiturates	Combination may increase CNS depression due to additive effect; caution is advised
Gabapentin (Neurontin)	Benzodiazepine (e.g., alprazolam, and diazepam)	Combination may increase CNS depression due to additive effect; caution is advised
Gabapentin (Neurontin)	Naproxen	Combination may increase gabapentin levels; caution is advised
Gabapentin (Neurontin)	Tramadol (Ultram)	Combination may increase risk of CNS depression and uncontrolled seizures; caution is advised
Lamotrigine	Phenobarbital	Combination may decrease lamotrigine levels; caution is advised
Ethosuximide	Azole antifungals (e.g., fluconazole)	Concurrent use may increase ethosuximide levels; monitor levels or use alternative drug
Ethosuximide	Erythromycin/clarithromycin	Combination may increase ethosuximide levels; monitor levels or use alternative drug such as azithromcyin
Ethosuximide	All benzodiazepines	Concurrent use may increase risk of CNS depression; caution is advised
Ethosuximide	Ciprofloxacin	Combination may increase ethosuximide levels. Caution is advised
Ethosuximide	Narcotic (e.g., codeine, hydrocodone, and oxycodone) combination with NSAIDs. Tramadol	Concurrent use may increase risk of CNS depression; use with caution
Ethosuximide	Tricyclic antidepressant	Concurrent use may alter seizure control and increase CNS depression; caution is advised
Phenobarbital	Azole antifungals (e.g., fluconazole, and ketoconazole)	Caution advised. Do not use these two drugs concurrently. Combination decrease antifungal levels

Table 8.8　*(cont'd)*

Drug	Dental drug	Management of interaction
Phenobarbital	Acetaminophen (alone or in combination with a narcotic including codeine, oxycodone, hydrocodone)	Combination may increase risk of acetaminophen liver toxicity; avoid using together
Phenobarbital	Local anesthetics/local anesthetics with epinephrine bupivacaine, lidocaine, mepivacaine, procaine, articaine (with EPI)	AVOID combination; use alternative. Combination use may increase risk of methemoglobinemia
Phenobarbital	Topical anesthetic (benzocaine)	Contraindicated if <1 years of age; caution advised with everyone else. Risk of methemoglobinemia
Phenobarbital	Benzodiazepines (alprazolam, midazolam, triazolam)	Concurrent use may decrease benzodiazepine levels and/or may increase CNS depression; Caution is advised
Phenobarbital	Tramadol (Ultram)	Combination may decrease tramadol levels and may alter seizure control. May increase CNS depression. Avoid using together
Phenobarbital	Buspirone (Zyban: smoking cessation)	Caution advised; concurrent use may decrease buspirone levels
Phenobarbital	Narcotics (e.g., codeine, hydrocodone, oxycodone, and meperidine)	Combination use may cause additive CNS and respiratory depression; caution advised
Phenobarbital	Systemic corticosteroids	Caution advised: concurrent use may decrease corticosteroid levels
Phenobarbital	Doxycycline	Caution advised; concurrent use may decrease doxycycline levels
Phenobarbital	Metronidazole	Caution advised; concurrent use may decrease metronidazole levels

Box 8.1　Common Oral Features in the Epileptic Patients.

- Drug-induced gingival enlargement usually appears in the anterior labial area
  - Reinforce optimum oral hygiene
  - Review for possible periodontal surgical intervention
  - Speak with physician about prescribing an alternative drug
- Oral soft tissue lacerations: tongue, cheek, lip
  - Check for sharp edges on restorations/prosthesis
  - Recommend mouth guard
- Broken teeth

Patients who have not had a seizure in years, whether taking medications or not, and do not have masticatory involvement are considered to have low dental risk factors and can be dentally treated the same as a patient without epilepsy. Patients who show hard and soft oral tissue injury may require adjustments in treatment. For example, if there are signs of attrition or abrasion, it is best to avoid ceramic or composite resin materials and to fabricate fixed prosthesis rather than removable, which can be displaced during a seizure (Karolyhazy et al. 2003). In these patients it is acceptable to place implants (Cune et al. 2009).

Patients taking carbamazepine must have regular blood tests to monitor bone marrow problems (e.g., agranulocytosis and thrombocytopenia). Monitor gingival enlargement in patients taking phenytoin and valproic acid.

Administration of local anesthetics (e.g., intravascular injection or overdose) is a frequent cause of a seizure. Nitrous oxide/oxygen can be administered. Moderate sedation or general anesthesia is another option.

The patient may be most comfortable if placed in a supine position in the dental chair, and make sure that all instruments and other objects are away from the patient if they should have a seizure.

Questions to ask the patient (Karolyhazy et al. 2003)

1. When did the last seizure occur?
2. What precipitates your seizures?
3. Do you know or feel when will you get a seizure?
4. Did you acquire any oral cavity injuries previously due to seizure?
5. What medications you take and how routinely you take your medications?
6. Have seizures affected your mastication and parafunctional habits (e.g., bruxism, clenching, abrasion, and attrition)?
7. How frequently do you take oral home care?
8. How frequently you visit the dentist?

Table 8.9 reviews the different dental problems that can occur in patients with epilepsy (Karolyhazy et al. 2003; Aragon and Burneo 2007).

Table 8.9   Dental concerns in the epileptic patient and their management.

Dental concern	Dental notes
Periodontal	Monitor for gingivitis and stomatitis (due to medications); soft and hard tissue injury
Prosthetics	Patients that have frequent (more than once a year) generalized tonic–clonic seizures may have more frequent injury to the masticatory apparatus and should not have ceramic/porcelain restorations. Fixed prostheses are preferred over removable appliances. Recommend a night guard. If removal dentures are prescribed, precision attachments is recommended to resist dislodgement during a seizure. For complete dentures, metal palates instead of acrylic or metal mesh embedded into acrylic palate are recommended
Operative/restorative	Monitor for dental caries (due to medication-induced xerostomia). Patients that show tooth abrasion or attrition may not be suitable for ceramic or composite resin restorations. Use of a rubber dam is helpful

References

Aragon, C.E. & Burneo, J.G. (2007) Understanding the patient with epilepsy and seizures in the dental practice. *Journal of the California Dental Association*, **73**, 71–76.

Chemaly, D., Lefrançois, A., & Pérusse, R. (2000) Oral and maxillofacial manifestations of multiple sclerosis. *Journal of the Canadian Dental Association*, **66**, 600–605.

Clarke, C.E. (203) Parkinson's disease. *Clinical Evidence*, **10**, 1582–1598.

Commission on Classification and Terminology of the International League Against Epilepsy (1989). Proposal for revised classification of epilepsies and epileptic syndromes. *Epilepsia*, **30 (4)**, 389–399.

Cune, M.S., Strooker, H., van der Reijden, W.A., de Putter, C., Laine, M.L., Verhoeven, J.W. (2009) Dental implants in persons with severe epilepsy and multiple disabilities: a long-term retrospective study.. *International Journal of Oral & Maxillofacial Implants*, **24 (3)**, 534–540.

Dickerson, L.M. (2005) Treatment of early Parkinson's disease. *American Family Physician*, **72**, 497–500.

Elemek, E. & Almas, K. (2013) Multiple sclerosis and oral health: an update. *New York State Dental Journal*, **79**, 16–21.

Factor, S. (2007) Levodopa. In: R. Pahwa & K.E. Lyons (eds). *Handbook of Parkinson's Disease*, 4th ed, pp.309–334. Informa Healthcare, New York.

Fischer, D.J., Epstein, J.B., & Klasser, G. (2009) Multiple sclerosis: an update for oral health care providers. *Oral Surgery Oral Medicine Oral Pathology Oral Radiology Endodontology*, **108 (3)**, 318–327.

Fiske, J., Griffiths, J., & Thompson, S. (2002) Multiple sclerosis and oral care. *Dental Update*, **29 (6)**, 273–283.

Ford, B. (2004-2005) Pain in Parkinson's disease. *Parkinson's Disease Foundation Newsletter, Winter* **2004-2005**.

Fox, E.J. (2010) Emerging oral agents for multiple sclerosis. *American Journal of Managed Care*, **16 (8 Suppl.)**, S219–S226.

Friedlander, A.H., Mahler, M., Norman, K.M. *et al.* (2009) Parkinson disease: systemic and orofacial manifestations, medical and dental management. *Journal of the American Dental Association*, **140**, 658–669.

Giron, L.T. Jr & Koller, W.C. (1996) Methods of managing levodopa-induced dyskinesias. *Drug Safety*, **14 (6)**, 365–374.

Goetz, C.G. (2013) Third World Parkinson Abstracts. *Medical therapy. Journal of Parkinson's Disease*, **3**, 3–240.

Goldenberg, M.M. (2012) Multiple sclerosis review. *Pharmacy and Therapeutics*, **37**, 175–184.

Gurbuz, T. (2011). Epilepsy and Oral Health, Novel Aspects on Epilepsy, Prof. Humberto Foyaca-Sibat (ed), ISBN: 978-953-307-678-2, InTech. http://www.intechopen.com/books/novel-aspects-on-epilepsy/epilepsy-and-oral-health [accessed on July 30, 2014].

Jankovic, J. (2008) Parkinson's disease: clinical features and diagnosis. *Journal of Neurology, Neurosurgery and Psychiatry*, **79 (4)**, 368–376.

Jenner, P., Morris, H.R., Robbins, T.W. *et al.* (2013) Parkinson's disease – the debate on the clinical phenomenology, aetiology, pathology and pathogenesis. *Journal of Parkinson's Disease*, **3**, 1–11.

Karolyhazy, K., Kovacs, E., Kivovics, P. *et al.* (2003) Dental status and oral health of patients with epilepsy: an epidemiologic study. *Epilepsia*, **44**, 1103–1108.

Klein, C. & Westenberger, A. (2012) Genetics of Parkinson's disease. *Cold Spring Harbor Perspectives in Medicine*, **2**, 1–16.

Luzzio, C. (2014) Multiple sclerosis. http://emedicine.medscape.com/article/1146199-overview#aw2aab6b2b2. Last updated: January 21, 2014 [accessed 28 January 2014].

McGrother, C.W., Dugmore, C., Phillips, M.J. *et al.* (1999) Multiple sclerosis, dental caries and fillings: a case-control study. *British Dental Journal*, **187**, 261–264.

Merello, M. (2008) Sialorrhoea and drooling in patients with Parkinson's disease: epidemiology and management. *Drugs & Aging*, **25**, 1007–1019.

National Institute for Health and Clinical Excellence (NICE) (2012) The epilepsies: the diagnosis and management of the epilepsies in adults and children in primary and secondary care. NICE, London UK. p. 117 (Clinical guideline; no. 137).

Noble, J.M. (2009) Dental health and Parkinson's disease. *Parkinson's Disease Foundation Newsletter*, Winter 2009.

Reich, M.J. & Campbell, P.R. (2010) The oral implications of MS. *Dimensions of Dental Hygiene*, **8** (1), 52–55.

Salat, D. & Tolosa, E. (2013) Levodopa in the treatment of Parkinson's disease: current status and new developments. *Journal of Parkinson's Disease*, **3**, 255–269.

Sapir, S., Ramig, L.O., & Fox, C. (2007) *Dopamine agonists*, 4th ed. R. Pahwa & K.E. Lyons, K.E. (eds). pp. 335–348. Informa Healthcare, New York.

Scully, C.C. & Shotts, R. (2001) The mouth in neurological disorders. *Practitioner*, **254**, 539,542–546, 548–549.

Street, V. & Stacy, M. (2007) Voice, speech, and swallowing disorders. In: R. Pahwa & K.E. Lyons, K.E. (eds). *Handbook of Parkinson's Disease*, 4th ed. pp. 451–474. Informa Healthcare, New York.

Takahashi, H. & Wakabayashi, K. (2001) The cellular pathology of Parkinson's disease. *Neuropathology*, **21**, 315–322.

Tullman, M.J. (2013) A review of current and emerging therapeutic strategies in multiple sclerosis. *The American Journal of Managed Care*, **19** (2 **Suppl.**), S21–S27.

Van Den Eeden, S.K., Tanner, C.M., Bernstein, A.L. *et al.* (2003) Incidence of Parkinson's disease: variation by age, gender, and race/ethnicity. *American Journal of Epidemiology*, **157**, 1015–1022.

Wakabayashi, K., Tanji, K., Mori, F., *et al.* (2007) The Lewy body in Parkinson's disease: molecules implicated in the formation and degradation of alpha-synuclein aggregates. *Neuropathology*, **27**, 494–506.

Chapter 9

Psychiatric disorders

Introduction	125
A. Antipsychotics	126
a. Typical antipsychotics	127
b. Atypical antipsychotics	128
c. Anticholinergic medications	128
B. Antidepressants	132
a. Monoamine oxidase inhibitors	133
b. Tricyclics and tetracyclics	134
c. Selective serotonin reuptake inhibitors	135
d. Selective serotonin norepinephrine reuptake inhibitors (SNRIs)	136
e. Others	136
f. Summary: Dental interactions and side effects	136
C. Mood stabilizers	138
a. Lithium	139
b. Valproic acid (Depakote)	140
c. Lamotrigine (Lamictal)	140
d. Carbamazepine (Tegretol)	141
e. Oxcarbazepine (Trileptal)	141
D. Alcohol and other drugs with addictive potential	142
a. Alcohol	142
b. Sedatives and hypnotics	143
c. Opioids	143
d. Cocaine	145
References	145

Introduction

Psychiatry is a unique and interesting field for many reasons. Take for instance the method of making a diagnosis. Unlike in every other field of medicine, the majority of diagnoses in psychiatry are made purely based on symptoms. There are no diagnostic blood tests or X-rays, and in many cases, patients with differing set of symptoms will fall under the same diagnostic category based on meeting criteria in the

The Dentist's Quick Guide to Medical Conditions, First Edition. Mea A. Weinberg, Stuart L. Segelnick, Joseph S. Insler, with Samuel Kramer.
© 2015 John Wiley & Sons, Inc. Published 2015 by John Wiley & Sons, Inc.

recently updated DSM 5 (Diagnostic and Statistical Manual of Mental Disorders (DSM) 5, a classification and diagnostic tool published by the American Psychiatric Association). This can pose a treatment quandary, as many have suggested that a diagnosis such as schizophrenia may actually be a heterogeneous disorder composed of several different conditions. A look at the history of the nomenclature in psychiatry will demonstrate that the names and applications of these medications frequently change and I would argue that this trend will continue in the future as new, more specific treatments emerge.

Since clinicians tend to organize medications based on their class name (e.g., antipsychotic) rather than by the disease they treat (e.g., schizophrenia), this will be done in this chapter; however, it must be kept in mind that there is no true antipsychotic, or mood stabilizer, or anything of the sort. These are names that were developed to both aid our conceptualization of these medications and promote their use in treating sick patients. While there is some correlation between the names of the medications and the symptoms they treat, the pharmacology and indications for treatment are far more complex than the names suggest. These names are vast oversimplifications of what the medications do. Additionally, a quick look at the history of the nomenclature in psychiatry will demonstrate that these classes and categorizations as well as the applications of these medications frequently change and will continue in the future as new, more specific treatments emerge.

A. Antipsychotics

Clinical synopsis

During the 1940s, researchers at Rhône-Poulenc, a French pharmaceutical company, discovered that phenothiazines, a class of chemicals well-known to the dyeing industry, could have medicinal value (López-Muñoz 2005). They were noted to have strong antiallergenic effects and categorized as antihistamines. Promethazine was among the phenothiazines discovered at this time, and in 1949, Dr. Henri-Marie Laborit, a French army surgeon who was investigating solutions for preventing postsurgical shock, started treating his patients with it. The prevailing theory at the time argued that shock, along with its accompanied hypotension, resulted from trauma such as surgery and could be mediated by an intense histaminic response (López-Muñoz 2005). Because promethazine worked as an antihistamine, Dr. Laborit saw this as an opportunity to prevent postsurgical shock, and he did so with reasonable success (López-Muñoz 2005). Interestingly, Dr. Laborit began to notice that his patients were much calmer after receiving promethazine. This observation was also noted by others, leading to its use in anesthesia, and ultimately in psychiatry (López-Muñoz 2005). In 1950, after some modifications, the researchers at Rhône-Poulenc developed chlorpromazine, the first antipsychotic and the medication that would become the driving force in the deinstitutionalization phase of the United States of America (Yohanna 2013).

Early clinicians described chlorpromazine as a revolutionary medicine in the field, likening it with penicillin (López-Muñoz 2005). It was categorized as a "pharmacological lobotomy" for its ability to produce calming effects in agitated patients without simply sedating them and was responsible for the release of thousands of chronically mentally ill and presumed untreatable psychiatric patients from long-term psychiatric hospitals (López-Muñoz 2005). The success of chlorpromazine led to the investigation of other antipsychotic agents. Most notably, in the late 1950s, haloperidol was developed, and then three decades later, the atypical antipsychotics emerged. Interestingly, with the exception of clozapine, the newer medications are not accepted to be any more effective than the older ones (Sadock *et al.* 2007). Therefore, prescribing practices are generally driven on a case-by-case basis with particular emphasis placed on both previous patient experience and potential adverse side effects.

As a result, clinicians are faced with the responsibility of becoming quite familiar with the pharmacology, laboratory monitoring, and drug interactions of these medications. Because there are many comparably effective choices, there is increased opportunity and thus an increased duty to find an agent that is appropriate and safe.

Antipsychotics are commonly classified into two main categories: typical and atypical. The typical antipsychotics, also known as the first-generation antipsychotics, work differently than the newer, atypical agents, and as a result they each carry with them a vastly different side effect profile. Whereas the older, typical agents are more likely to cause extrapyramidal symptoms (EPS) such as tardive dyskinesia (a repetitive, involuntary muscle tremor), and parkinsonism, the newer agents are much more likely to cause metabolic side effects such as weight gain and exacerbation of diabetes (American Psychiatric Association 2006; Sadock *et al.* 2007; Stahl 2008). It appears that our society has made the determination that the metabolic side effects are preferable, or at least this is what our prescribing practices would argue. Since the introduction of the atypical agents, their use has increased exponentially. In fact, in 2013, the highest grossing medication in USA was aripiprazole (Abilify), an atypical antipsychotic medication (Lowes 2013).

Mechanisms of psychosis and schizophrenia

Schizophrenia is a complex illness that can present in vastly different ways. In deconstructing the illness, clinicians will often divide it into positive and negative symptoms, the former being more easily treatable and the latter more functionally debilitating and resistant to pharmacological treatment (Grant and Beck 2009). Delusions and hallucinations are examples of positive symptoms, and there is evidence to support that the manifestation of positive psychotic symptoms occurs secondary to increased dopaminergic activity in the mesolimbic pathway of the brain (Stahl 2008). Thus, treatment of psychosis generally involves medications that target this pathway and dopamine hypersensitivity. It should be noted that there are several dopaminergic pathways in the brain and that the effects of these antipsychotic medications are not specific to one area. Thus, when medications that decrease dopaminergic activity are given, they exert this effect not only at the mesolimbic areas but also in the mesocortical, nigrostriatal, and tuberoinfundibular pathways as well, and by these mechanisms lead to many unwanted side effects (Stahl 2008).

a. Typical antipsychotics

Table 9.1 lists the most commonly prescribed typical antipsychotics and Table 9.2 lists the most commonly prescribed atypical antipsychotics. Typical antipsychotics are classified according to potency which further delineates expected side effects.

Table 9.1   Commonly prescribed typical antipsychotics.

Medication	Brand name	Potency
Chlorpromazine	Thorazine	Low
Fluphenazine	Prolixin	High
Haloperidol	Haldol	High
Loxapine	Loxitane	Medium
Perphenazine	Trilafon	Medium
Pimozide	Orap	High
Prochlorperazine	Compazine	High
Thiothixene	Navane	Medium
Thioridazine	Mellaril	Low
Trifluoperazine	Stelazine	High

Table 9.2   Commonly prescribed atypical antipsychotics (Cullen *et al.* 2008).

Medication (generic)	Brand name	FDA approved
Aripiprazole	Abilify	2002
Asenapine	Saphris	2009
Clozapine	Clozaril	1990
Iloperidone	Fanapt	2009
Lurasidone	Latuda	2010
Olanzapine	Zyprexa	1996
Olanzapine/fluoxetine	Symbyax	2009
Paliperidone	Invega	2006
Quetiapine	Seroquel	1997
Risperidone	Risperdal	1993
Ziprasidone	Geodon	2001

Looking further at the pharmacological properties of typical antipsychotics, all involve blockade at the dopamine-2 (D2) receptor (Stahl 2008). As previously noted, this is what gives the medications their ability to block psychotic symptoms and also explains the etiology of some of their side effects. A closer look at the pharmacodynamics of these medications shows that they act not only on the D2 receptor but also on several other receptors. These receptors, which include the muscarinic cholinergic receptor, histamine-1 receptor, and alpha-1 receptor, give further insight into our understanding of these medications and their clinical impact.

To compare low and high potency agents, let us take a look at two of the most well-known typical antipsychotics today: chlorpromazine was the first one discovered, and haloperidol is perhaps the most widely recognized. Both have a high affinity for the D2 receptor, but chlorpromazine (unlike haloperidol) also has a high affinity for blocking the muscarinic cholinergic receptor as well as the histaminic and alpha-1 receptor. As a result, chlorpromazine is much more likely than haloperidol to cause sedation, dry mouth, blurry vision, and constipation (Sadock *et al.* 2007; Stahl 2008).

b.   *Atypical antipsychotics*

The atypical antipsychotics work via different pharmacodynamics. Most have some level of D2 receptor antagonism, but unlike the typical agents, many work as serotonin antagonists as well (Stahl 2008). This serotonin antagonism can lead to increased dopamine release in certain areas (such as the substantia nigra), and may be the mechanism responsible for the decreased EPS.

The atypical agents are not without concerning side effects. Atypical antipsychotics are classified according to their receptor (dopamine, serotonin, and histamine; alpha adrenergic; and muscarinic cholinergic)-binding profiles, which will dictate their potential to cause different adverse side effects. The major side effects seen in the atypical antipsychotics are weight gain, dyslipidemia, and the exacerbation or development of diabetes (American Psychiatric Association 2006; Sadock *et al.* 2007). Studies have shown that these changes can raise the risk of cardiac disease, and thus, in certain patients with risk factors, atypical antipsychotics can raise the risk of premature death (Stahl 2008).

c.   *Anticholinergic medications*

It has been proposed that dopamine inhibits the release of acetylcholine. Therefore, medications that block dopamine (antipsychotics), reduce this inhibition, and lead to increased acetylcholine activity.

This process has been implicated in the development of extrapyramidal side effects (Stahl 2008). Because of this proposed mechanism, extrapyramidal side effects are often treated with anticholinergic medications (American Psychiatric Association 2006; Sadock *et al.* 2007; Stahl 2008). Additionally, it should be noted that antipsychotic medications with a built-in high affinity for the muscarinic cholinergic receptor, such as chlorpromazine, are less likely to cause EPS compared to those that have a low affinity for the receptor, such as haloperidol (Stahl 2008).

As a result, it can be quite common to see dental patients with psychiatric illness who are prescribed anticholinergic medication. These include benztropine, trihexyphenidyl, and diphenhydramine. As previously discussed, these medications target the muscarinic cholinergic receptor; decrease the release of postsynaptic acetylcholine; and lead to side effects like dry mouth, blurry vision, and sedation (Stahl 2008).

Drug interactions and adverse side effects

The interactions and side effects portions of this chapter are perhaps the most important, as this is where the practice of dentistry and psychiatry have the greatest overlap. By developing a good understanding of the concerning aspects of psychotropic medications and the exacerbation or potentiation that commonly used dentistry medications can lead to, we can decrease the likelihood of iatrogenic complications and improve patient care.

It has been reported that medications used in the treatment of schizophrenia are significantly more likely to be associated with adverse drug interactions when compared with other types of medications (Sun *et al.* 3013). This further supports the importance of familiarizing oneself with these medications. There are several adverse side effects and drug interactions involving antipsychotic medications, and the next section will serve to elucidate those that are clinically relevant.

Neuromuscular side effects and oral hygiene

Extrapyramidal symptoms, which include parkinsonism and tardive dyskinesia, refer to tremors that result from the use of any antipsychotic medications (American Psychiatric Association 2006; Sadock *et al.* 2007). This disruption in neuromuscular control can make life quite challenging for patients and can even contribute to poor dental health (Tani *et al.* 2012). When antipsychotic medications lead to tremors, this not only interferes with patients' ability to brush their teeth but it has also been found to be associated with an increased risk of caries (Tani *et al.* 2012).

Other mechanisms of increased periodontal disease among patients with schizophrenia include fewer dental office visits (Tani *et al.* 2012) and dry mouth or xerostomia as a result of antipsychotic use (Eltas *et al.* 2013). Anticholinergic medications carry a significant risk of xerostomia as well, which if left untreated can lead to dental and root caries, candidiasis, and many other complications (Keene *et al.* 2003).

Cigarette smoking, which is seen in well over half of the patients with schizophrenia, is also a major factor in the increased incidence of periodontal disease (Eltas *et al.* 2013). Interestingly, it is also one of the most relevant inducers of cytochrome P450, which will be discussed below.

Cytochrome P450 enzymes

Most antipsychotic medications are metabolized via the enzymes of the hepatic cytochrome P450 system (Sandson *et al.* 2005). Therefore, caution must be used when taken with other medications that either induce or inhibit this system (Sandson *et al.* 2005).

Ketoconazole, itraconazole, and fluconazole are all antifungals that may be used in dentistry, and it should be noted that they each have the potential to increase plasma levels of some antipsychotic medication through their inhibition of cytochrome P450 (Guo *et al.* 2012; Mahatthanatrakul *et al.* 2012; Llerena *et al.* 2013). Changes in plasma levels can put a patient at increased risk of relapse, or increased risk of an adverse drug reaction, and so awareness of this impact is important (Llerena *et al.* 2013). Additionally, I would argue that it is important to communicate with the treating psychiatrist when such a medication is started so that the appropriate dose correction can be implemented.

Ciprofloxacin, a fluoroquinolone antibiotic, also leads to increased plasma levels of antipsychotics through inhibition of the cytochrome P450 (Brouwers *et al.* 2009). This can be quite relevant clinically. When taken concomitantly with clozapine, for example, significantly elevated clozapine levels have been reported, along with severe adverse effects (Brouwers *et al.* 2009). Fluoroquinolones have additionally been reported to lead to neuropsychiatric sequelae in both healthy and susceptible individuals (Tomé and Filipe 2011). This is quite rare, but nevertheless clinicians should be aware when considering their prescribing options.

Macrolide antibiotics such as clarithromycin and erythromycin also act as inhibitors of the cytochrome P450 system and have been reported to induce dangerously high levels of clozapine when taken together (Von rosensteil and Adam 1995; Cohen *et al.* 1996).

There are other medications commonly used in dentistry that may contribute to alterations in plasma levels. It is recommended that the clinician always evaluate for drug–drug interactions prior to prescribing a new agent. Even cigarettes, for example, can profoundly change the plasma levels of certain medications. Clozapine is metabolized via CYP1A2, and thus, patients who are smokers will have reduced clozapine plasma levels. Should they stop smoking, particularly if it is done abruptly, it can lead to vastly increased plasma levels and put them at increased risk of an adverse event such as seizures or even agranulocytosis (American Psychiatric Association 2006). Generally, it is recommended that if a patient is interested in smoking cessation, the dentist should communicate with the psychiatrist so that the clozapine dose can be properly decreased in order to maintain a therapeutic and safe level.

Agranulocytosis

Agranulocytosis is a rare condition referring to a significant reduction in or absence of granulocytes that can lead to neutropenia and put patients at risk for life-threatening infections (Sadock *et al.* 2007). While there are many mechanisms that can contribute to agranulocytosis, most cases are associated with medication use (Kaufman *et al.* 1996). In psychiatry, the highest risk is seen with the atypical antipsychotic clozapine (American Psychiatric Association 2006; Sadock *et al.* 2007).

Clozapine is unique among the antipsychotics for many reasons. It is not thought to cause EPS, and some have even argued that it can ameliorate symptoms in patients already suffering from EPS (Shapleske *et al.* 1996). It is also considered the most effective antipsychotic available when it comes to treating symptoms of schizophrenia (American Psychiatric Association 2006). Most patients with schizophrenia never take it, however, due to its increased risk of life-threatening side effects. This includes seizures (2%), agranulocytosis (0.5–1%), and, in rare instances, myocarditis and cardiomyopathy (American Psychiatric Association 2006). While there is a dose-related association with seizures that clinicians must recognize, it is the risk of agranulocytosis that prompted a standardized titration process to maintain patient safety (American Psychiatric Association 2006). To reduce the risk of adverse events, it is recommended to titrate very slowly. This is regulated by the Clozapine Registry, a database created to ensure that clinicians monitor patients appropriately while prescribing clozapine (American Psychiatric Association 2006).

The risk of agranulocytosis is particularly high during the beginning of treatment, which is why weekly blood monitoring is required for all patients taking it during the first 6 months of treatment (American Psychiatric Association 2006). While weekly blood draws can obviously be a nuisance, they are absolutely necessary, and there is strong evidence to support their use. There has been a significant decline in clozapine-associated agranulocytosis as well as clozapine-associated fatalities following the implementation of the monitoring system (American Psychiatric Association 2006). Psychiatrists are quite familiar with this practice and the importance of understanding the risks of clozapine, but it is equally as important that dentists and other clinicians are aware in order to minimize the risk of agranulocytosis, seizures, and other sequelae.

While dentists do not generally prescribe medications that can induce neutropenia, it is essential to be aware of the risk and to take the appropriate precautions if it turns out that someone is neutropenic. Nearly every dental procedure has the potential to increase a patient's exposure to pathogens, and so it is essential that immunocompromised patients not be unnecessarily put at risk. Furthermore, there are reported cases of medications used in dentistry (such as penicillin and naproxen) that have been connected with agranulocytosis, and so caution is advised as the literature depicts a cumulative risk when multiple offenders are taken concomitantly (Henderson and Borba 2001).

QT interval prolongation and Torsades de Pointes

Prolongation of the QT interval is a serious side effect associated with many medications. This includes all the antipsychotics, though some (such as ziprasidone) carry a greater risk than others. There is an established connection between QT prolongation and the risk of Torsades de Pointes, a potentially fatal arrhythmia. While some persons are born with a predisposition of developing this fatal arrhythmia, in the majority of cases, it is acquired through the use of certain medications (Cubeddu 2009). Because most cases are iatrogenic and preventable, this further places the burden on the clinician to ensure their patient is not unnecessarily or inappropriately exposed to a potentially lethal cocktail of medication.

There are several monitoring guidelines that are in place for psychiatrists to minimize the risk of Torsades de Pointes, but it is extremely important that all clinicians are aware of the risks and take the necessary precautions to minimize this adverse and often preventable outcome. While a host of variables including sex, and electrolytes, play a role in determining one's chance of developing Torsades de Pointes, it is the length of the QT interval that is the strongest marker and carries the most weight in predicting one's risk (Cebeddu 2009).

Because an increased heart rate will decrease the QT interval, the QTc, or rate-corrected value, is used when examining a patient's EKG (Cebeddu 2009). While there is no consensus regarding what value becomes concerning, there is literature supporting a decreased risk and lower level of concern in men with QTc values <450 ms and women with values <470 ms (Cebeddu 2009).

The astute dentist may be wondering at this point whether the previously listed medications that inhibit the metabolism of the antipsychotics, resulting in higher plasma levels, place patients at greater risk of Torsades de Pontes. In fact, this has been found to be true. Not only is there an increased risk of Torsades de Pointes in patients who take medications that inhibit the metabolism of antipsychotics but there is also an increased risk in patients who take more than one QT-prolonging medication (De Bruin *et al.* 2007; Cebeddu 2009). As it turns out, there are medications commonly used in dentistry that do both.

Macrolide antibiotics such as erythromycin and clarithromycin as well as fluoroquinolones such as ciprofloxacin inhibit the metabolism of antipsychotics and act as QT-prolonging drugs (Cebeddu 2009). Therefore, clinicians should be cautious when starting them in patients who are already on QT-prolonging medications such as antipsychotics. In fact, some clinicians advocate that patients should not be started on any QT-prolonging agent without first ruling out a history of Torsades de Pointes, checking an EKG, and making sure to correct any electrolyte disturbances such as hypokalemia (Cebeddu 2009). Other notable QT-prolonging drugs used in dentistry include chloral hydrate, azithromycin, and epinephrine (Karp and Moss 2006).

Weight gain and dyslipidemia and glucose abnormalities

While the typical antipsychotics are notorious for causing EPS, the atypical agents are more likely to lead to significant weight gain, poor glucose control, elevated cholesterol and/or triglycerides (American Psychiatric Association 2007; Sadock *et al.* 2007; Stahl 2008). Since there is a direct relationship between diabetes and periodontal disease, it is important for the dentist to be aware of these abnormalities.

Diagnostics/lab values

Lab testing is generally divided into baseline testing and routine monitoring after initiating treatment with medication. While the responsibility of the recommendations listed below falls on the psychiatrist, it is a good idea for the dentist to be familiar with these guidelines.

Baseline testing

According to the American Psychiatric Association (APA) Practice Guidelines, all patients should have their weight and BMI measured in addition to having vitals taken at their initial presentation. In addition, basic laboratory studies should be done and should include a complete blood count (CBC), a chemistry panel, a rapid plasma reagin (RPR) to rule out syphilis, screening for diabetes, and a lipid panel. Because antipsychotic medication can prolong the QTc interval and put patients at risk of Torsades de Pointes, many clinicians will get an EKG prior to initiating treatment. According the APA Guidelines, clinicians should check a baseline EKG prior to initiation of thioridazine, mesoridazine, and pimozide (American Psychiatric Association 2006). If there are cardiac risk factors present, then it is recommended to get an EKG at baseline prior to starting ziprasidone.

It is also recommended to do an assessment looking at symptoms of hyperprolactinemia as well as tardive dyskinesia and other signs of EPS (American Psychiatric Association 2006).

Routine monitoring

Patients on antipsychotic medication should be monitored regularly during their subsequent visits for signs of illness and side effects due to their medications. The APA Practice Guidelines state that BMI should be measured at each visit for the first 6 months and every 3 months after that. CBC monitoring is crucial for patients on clozapine and must be monitored weekly for the first 6 months and every other week after that (Sadock *et al.* 2007). The Clozapine National Registry ensures that these strict guidelines are followed in order to maintain patient safety. After 1 year of treatment without concerning lab values, a patient may be switched to monthly CBC draws according to the national monitoring guidelines (American Psychiatric Association 2006).

Blood chemistry is recommended annually, and monitoring for diabetes (either fasting blood sugar or HgA1C) should be done 4 months after starting an antipsychotic medication and yearly after that APA guidelines reference. Lipids should be checked at least every 5 years, and EKG should be rechecked periodically in patients taking antipsychotics.

B. Antidepressants

Clinical synopsis

On March 4th, 1984, an 18-year-old college student named Libby Zion was admitted to New York Hospital with flu-like symptoms (Asch and Parker 1988). She was initially given meperidine to treat her pain for what appeared to be a simple illness, but to her physician's surprise, Mrs. Zion's condition quickly deteriorated. She became agitated with unusual muscle twitches, and her temperature skyrocketed to nearly 108 degrees Fahrenheit. These symptoms ultimately led to her death, and shook the nation as a bitter fight ensued between her father and the hospital in one of the most important and influential medical cases in the history of American medicine. Her father's anger and persistence inspired an investigation into the organization of the contemporaneous hospital and medical education system, which led to major policy changes that remain to this day (Asch and Parker 1988; Boyer 2005).

As it turns out, Libby Zion had a history of depression, which was being treated with the medication known as phenelzine. Many (including her father) postulated that the meperidine induced a dangerous chemical reaction with the phenelzine, leading to toxic levels of serotonin and directly resulting her death (Boyer 2005). This story, as harrowing as it is, serves not only as valuable reminder of the dangers of medication interactions, but also of the responsibility that we as clinicians face when treating patients. "First do no harm" is nothing new, but when looking at the dearth of potential interactions that litter the field of dentistry, one realizes how challenging this proverb can be. At the risk of sounding redundant, I would like to reiterate the importance of knowing the clinically relevant medications interactions in dentistry, and hope this chapter serves as a guide to accomplishing this task and improving patient care. Though serotonin may be implicated in the death of Libby Zion, it is the neurotransmitter targeted by nearly all antidepressants and plays a critical role in the prevailing theory of depression (American Psychiatric Association 2006; Stahl 2008). Understanding the mechanism, and treatment of the illness is an essential tool for treating patients with depression, and avoiding iatrogenic complications.

Advances in the biological treatment of depression gained momentum shortly after World War II. It was during this time that researchers began talking of a chemical theory of depression. As is often the case in medicine the most significant advancement came quite serendipitously, when in 1952 one of the tuberculosis medications known as iproniazid was observed to have an energizing effect that could potentially be used to treat depression (Fangmann *et al.* 2008).

Iproniazid's therapeutic effect on mood was attributed to its action as a monoamine oxidase inhibitor (MAOI) (Fangmann *et al.* 2008). This discovery would pave the way to the monoamine theory of depression and the discovery and development of newer antidepressants to target the neurotransmission of the specific monoamines (serotonin, norepinephrine and dopamine). Proponents of this theory argued that depression results from low levels of these neurotransmitters and that by inhibiting their depletion, one could correct this imbalance (Stahl 2008). Our bodies naturally catalyze the oxidative deamination of monoamines via monoamine oxidase, and so if this process were to be inhibited by an MAOI, for example, this would lead to substantially higher levels of monoamines (Tipton *et al.* 2004).

It should be noted that the contemporary theory of depression is more complex and that the efficacy of antidepressants is generally attributed to neuroplastic changes that occur in response to increased amine levels via mechanisms such as receptor downregulation (Stahl 2008). Evidence in favor of this theory developed from the observation that monoamine levels rise quite quickly after starting an antidepressant, whereas symptom relief is not typically seen for several weeks (Stahl 2008). On the other hand, the side effects typically occur early in the course of treatment and can be directly attributed to changes in monoamine levels.

a. Monoamine oxidase inhibitors

Among the clinically available antidepressants, MAOIs were discovered first (as mentioned previously) when physicians noticed patients receiving iproniazid began to feel more energized. Other MAOIs quickly followed, and today there are several that may be used in clinical practice. They work by irreversibly inhibiting monoamine oxidase and thus preventing the breakdown of monoamines like serotonin, norepinephrine, and dopamine. Table 9.3 lists the currently available MAOIs and should be used for reference.

MAOIs are not commonly prescribed and are not considered first-line treatment due to the risk of life-threatening side effects (Sadock *et al.* 2007). Additionally, patients must follow a strict special diet

Table 9.3 Clinically available monoamine oxidase inhibitors.

Medication (generic)	Brand name
Phenelzine	Nardil
Isocarboxazid	Marplan
Tranylcypromine	Parnate
Selegiline	Eldepryl

while taking an MAOI. Because MAOIs inhibit the breakdown of the monoamine tyramine, foods rich in tyramine must be avoided to prevent a tyramine-induced hypertensive crisis. It is similarly advised that patients avoid other sympathomimetic amines like ephedrine, pseudoephedrine, and dextromethorphan when taking MAOIs (Sadock *et al.* 2007). Therefore, MAOIs are generally reserved for treatment-resistant cases or a particular type of depression known as atypical depression (Sadock *et al.* 2007).

Another life-threatening side effect that occurs with MAOIs is serotonin syndrome or serotonin toxicity, which is a potentially fatal event that occurs when one or more serotonergic medications lead to significantly dangerous increases in the level of serotonin in the central nervous system (CNS) (Volpi-abadie *et al.* 2013; Buckley *et al.* 2014). While nearly all antidepressants carry the risk of inducing serotonergic toxicity (particularly when combined with other serotonergic medications), the risk is greatest among the MAOIs (Güzelcan and Kleinpenning 2006; Buckley *et al.* 2014).

As a result of these risks, patients are advised not to start a tyramine-rich diet for at least 2 weeks after discontinuing an MAOI (Sadock *et al.* 2007). The same caution is advised with regards to changing from or to an MAOI. There is a 2-week washout period recommended when switching from an MAOI to another antidepressant (and vice versa) (American Psychiatric Association 2006). The exception to this rule applies to a switch from fluoxetine to an MAOI, where because of the long half-life a washout period of 5 weeks is recommended (American Psychiatric Association 2006).

Dental drug interactions: MAOIs

Although it may be controversial, current literature asserts that local anesthetics with epinephrine are not contraindicated with MAOIs and this interaction may have been slightly overestimated (Yagiela *et al.* 1985; Goulet *et al.* 1992; Yagiela 1999; Lambrecht *et al.* 2013). Remember, epinephrine is metabolized primarily by catechol-O-methyltransferase (COMT) and by reuptake into the neuron. Thus, while MAOIs can cause a slight cardiovascular effect when epinephrine is injected, the MAOIs are less effective in prolonging or potentiating the action of exogenous catecholamines such as epinephrine (Goulet *et al.* 1992).

b. Tricyclics and tetracyclics

The tricyclic and tetracyclic antidepressants came into use shortly after the MAOIs around the mid-1950s (Sadock *et al.* 2007). While their mechanism of action involves inhibition of the reuptake of both norepinephrine and serotonin, many of the adverse side effects can be attributed to their histaminergic, cholinergic, and alpha blockade (American Psychiatric Association 2006; Becker 2008). They are generally considered to be equally effective antidepressants compared with the other classes, though some patients may receive added benefit if chronic pain is also a significant symptom (Sadock *et al.* 2007). Amitriptyline is frequently prescribed to patients with nocturnal bruxism or facial pain. Like MAOIs, TCAs are not considered first line due to the substantial side-effect profile (Sadock *et al.* 2007).

Table 9.4 Common tricyclic antidepressants.

Medication (generic)	Brand name
Imipramine	Tofranil
Amitriptyline	Elavil
Trimipramine	Surmontil
Doxepin	Sinequan
Clomipramine	Anafranil
Desipramine	Norpramin
Nortriptyline	Aventyl, Pamelor
Protriptyline	Vivactil
Amoxapine	Asendin
Maprotiline	Ludiomil

The following are interactions of dental drugs with tricyclic antidepressants:

1. Epinephrine: Tricyclic antidepressants (TCAs), such as amitriptyline (Elavil) and clomipramine (Anafranil), work by inhibiting the reuptake of norepinephrine from the synapse by blocking the noradrenergic reuptake pump allowing more of norepinephrine to stay in the neuronal synapse. Injected epinephrine can be terminated by two ways: metabolized by COMT and neuronal reuptake by the noradrenergic reuptake pump, the same pump that takes up norepinephrine. Thus, if the pump is not removing epinephrine from the synapse, it will accumulate. The amount of epinephrine should be limited to two cartridges of 1:100,000 (Goulet *et al.* 1992). TCAs block the α-adrenergic receptors, which cause vasoconstriction in smooth muscles, allowing epinephrine to stimulate the β-adrenergic receptors causing vasodilation instead of vasoconstriction. This results in hypotension and tachycardia (Lambrecht *et al.* 2013). In addition, there is an increased risk of systemic toxicity with the epinephrine because the blood flow at the injection site increases allowing the local anesthetic to enter the circulation (Lambrecht *et al.* 2013).
2. Erythromycin or clarithromycin or ciprofloxacin: When taken with TCAs can cause increased serum levels of the TCA due to inhibition of its biotransformation by inhibiting CYP3A4 and CYP1A2 isoenyzmes. Adverse effects seen include excessive anticholinergic and $α_1$-adrenergic blocking activities causing xerostomia, constipation, increased intraocular pressure, tachycardia, dysrhythmias, confusion, and orthostatic hypotension (Wynn 1992; Lambrecht *et al.* 2013).
3. "Azole" antifungal agents [e.g., fluconazole (Diflucan)]: St. John's wort can reduce the effects of the antifungal drug (Lambrecht *et al.* 2013).
4. Erythromycin: St. John's wort, a nutraceutical, induces the biotransformation of erythromycin reducing its antibiotic effect (Lambrecht *et al.* 2013) (Table 9.4).

c. Selective serotonin reuptake inhibitors

Selective serotonin reuptake inhibitors (SSRIs) are widely considered the first line of treatment when it comes to treating depression due to their comparable efficacy with that of other antidepressants, while having a substantially safer side-effect profile (Sadock *et al.* 2007). They were first discovered in 1987 with the advent of fluoxetine (Prozac), and since then, they have become a staple in the treatment of various mental illnesses including anxiety and other disorders (Sadock *et al.* 2007). Table 9.5 lists available SSRIs.

Table 9.5 Currently available selective serotonin reuptake inhibitors.

Medication (generic)	Brand name
Fluoxetine	Prozac
Sertraline	Zoloft
Citalopram	Celexa
Escitalopram	Lexapro
Fluvoxamine	Luvox
Paroxetine	Paxil

Dental drug–SSRI interactions

One concern regarding SSRIs in dental practice is their ability to inhibit platelet aggregation by inhibiting the formation of thromboxane A_2, which could contribute to increased bleeding risk, including gastrointestinal bleeding. This risk is increased when taken with nonsteroidal anti-inflammatory drugs (NSAIDs), particularly in patients with peptic ulcer disease or other known bleeding risks (Becker 2008).

d. Selective serotonin norepinephrine reuptake inhibitors (SNRIs)

The SNRIs work to block the reuptake of serotonin and norepinephrine (like TCAs); however, unlike the TCAs, the SNRIs have relatively few side effects or serious interactions due to their more selective mechanism (Sadock *et al.* 2007; Becker 2008). The SNRIs include venlafaxine (Effexor), duloxetine (Cymbalta), and desvenlafaxine (Pristiq). Like the SSRIs, caution must be used in certain at-risk patients when combining SNRIs with NSAIDs, as both can inhibit platelet aggregation (Sadock *et al.* 2007).

e. Others

Bupropion (Wellbutrin) is an antidepressant that works by blocking the reuptake of dopamine and norepinephrine (Sadock *et al.* 2007). Bupropion is distinguished for its common use as an adjunctive treatment for depression in conjunction with other antidepressants, as well as its benign side-effect profile. Bupropion (Zyban) is also prescribed for smoking cessation with a starting dose of 150 mg daily for 3 days, and then the dose is increased to 150 mg twice a day for 7–12 weeks (Sadock *et al.* 2007).

f. Summary: Dental interactions and side effects

There are several serious interactions that the dentist must be mindful of when treating a patient on antidepressants. The severity can range from xerostomia and orthostatic hypotension, which may be seen in several of the antidepressants, to the life-threatening serotonin syndrome (Sadock *et al.* 2007).

Serotonin syndrome

As previously noted, serotonin syndrome (also commonly referred to as serotonin toxicity in the literature) is a potentially fatal condition resulting from increased serotonergic activity in the CNS following the administration of one or more serotonergic agents. It is notable for the role in the death of Libby Zion and should be viewed as an iatrogenic condition that can be avoided with an appropriate knowledge of pharmacologic interactions and good prescribing practices (Buckley *et al.* 2014).

Serotonin syndrome is characterized by altered mental status (confusion and agitation), neuromuscular changes (myoclonus and rigidity), and autonomic changes (fever, tachycardia, and diaphoresis) (American Psychiatric Association 2006; Sadock *et al.* 2007; Buckley *et al.* 2014). If it is not recognized and treated quickly, it can lead to severe complications and death (Buckley *et al.* 2014).

While it can occur in patients taking a single serotonergic medication, this is the exception and not the rule (American Psychiatric Association 2006). It is important to know which medication combinations can be problematic in order to avoid unnecessary risk. Patients on MAOIs have the highest risk, and extreme caution must be used prior to prescribing any medication where there is a concern for an interaction. This includes several pain medications (fentanyl, meperidine, and tramadol), decongestants, as well as others (Becker 2008; Buckely *et al.* 2014). The best course of action is to familiarize oneself with all the MAOIs (see Table 9.3) and check for interactions prior to starting any new medication.

For SSRIs, SNRIs, and TCAs, the risk of serotonin toxicity is less; however, there are reported cases when taken with certain pain medications such as tramadol, dextromethorphan, fentanyl, meperidine, and even oxycodone (Karunatilake and Buckley 2006; Sadock *et al.* 2007; Buckely *et al.* 2014). Caution is advised when prescribing any opioid analgesic, and patients should be educated on relevant symptoms. Some have noted morphine to carry a lower risk due to its nonserotonergic activity (Sadock *et al.* 2007; Rastogi *et al.* 2011).

Cytochrome P450

Many antidepressants inhibit the metabolism of other medications through the cytochrome P450 enzyme. Caution is advised when prescribing certain benzodiazepines (such as alprazolam, midazolam, and triazolam) concomitantly with the SSRIs fluvoxamine, paroxetine, and fluoxetine as this can lead to increased benzodiazepine plasma levels, due to inhibition via CYP3A4 (Sadock *et al.* 2007; Moffa Jr. 2010). Nefazodone (Serzone) is a strong inhibitor of CYP3A4, which can lead to increased levels of benzodiazepines as well (American Psychiatric Association 2006). A major interaction of nefazodone occurs with the macrolide antibiotics clarithromycin and erythromycin, and this practice should be avoided (Ray *et al.* 2004). When taken together, dangerously high levels of clarithromycin or erythromycin may result, putting the patient at risk for a fatal arrhythmia (Ray *et al.* 2004; American Psychiatric Association 2006).

The inhibition of the metabolism of certain pain medications can lead to reduced pain control in certain patients. For example, bupropion and certain SSRIs such as paroxetine, fluvoxamine, and fluoxetine will limit the effectiveness of opiates such as hydrocodone, oxycodone, and codeine by inhibiting their conversion to their active metabolites via CYP2D6 (Sadock *et al.* 2007; Becker 2008). An alternative treatment suggested by Becker is to give morphine in these cases (Becker 2008).

Plasma levels of antidepressants can similarly be affected by other medications. Toxic levels of citalopram (Celexa) have been reported due to fluconazole's inhibition via CYP2C19 (Levin *et al.* 2008). Fluvoxamine is metabolized via CYP3A4, and so inhibitors of the isoenzyme such as some of the macrolides and antifungals must be used with caution (Becker 2008). Because of the concern for dangerous interactions, it is generally good practice for the clinician to check prior to starting a medication that is known to significantly affect the cytochrome P450 system.

Cardiac risks

In the past, one major concern among dentists was the use of epinephrine or other sympathomimetic agents in patients on antidepressants such as MAOIs and TCAs. They theorized that the increased norepinephrine levels could increase the risk of cardiac complications, but though there may be some concerns, the risk generally appears to be more theoretical than clinically relevant (Yagiela 1999; Becker 2008). Nevertheless, Becker suggests using caution and rechecking vital signs often when using sympathomimetics in patients on TCAs (Becker 2008).

Another cardiac concern is illustrated by Cubeddu who notes that the TCAs and other "drugs with antidepressant properties may also prolong the QT interval; among them: desipramine, imipramine, doxepin" and others (Cubeddu 2009). While there have been studies implicating SSRIs as well, generally, the risk is thought to be greater and more clinically relevant with the TCAs (American Psychiatric Association 2006; Sadock *et al.* 2007; Alvarez and Pahissa 2010; Lam 2013).

TCAs act in a similar fashion to class IA antiarrhythmic medications like quinidine, and the cardiac risk is cumulative when combined with other antiarrhythmic agents (American Psychiatric Association 2006; Cubeddu 2009; Lam 2013). Therefore, starting another QT-prolonging agent such as erythromycin or clarithromycin in patients taking a TCA should be avoided, and if deemed medically necessary, it should only be done under close medical supervision (Yap and Camm 2004; American Psychiatric Association 2006; Cubeddu 2009; Alvarez and Pahissa 2010; Moffa 2010; Lam 2013).

Other risks and interactions

Tricyclics and tetracyclics as well as MAOIs can be sedating and lead to confusion with increasingly high doses. When combined with other CNS depressants, there is an increased risk of adverse events such as falls or altered mentation, particularly if substances such as alcohol or barbiturates are involved (Sadock *et al.* 2007).

Lab tests/monitoring

Most antidepressants do not require routine monitoring, though there are some exceptions. Because hypertension can occur in patients taking venlafaxine, it is generally recommended to monitor the blood pressure (Sadock *et al.* 2007).

TCAs are unique among the antidepressants in that it is recommended to get plasma levels during their use (Sadock *et al.* 2007). According to the APA Guidelines, EKG monitoring is recommended in patients taking TCAs, and a baseline EKG should be checked in patients with risk factors or in anyone over 50 years of age prior to initiating treatment (American Psychiatric Association 2006).

C. Mood stabilizers

In the late 1940s, while experimenting with the urine of manic patients and injecting it into guinea pigs, an Australian psychiatrist by the name of John Cade discovered the mood-stabilizing effects of lithium (Burrows and Tiller 1999). Patients who had been suffering with manic symptoms for years suddenly became more reserved within just a few days of treatment. Despite his success, because Dr. Cade was considered a nonentity with unpolished research techniques, lithium would not gain approval in the USA until 1970—more than 20 years after his first reported success (Burrows and Tiller 1999; Sadock *et al.* 2007).

While the efficacy of lithium was gaining importance, concerns about toxicity started to emerge. Cade began to notice that lithium was not nearly as safe as he had originally thought, and several of his patients ended up dying from toxicity (Burrows and Tiller 1999). As it turned out, the plasma levels required for successful treatment differed only slightly from those considered toxic levels, and so an individualized regimen was deemed necessary due to the low therapeutic index (Burrows and Tiller 1999; American Psychiatric Association 2006; Sadock *et al.* 2007).

Presently, there are several available treatments for bipolar disorder, but to this day, nothing has surpassed the efficacy of lithium (American Psychiatric Association 2006; Sadock *et al.* 2007). Fortunately, one thing that has changed is the ability and requirement to monitor and ensure the safety of patients who take lithium and other mood stabilizers.

a.   Lithium

Lithium is an effective treatment during the acute and maintenance stages of bipolar disorder, but due to its narrow therapeutic index, heavy side-effect profile, and significant drug–drug interactions, it must be used with great caution (American Psychiatric Association 2006; Sadock *et al.* 2007; Stahl 2008).

Interaction and side effects

It is quite common for patients taking lithium to experience adverse side effects. The APA Guidelines report that up to 75% of patients will develop side effects during lithium treatment. These include sedation, confusion, memory deficits, polyurina, polydipsia, tremors, gastrointestinal issues, xerostomia, and many others (American Psychiatric Association 2006; Sadock *et al.* 2007; Stahl 2008).

In addition to the minor adverse side effects, there are several major and potentially life-threatening side effects that can occur with lithium use. Because lithium is renally excreted, many of the major side effects result from anatomical and functional changes in the kidney. These include nephrogenic diabetes insipidus, chronic renal insufficiency, and even irreversible renal failure requiring hemodialysis. Typically, these changes are seen with either toxic levels or prolonged use (more than 10 years) (American Psychiatric Association 2006; Sadock *et al.* 2007; Stahl 2008). Other notable major side effects include hypothyroidism and cardiac conduction abnormalities, which can be particularly worrisome in patients with electrolyte abnormalities (American Psychiatric Association 2006; Sadock *et al.* 2007). While both the minor and the major side effects may occur with therapeutic drug levels, the risk is substantially greater with higher plasma levels and so it is essential to be familiar with medications that interfere with renal excretion (American Psychiatric Association 2006).

NSAIDs are a first-line treatment for pain and often prescribed or purchased without hesitation, but while aspirin may be taken safely in patients taking lithium, all other NSAIDs should be avoided as concomitant use can lead to a dangerous increase in lithium levels (Haas 1999; Sadock *et al.* 2007).

Metronidazole and tetracyclines have also been reported to decrease the excretion of lithium and place patients at risk for toxic levels (Teicher *et al.* 1987; Hersh 1999; Sadock *et al.* 2007). It is generally best to avoid these, but if one is started, it is extremely important to notify the psychiatrist so that the lithium levels can be appropriately monitored.

Lab tests/monitoring

Baseline testing: Because of the potential for adverse events, there are several guidelines recommended when prescribing lithium (American Psychiatric Association 2006). A medical history and physical exam should be performed and may be used to rule out preexisting kidney and thyroid disease. BUN, creatinine, thyroid function, and a pregnancy test should be given prior to initiating treatment, and in certain patients a CBC and/or an EKG as well (American Psychiatric Association 2006).

Routine monitoring: Patients on lithium should have their plasma levels and kidney function checked at least every 6 months and more frequently when first starting treatment (American Psychiatric Association 2006). Thyroid function should be monitored periodically as well. The APA Guidelines recommend that monitoring be done about every 6 months (American Psychiatric Association 2006).

b. Valproic acid (Depakote)

Valproic acid (or valproate) is an approved medication for the acute and maintenance treatment of patients with bipolar disorder (American Psychiatric Association 2006; Sadock *et al.* 2007).

Interaction and side effects

There are many concerning side effects that clinicians should be familiar with when treating patients with valproic acid. Hair loss, tremors, weight gain, and sedation can all be quite common (Sadock *et al.* 2007). The major side effects are less common but include hepatotoxicity, thrombocytopenia, and pancreatitis. Like lithium, and all other mood stabilizers, valproic acid is teratogenic and should be avoided during pregnancy (American Psychiatric Association 2006; Sadock *et al.* 2007).

Because of its tendency to cause sedation and somnolence, caution is advised when taking with other CNS depressants (Sadock *et al.* 2007). This concern is magnified with the coadministration of certain substrates due to valproic acid's significant inhibition of the cytochrome P450 system as well as its ability to disrupt protein binding (Sadock *et al.* 2007; Becker 2008). As a result, significantly elevated benzodiazepine levels have been reported with valproic acid use, and caution is advised when prescribing benzodiazepines concomitantly (Dhillon and Richens 1982; Perucca 2001, 2006; Becker 2008).

Clinicians should also be aware that certain medications might lead to clinically relevant increases in plasma levels of valproic acid. This has been reported with the use of macrolides like erythromycin, as well as with aspirin, (Von rosensteil and Adam 1995; Sandson *et al.* 2006; Becker 2008; Desai 2008).

Lab tests/monitoring

Baseline testing: Due to concerns of hepatotoxicity and thrombocytopenia, it is recommended that patients have a baseline CBC and liver function tests measured prior to initiating treatment (Sadock *et al.* 2007).

Routine monitoring: Because mild thrombocytopenia and mild elevation in liver enzymes do not reliably predict life-threatening conditions such as bone marrow suppression and hepatic failure, respectively, most experts stress the importance of educating patients on concerning symptoms in lieu of routine blood work (American Psychiatric Association 2006; Sadock *et al.* 2007). Still, it is common practice to monitor liver function and complete blood work around 6 month intervals (American Psychiatric Association 2006; Sadock *et al.* 2007).

c. Lamotrigine (Lamictal)

Lamotrigine is a mood stabilizer with good efficacy in treating bipolar depression (American Psychiatric Association 2006; Sadock *et al.* 2007).

Interactions and side effects

Compared with lithium and valproic acid, lamotrigine is better tolerated and has relatively few side effects (Sadock *et al.* 2007). There is no monitoring required, and while there are significant interactions that may occur with other psychotropic medications such as carbamazepine and valproic acid, there are relatively few concerns in dentistry (Sadock *et al.* 2007).

One potentially relevant interaction could occur in the setting of pain control. The use of acetaminophen may significantly decrease lamotrigine levels and lead to decreased efficacy (Becker 2008). This could be additionally problematic in theory should the patient suddenly stop the acetaminophen as this could lead to a faster titration of Lamictal, which has been associated with increased risk of Stevens–Johnson syndrome (American Psychiatric Association 2006; Sadock *et al.* 2007).

d. Carbamazepine (Tegretol)

Carbamazepine was approved by the FDA as a treatment for bipolar disorder in 2004 (Sadock *et al.* 2007). While there is literature supporting its efficacy, it is as not as well established as valproic acid and lithium, and so it is generally not considered a first-line choice (American Psychiatric Association 2006). Carbamazepine is also indicated for trigeminal neuralgia.

Interactions and side effects

Carbamazepine is notable for its significant interaction with other medications through the cytochrome P450 system. Significant decreases in plasma levels of acetaminophen, alprazolam, clonazepam, and doxycycline have all been reported when taken concomitantly with carbamazepine (Sadock *et al.* 2007). On the other hand, it may also experience clinically relevant metabolic disruptions (O'connor and Fris 1994). When taken with erythromycin, clarithromycin, ketoconazole, itraconazole, or propoxyphene, carbamazepine levels may be significantly increased, and there have been reports of severe toxicity (O'connor and Fris 1994; Von rosensteil and Adam 1995; Hersh 1999; Sadock *et al.* 2007; Becker 2008; Desai 2008). As a result, avoiding these agents is recommended, but if medically necessary, then an adjustment in the dose of carbamazepine may be indicated (O'connor and Fris 1994; Von rosensteil and Adam 1995).

Lab tests/monitoring

While not required, because there is a risk of blood dyscrasias, it is good practice to check blood periodically and monitor for signs and symptoms of aplastic anemia or agranulocytosis (American Psychiatric Association 2006; Sadock *et al.* 2007). Additionally, obtaining plasma levels may be of use at times due to variations in individual metabolism, as well as certain drug interactions (O'connor and Fris 1994).

e. Oxcarbazepine (Trileptal)

Oxcarbazepine is similar in structure to carbamazepine, but due to the lack of studies, the efficacy is not well established in bipolar disorder (American Psychiatric Association 2006; Sadock *et al.* 2007).

Interactions and side effects

While there is a lower risk of blood dyscrasias compared with that of carbamazepine, up to 5% of patients may develop hyponatremia (American Psychiatric Association 2006; Sadock *et al.* 2007).

Oxcarbazepine is metabolized by cytochrome P450, and can lead to decreased plasma levels of anticoagulants and birth control (like carbamazepine), as well as some benzodiazepines through CYP3A4 (Baruzzi *et al.* 1994; American Psychiatric Association 2006; Sadock *et al.* 2007). Unlike carbamazepine, when taken with erythromycin, there was not a clinically relevant alteration in metabolism (Baruzzi *et al.* 1994).

Lab tests/monitoring

Laboratory tests are not required, but due to the risk of hyponatremia and its sequelae, checking electrolytes early in treatment is recommended (Sadock *et al.* 2007).

D.   Alcohol and other drugs with addictive potential

Substance abuse and mental illness often go hand in hand, and it is always important to ask about substance use when evaluating and treating a dental patient. Substances such as methamphetamine and tobacco, for example, will contribute to significant periodontal disease, while others such as alcohol may interact with prescription medications.

a.   Alcohol

Alcohol is a CNS depressant, which can be problematic when taken with other sedating medications such as pain medications, antihistamines, muscle relaxants, or sedative/hypnotics (Fangmann *et al.* 2008). It also can affect the metabolism of other medications. In chronic users, for example, the liver changes at a cellular level, increasing the activity of CYP2E1 in order to better tolerate heavy drinking (Fangmann *et al.* 2008). This correlates with faster metabolism of certain chemicals like acetaminophen when sober, but when acutely intoxicated, there is a risk for acetaminophen (and other chemical) toxicity due to the competition for the same enzyme (Fangmann *et al.* 2008). As a result, caution is advised with the use of acetaminophen in patients with heavy alcohol use, particularly if there are signs of significant liver damage such as cirrhosis. It is extremely important to keep in mind that some medications (such as Percocet) contain acetaminophen and that this can accumulate and lead to toxicity (Fangmann *et al.* 2008). In patients with opioid dependence who may require higher doses of opioids to treat their pain, this risk could be even higher (Center for Substance Abuse Treatment 2004). Therefore, it is important to inform patients with alcohol dependence and/or liver damage about these concerns and to use acetaminophen sparingly if at all in this population.

There are several medications that may be prescribed by a physician (often a psychiatrist) to aid in patients who suffer from alcoholism. These medications include naltrexone, baclofen, acamprosate, and disulfiram to name a few. Disulfiram is of clinical significance as it, like metronidazole, inhibits the metabolism of alcohol causing a buildup of acetaldehyde. This buildup of acetaldehyde leads to an increase in the unpleasant side effects associated with alcohol and is the rationale for its treatment as an agent to curtail abuse (Fangmann *et al.* 2008). Because both disulfiram and metronidazole inhibit the metabolism of alcohol, this can lead to dangerous side effects (such as psychosis or confusion referred to as "disulfiram reaction") when used together, and this practice should be avoided (Rothstein and Clancy 1969). Similarly, it is important to warn patients about the dangers of drinking alcohol while taking metronidazole, and if there is a concern about heavy drinking, then an alternative agent is likely a better choice.

In addition to several drug–drug interactions, chronic alcohol use has been associated with moderately increased severity of periodontal diseases (Tezal *et al.* 2001). Moreover, an animal study suggests that the simultaneous use of alcohol and nicotine may have a synergistic effect in the progression of periodontitis (Pereira Vasconcelos *et al.* 2013).

b. Sedatives and hypnotics

Benzodiazepines are commonly prescribed in both psychiatry and dentistry. While there are many benefits of benzodiazepines, clinicians must exercise caution in order to minimize the risk of abuse, and adverse events. The risk of CNS and respiratory depression can be cumulative when mixed with other sedating agents such as alcohol and opioids (Moore 1999; Sadock *et al.* 2007). Additionally, certain medications such as macrolides and antifungals may substantially increase plasma levels through inhibition of CYP3A4, putting patients further at risk (Moore 1999). This has been observed to have clinical significance with midazolam, triazolam, and alprazolam, and so this practice should be avoided, particularly since there are alternative benzodiazepines (such as lorazepam) that may be used that are not subject to the same interaction (Von rosensteil and Adam 1995; Moore 1999; Becker 2008).

c. Opioids

The use of illicit opioids has steadily increased over the last 20 years and has become an increasingly common issue in dentistry. It is quite common for patients to complain of pain; however, many clinicians are uncomfortable prescribing pain medication to patients with a history of opioid dependence or any history of substance abuse (Alford *et al.* 2006). Moreover, research shows that patients with a physiological dependence on opioids develop hyperalgesia, or increased sensitivity to pain, and this can further complicate the issue of appropriate pain control (Pud *et al.* 2006).

Dentists must be cognizant of the fact that many patients take opioids daily as prescribed by their psychiatrists in what is referred to as maintenance therapy. This practice is supported by strong evidence showing improved outcomes among patients who are deemed appropriate candidates (Alford *et al.* 2006; Mattick *et al.* 2009). Maintenance therapy "decreases opioid and other drug abuse, increases treatment retention, decreases criminal activity, improves individual functioning, and decreases HIV seroconversion" (Alford *et al.* 2006). The maintenance therapies available include methadone, buprenorphine (the primary component of suboxone) and naltrexone. Both methadone and buprenorphine act as opioid agonists to keep cravings at bay, while naltrexone acts as an antagonist, blocking the effects of exogenous opioids.

It is extremely important to become familiar with the intricacies of opioid dependence, its treatment, and how it relates to pain control in the dental patient. There are many assumptions that clinicians make, and each has the potential to lead to poor care and poor pain control (Alford *et al.* 2006). Alford *et al.* breaks down the common "misconceptions" of healthcare workers regarding patients receiving pain maintenance and is a great read for a more in-depth understanding when it comes to reasonable and appropriate treatment (Alford *et al.* 2006). First and foremost, it is important to understand that while maintenance therapies provide good treatment for addiction, their ability to treat acute pain has serious limitations. The analgesic effects are quite short-lived (just a few hours after taking them) compared with their effects on opioid withdrawal (which lasts 24–48 h), and so someone on maintenance therapy who takes the medication once a day cannot be expected to experience substantial analgesia from maintenance therapy alone (Alford *et al.* 2006).

Another point Alford and others make is with respect to the tolerance in opioid-dependent patients (Mitra and Sinatra 2004; Alford *et al.* 2006). While clinicians are often hesitant to give additional opioids citing concerns of respiratory and CNS depression, studies show that physiological dependence provides patients with a degree of tolerance to both (Alford *et al.* 2006). On the other hand, dependence will also lead to tolerance of the analgesic effects of opioids, and this is not seen in just one type of opioid. Cross-tolerance occurs, leading patients to experience less analgesic effects from different classes of opioids. This means that dependent patients will require much higher doses to achieve the same level of pain control as would be expected in an opioid-naive patient (Alford *et al.* 2006). While this may be true for patients who are not in pain, for opioid dependent patients.

There is also a fear that by treating acute pain with opioid analgesics, one could contribute to a relapse. Though the literature is sparse, there is evidence demonstrating no increased risk of relapse, and in fact, some have argued a decreased risk (Kantor *et al.* 1980).

Keeping these concepts in mind can serve as a valuable tool in the approach to proper pain management of the dental patient. While pain management can be complicated, there are several principles that one should follow. It is good practice to collaborate with the outpatient providers and/or methadone maintenance program to discuss treatment options as well as to report any new medications given that may show up in patients' toxicology screens. The best initial approach may involve non-opioid analgesics. If there is concern that this will not provide sufficient pain control, or if the patient does not experience adequate relief, opioid analgesics should be considered (Center for Substance Abuse Treatment 2004). For patients on methadone, this type of acute pain may be treated with short-term opioid agonist therapy (Alford *et al.* 2006).

For patients on buprenorphine, there are a number of different approaches, but caution should be advised if an adjunctive opioid analgesic is chosen (Alford *et al.* 2006). According to the *Clinical Guidelines for the use of buprenorphine in the Treatment of Opioid Addiction*, it is generally recommended that buprenorphine be discontinued in patients who will be receiving other opioid analgesics (Center for Substance Abuse Treatment 2004). Though it is not unheard of to give short-acting opioids to treat pain in a patient on maintenance therapy (Mitra and Sinatra 2004; Alford *et al.* 2006), the mechanism of action of buprenorphine can make this problematic, and so it is prudent to collaborate with other practitioners prior to undertaking this approach. Buprenorphine is unique for its high affinity and partial agonist activity at the μ receptor, which limits the effectiveness of other opioid analgesics. As a result, higher doses of analgesics will be required to achieve appropriate pain control when taken concomitantly with buprenorphine (Mitra and Sinatra 2004). If a patient were to suddenly stop taking buprenorphine while taking high doses of other analgesics, this would pose a serious risk as the patient would now be at risk for CNS and respiratory depression, and so patients must be cautioned not to abruptly discontinue their outpatient regimen (Alford *et al.* 2006).

Another approach to pain control supported in the literature would be to increase the frequency at which the buprenorphine is taken (Alford *et al.* 2006). To be clear, this must be addressed with the primary prescriber, and not taken on solely by the dentist. As previously mentioned, the analgesic effects are short-lived, and so shortening the duration between doses may provide some benefit (Alford *et al.* 2006).

Because naltrexone binds to the μ-opioid receptor with such strength, short-acting opioids will provide little relief in patients on naltrexone maintenance. Therefore, experts recommend either stopping it 48–72 h prior to a known procedure that will require significant pain control or using non-opioids to manage pain (Vickers and Jolly 2006).

Clinicians should remember that certain opioids such as methadone prolong the QTc interval, and as mentioned in the previous section, this can be problematic due to the associated risk of Torsades de Pointes. Thus, great caution must be taken not to give other QT-prolonging agents or medications that significantly inhibit the metabolism of methadone (Thanavaro and Thanavaro 2011). Methadone is metabolized via the isoenzyme CYP3A4 of the cytochrome P450 system, and so certain antibacterial and antifungal agents can be quite risky when taken by patients on methadone maintenance (Thanavaro and Thanavaro 2011). The antifungals ketoconazole and itraconazole are particularly strong inhibitors and should be used with great care (Wolbrette 2004). The macrolides erythromycin and clarithromycin are not only strong inhibitors but also act as QT-prolonging agents themselves (Center for Substance Abuse Treatment 2004). Similarly, there are reports of fluoroquinolones such as ciprofloxacin inducing dangerous increases in methadone levels (Galanter *et al.* 2008). Therefore, when considering an antibacterial or antifungal agent in patients on methadone maintenance, an alternative and comparably effective choice may be more prudent. If the clinical situation strongly calls for one of these agents, experts recommend that clinicians check a recent EKG, take an appropriate cardiac history, and check for any lab abnormalities to further evaluate the safety prior to proceeding (Cubeddu 2009). Clinicians should coordinate with the Methadone Program as well as a reduction in the dose may be appropriate.

d. Cocaine

Adrenergic vasoconstrictors (e.g., epinephrine) must not be used <24 h after cocaine use as this could lead to significant cardiac complications (Yagiela 1999). While patients are often not forthcoming with regards to their substance use, physical agitation, psychomotor agitation, and nasal septum damage are all signs to monitor for, and any elective procedure should be postponed if intoxication is suspected (Yagiela 1999).

Dental notes

There are several interactions that may occur when treating psychiatric patients in the dental office. These are all of clinical importance and should be considered prior to initiating any kind of intervention.

- Cytochrome P450 interactions involving antibiotics, antifungals, and other medications.
- Prolonged QTc and increased risk of Torsades de Pointes.
- Serotonin syndrome with the use of certain pain medications.
- Lithium toxicity with the use of metronidazole, analgesics (NSAIDs), and other medications.
- Significant interactions in patients using alcohol and/or other substance with potential for abuse.

References

Alford, D.P., Compton, P., & Samet, J.H. (2006) Acute pain management for patients receiving maintenance methadone or buprenorphine therapy. *Annuals of Internal Medicine*, **144** (**2**), 127–134.

Alvarez, P.A. & Pahissa, J. (2010) QT alterations in psychopharmacology: proven candidates and suspects. *Current Drug Safety*, **5** (**1**), 97–104.

American Psychiatric Association Practice Guidelines for the Treatment of Psychiatric Disorders (2006). http://www.appi.org/searchcenter/pages/SearchDetail.aspx?ItemId=2385 [accessed on March 8, 2014].

Asch, D.A. & Parker, R.M. (1988) The Libby Zion case. One step forward or two steps backward?. *The New England Journal of Medicine*, **318** (**12**), 771–775.

Baruzzi, A., Albani, F., & Riva, R. (1994) Oxcarbazepine: pharmacokinetic interactions and their clinical relevance. *Epilepsia*, **35** (**Suppl. 3**), S14–S19.

Becker, D.E. (2008) Psychotropic drugs: implications for dental practice. *Anesthesia Progress*, **55** (**3**), 89–99.

Boyer, E.W. (2005) The serotonin syndrome. *The New England Journal of Medicine*, **352**, 1112–1120.

Brouwers, E.E., Söhne, M., Kuipers, S., *et al.* (2009) Ciprofloxacin strongly inhibits clozapine metabolism: two case reports. *Clinical Drug Investigation*, **29** (**1**), 59–63.

Buckley, N.A., Dawson, A.H., & Isbister, G.K. (2014) Serotonin syndrome. *British Medical Journal*, **348**, g1626.

Burrows, G.D. & Tiller, J.W. (1999) Cade's observation of the antimanic effect of lithium and early Australian research. *Australian & New Zealand Journal of Psychiatry*, **33** (**Suppl.**), S27–S31.

Cubeddu, L.X. (2009) Iatrogenic QT abnormalities and fatal arrhythmias: mechanisms and clinical significance. *Current Cardiology Reviews*, **5** (**3**), 166–176.

Center for Substance Abuse Treatment (2004) *Clinical Guidelines for the Use of Buprenorphine in the Treatment of Opioid Addiction.* Treatment Improvement Protocol(TIP) Series 40. DHHS Publication No. (SMA)04-3939. Substance Abuse and Mental Health Services Administration, Rockville, MD.

Cohen, L.G., Chesley, S., Eugenio, L., *et al.* (1996) Erythromycin-induced clozapine toxic reaction. *Archives of Internal Medicine*, **156** (**6**), 675–677.

Cullen, K.R., Kumra, S., Westerman, M. *et al.* (2008) Atypical antipsychotics for treatment of schizophrenia spectrum disorders. Psychiatric Times, March 1. Retrieved from http://www.psychiatrictimes.com/schizophrenia/content/article/10168/1147536 [accessed on July 30, 2014].

De Bruin, M.L., Langendijk, P.N., Koopmans, R.P., *et al.* (2007) In-hospital cardiac arrest is associated with use of non-antiarrhythmic QTc-prolonging drugs. *British Journal of Clinical Pharmacology*, **63** (**2**), 2216–2223.

Desai, J. (2008) Perspectives on interactions between antiepileptic drugs (AEDs) and antimicrobial agents. *Epilepsia*, **49** (**Suppl. 6**), 47–49.

Dhillon, S. & Richens, A. (1982) Valproic acid and diazepam interaction in vivo. *British Journal of Clinical Pharmacology*, **13** (**4**), 553–560.

Eltas, A., Kartalcı, S., Eltas, S.D., *et al.* (2013) An assessment of periodontal health in patients with schizophrenia and taking antipsychotic medication. *International Journal of Dental Hygiene*, **11** (**2**), 78–83.

Fangmann, P., Assion, H.J., & Juckel, G. (2008) Half a century of antidepressant drugs: on the clinical introduction of monoamine oxidase inhibitors, tricyclics, and tetracyclics. Part II: tricyclics and tetracyclics. *Journal of Clinical Psychopharmacology*, **28** (**1**), 1–4.

Galanter, M. & Kleber, H.D. (2008) The American Psychiatric Publishing Textbook of Substance Abuse Treatment. *American Psychiatric Pub.*

Goulet, J.-P., Perusse, R., & Turcotte, J.-Y. (1992) Contraindications to vasoconstrictors in dentistry: Part III. *Oral Surgery, Oral Medicine, Oral Pathology*, **74**, 692–697.

Grant, P.M. & Beck, A.T. (2009) Defeatist beliefs as a mediator of cognitive impairment, negative symptoms, and functioning in schizophrenia. *Schizophrenia Bulletin*, **35** (**4**), 798–806.

Guo, J.J., Wu, J., Kelton, C.M., *et al.* (2012) Exposure to potentially dangerous drug-drug interactions involving antipsychotics. *Psychiatric Services*, **63** (**11**), 1080–1088.

Güzelcan, Y. & Kleinpenning, A.S. (2006) Life-threatening serotonin syndrome following a single dose of a serotonin reuptake inhibitor during maintenance therapy with a monoamine oxidase inhibitor. *Nederlands Tijdschrift Voor Geneeskunde*, **150** (**31**), 1748.

Haas, D.A. (1999) Adverse drug interactions in dental practice: interactions associated with analgesics, Part III in a series. *Journal of the American Dental Association*, **130** (**3**), 397–407.

Henderson, D.C. & Borba, C.P. (2001) Trimethoprim-sulfamethoxazole and clozapine. *Psychiatric Services*, **52** (**1**), 111–112.

Hersh, E.V. (1999) Adverse drug interactions in dental practice: interactions involving antibiotics. Part II of a series. *Journal of the American Dental Association*, **130** (**2**), 236–251.

Kantor, T.G., Cantor, R., & Tom, E. (1980) A study of hospitalized surgical patients on methadone maintenance. *Drug and Alcohol Dependence*, **6** (**3**), 163–173.

Karp, J.M. & Moss, A.J. (2006) Dental treatment of patients with long QT syndrome. *Journal of the American Dental Association*, **137** (**5**), 630–637.

Karunatilake, H. & Buckley, N.A. (2006) Serotonin syndrome induced by fluvoxamine and oxycodone. *Annuals of Pharmacotherapy*, **40** (**1**), 155–157.Kaufman, D.W., Kelly, J.P., Jurgelon, J.M., *et al.* (1996) Drugs in the aetiology of agranulocytosis and aplastic anaemia. *European Journal of Haematology*, **60** (**Suppl.**), 23–30.

Keene, J.J., Galasko, G.T., & Land, M.F. (2003) Antidepressant use in psychiatry and medicine: importance for dental practice. *Journal of the American Dental Association*, **134** (**1**), 71–79.

Lam, R.W. (2013) Antidepressants and QTc prolongation. *Journal of Psychiatry & Neuroscience*, **38** (**2**), E5–E6.

Lambrecht, T.J., Greuter, C., & Surber, C. (2013) Antidepressants relevant to oral and maxillofacial surgical practice. *Annual of Maxillofacial Surgery*, **3**, 160–166.

Llerena, A., Berecz, R., Peñas-lledó, E., *et al.* (2013) Pharmacogenetics of clinical response to risperidone. *Pharmacogenomics*, **14** (**2**), 177–194.

López-Muñoz, F. (2005) History of the discovery and clinical introduction of chlorpromazine. *Annals of Clinical Psychiatry*, **17**, 113–135.

Lowes, R. (2013) Top selling drugs through September Reported. *Medscape*, October 31. http://www.medscape.com/viewarticle/813571 [accessed July 27, 2014].

Mahatthanatrakul, W., Sriwiriyajan, S., Ridtitid, W., *et al.* (2012) Effect of cytochrome P450 3A4 inhibitor ketoconazole on risperidone pharmacokinetics in healthy volunteers. *Journal of Clinical Pharmacy and Therapeutics*, **37** (**2**), 221–225.

Mattick, R.P., Breen, C., Kimber, J., *et al.* (2009) Methadone maintenance therapy versus no opioid replacement therapy for opioid dependence. *Cochrane Database Systematic Reviews*, (**3**), CD002209.

Mitra, S. & Sinatra, R.S. (2004) Perioperative management of acute pain in the opioid-dependent patient. *Anesthesiology*, **101** (**1**), 212–227.

Moffa, Jr., D. (2010). Preventing toxic drug interactions and exposures. *Disease Management Project*. http://www.clevelandclinicmeded.com/medicalpubs/diseasemanagement/ [accessed on March 7, 2014].

Moore, P.A. (1999) Adverse drug interactions in dental practice: interactions associated with local anesthetics, sedatives and anxiolytics. Part IV of a series. *Journal of the American Dental Association*, **130** (**4**), 541–554.

O'connor, N.K. & Fris, J. (1994) Clarithromycin-carbamazepine interaction in a clinical setting. *The Journal of the American Board of Family Practice*, **7** (**6**), 489–492.

Pereira Vasconcelos, D.F., Dias da Sliva, M.A., Rocha Marques, M., *et al.* (2013) Effects of simultaneous nicotine and alcohol use in periodontitis progression in rats: a histomorphometric study. *Journal of Clinical and Experimental Dentistry*, **5**, e95–e99.

Perucca, E. (2001) Clinical pharmacology and therapeutic use of the new antiepileptic drugs. *Fundamental & Clinical Pharmacology*, **15** (**6**), 405–417.

Perucca, E. (2006) Clinically relevant drug interactions with antiepileptic drugs. *British Journal of Clinical Pharmacology*, **61** (**3**), 246–255.

Pud, D., Cohen D., Lawental, E., *et al.* (2006) Opioids and abnormal pain perception: new evidence from a study of chronic opioid addicts and healthy subjects. *Drug and Alcohol Dependence*, **82** (**3**), 218–223.

Rastogi, R., Swarm, R.A., & Patel, T.A. (2011) Case scenario: opioid association with serotonin syndrome: implications to the practitioners. *Anesthesiology*, **115** (**6**), 1291–1298.

Ray, W.A., Murray, K.T., Meredith, S., *et al.* (2004) Oral erythromycin and the risk of sudden death from cardiac causes. *The New England Journal of Medicine*, **351** (**11**), 1089–1096.

Rothstein, E. & Clancy, D.D. (1969) Toxicity of disulfiram combined with metronidazole. *New England Journal of Medicine*, **280** (**18**), 1006–1007.

Sadock, B.J., Kaplan, H.I., & Sadock, V.A. (2007) *Kaplan & Sadock's Synopsis of Psychiatry, Behavioral Sciences/Clinical Psychiatry*. Lippincott Williams & Wilkins, Philadelphia, PA.

Sandson, N.B., Armstrong, S.C., & Cozza, K.L. (2005) An overview of psychotropic drug-drug interactions. *Psychosomatics*, **46** (**5**), 464–494.

Sandson, N.B., Marcucci, C., Bourke, D.L., *et al.* (2006) An interaction between aspirin and valproate: the relevance of plasma protein displacement drug-drug interactions. *American Journal of Psychiatry*, **163** (**11**), 1891–1896.

Shapleske, J., Mickay, A.P., & Mckenna, P.J. (1996) Successful treatment of tardive dystonia with clozapine and clonazepam. *British Journal of Psychiatry*, **168** (**4**), 516–518.

Stahl SM. (2008) *Stahl's Essential Psychopharmacology, Neuroscientific Basis and Practical Applications*. Cambridge University Press, Cambridge.

Sun, J., Zhao, M., Fanous, A.H., *et al.* (2013). Characterization of schizophrenia adverse drug interactions through a network approach and drug classification. *Biomed Research International*, 2014, 258784.

Tani, H., Uchida, H., Suzuki, T., *et al.* (2012) Dental conditions in inpatients with schizophrenia: a large-scale multi-site survey. *BMC Oral Health*, **12**, 32–38.

Teicher, M.H., Altesman, R.I., Cole, J.O., *et al* (1987). Possible nephrotoxic interaction of lithium and metroni-dazole. *Journal of the American Medical Association*, **257** (**24**), 3365–3366.

Tezal, M., Grossi, S.G., Ho, A.W., *et al*. (2001) The effect of alcohol consumption on periodontal disease. *Journal of Periodontology*, **72**, 183–189.

Thanavaro, K.L. & Thanavaro, J.L. (2011) Methadone-induced torsades de pointes: a twist of fate. *Heart & Lung*, **40** (**5**), 448–453.

Tipton, K.F., Boyce, S., O'sullivan, J., *et al*. (2004). Monoamine oxidases: certainties and uncertainties. *Current Medicinal Chemistry*, **11** (**15**), 1965–1982.

Tomé, A.M. & Filipe, A. (2011) Quinolones: review of psychiatric and neurological adverse reactions. *Drug Safety*, **34** (**6**), 465–488.

Vickers, A.P. & Jolly, A. (2006) Naltrexone and problems in pain management. *British Medical Journal*, **332** (**7534**), 132–133.

Volpi-abadie, J., Kaye, A.M., & Kaye, A.D. (2013) Serotonin syndrome. *Ochsner Journal*, **13** (**4**), 533–540.

Von Rosensteil, N.A. & Adam, D. (1995) Macrolide antibacterials. Drug interactions of clinical significance. *Drug Safety*, **13** (**2**), 105–122.Wolbrette, D.L. (2004) Drugs that cause Torsades de pointes and increase the risk of sudden cardiac death. *Current Cardiology Reports*, **6** (**5**), 379–384.

Wynn, R.L. (1992) Antidepressant medications. *General Dentistry*, **40**, 192–197.

Yagiela, J.A. (1999) Adverse drug interactions in dental practice: interactions associated with vasoconstrictors. Part V or a series. *Journal of the American Dental Association*, **130**, 701–709.

Yagiela, J.A., Duffin, S.R., & Hunt, L.M. (1985) Drug interactions and vasoconstrictors used in local anesthetic solutions. *Oral Surgery, Oral Medicine, Oral Pathology*, **59**, 565–571.

Yap, Y.G. & Camm, A.J. (2003) Drug induced QT prolongation and torsades de pointes. *Heart*, **89** (**11**), 1363–1372.

Yohanna, D. (2013) Deinstitutionalization of people with mental illness: causes and consequences. *Virtual Mentor*, **15** (**10**), 886–891.

Chapter 10

Hematologic disorders and drugs that cause bleeding

A. Brief overview of the coagulation process	149
a. Thrombocytopenia	152
b. Thrombocytopathy	153
c. Antiplatelet medications	153
B. Bleeding disorders: Coagulation disorders	154
a. von Willebrand disease	154
b. Hemophilias	155
c. End-stage liver disease	156
d. Anticoagulation medications	157
References	167

A.   Brief overview of the coagulation process

The hemostatic system comprises platelets, coagulation factors, and endothelial cells lining the blood vessels (http://emedicine.medscape.com/article/201722-overview). Platelets are synthesized in the bone marrow and circulate in blood. All coagulation or clotting factors except von Willebrand factor (vWF) are synthesized in the liver. Blood vessels are lined with a layer of endothelial cells that allows blood to flow in its liquid state while keeping the clotting components circulating in an inactive state (Israels *et al.* 2006; D'Amato-Palumbo 2012). It is the resistance of the endothelial cells in the lining of the blood vessels which prevents thrombosis; however, hemostasis occurs when there is a disturbance of the continuity of this endothelial lining due to an injured or damaged blood vessel. At this point starts the coagulation cascade, which is a series of reactions that eventually lead to clot formation at the site of blood vessel injury. In certain individuals, if this normal system of clot formation is defective, either hypercoagulability or bleeding condition, abnormal clotting or blood loss occurs.

There are four phases of coagulation: vascular phase, platelet phase, coagulation phase, and fibrinolytic phase. The vascular phase occurs following blood vessel injury (*bleeding*) or damage resulting in *vasoconstriction* followed by platelet adherence to the tissues, specifically collagen. In turn, adenosine diphosphate is released, which causes the platelets to become sticky resulting in a *platelet plug*. This is the platelet phase and the initial step in preventing bleeding and blood loss. The coagulation phase, which is activated within minutes after injury, results in the formation of a clot. The coagulation cascade involves the conversion of soluble fibrinogen into insoluble fibrin

The Dentist's Quick Guide to Medical Conditions, First Edition. Mea A. Weinberg, Stuart L. Segelnick, Joseph S. Insler, with Samuel Kramer.
© 2015 John Wiley & Sons, Inc. Published 2015 by John Wiley & Sons, Inc.

(*fibrin clot*) through the action of thrombin, a precursor to prothrombin via prothrombin-converting factor. The production of prothrombin-converting factor can occur either as a result of an extrinsic mechanism or pathway that is activated when the blood vessels and tissues are damaged or as the result of the actions on an intrinsic mechanism or pathway that is present within the blood itself and is activated when the blood is traumatized. In the extrinsic pathway, tissue thromboplastin is released from damaged tissues and does not require contact activation. The extrinsic pathway involves factors VII, XIII, and X. The intrinsic pathway involves factors VIII, IX, X, XII, and XI and is a slower pathway than the extrinsic pathway. It is the activation of factor X that starts the common pathway. The fourth and last phase of hemostasis is fibrinolysis, which is the way of disposing fibrin after it has done its function (Patton 2003). Figure 10.1 shown is a short schematic representation of the coagulation cascade.

During the fibrinolytic phase, fibrin is broken down and removed after hemostasis is complete. Wound healing occurs during this phase (Patton 2003).

Diagnostics/lab values

In patients with a suspected bleeding disorder, the first steps are to review the medical history and the systems including extra- and intraoral tissues. The CBC values should be reviewed including platelets.

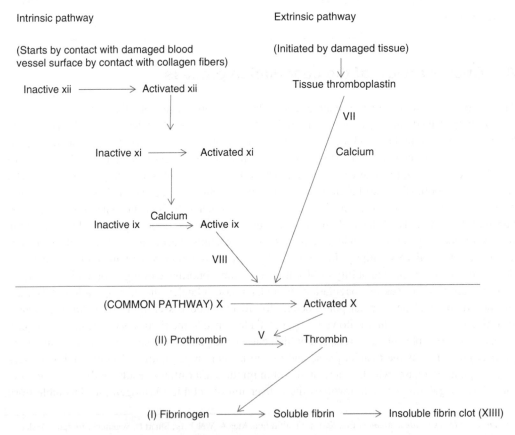

Figure 10.1   Brief schematic of the coagulation cascade.
Source: Patton 2003, Figure 17.2, p. 457. Reproduced with permission of PMPH-USA.

Platelet count: A normal range is 150,000–400,000 cells/mm^3 (Patton and Ship 2003). It is used to diagnose thrombocytopenia. Bleeding essentially occurs when the coagulation factors are not intact or platelet count is low. Since all coagulation factors except factor VIII (vascular endothelium) are synthesized in the liver, patients with end-stage liver disease will present with bleeding problems. Some patients with bleeding disorders may not have a problem with platelets, while some will have low platelets and some will have high platelets. There are bleeding problems with platelets <50,000, and patients will require a platelet transfusion. Patients with high platelets can be treated in the dental office without any problems (Patton and Ship 1994).

Bleeding time: The Ivy bleeding time (BT) is the time required for blood to stop flowing from a small wound. The BT is approximately 1–6 min. Prolonged BT may indicate thrombocytopenia or von Willebrand disease (vWD). A normal BT does not predict the safety of surgical procedures, and an abnormal BT does not predict excessive bleeding will occur. Assessment of the BT is extremely variable due to technical factors and is not sensitive when performing the test. Thus, the BT is not recommended as a pre-operative screening test and should not be used to evaluate bleeding disorders. The Platelet Function Analyzer (PFA-100) is an alternative technology that assesses platelet function with greater sensitivity and reproducibility than the BT (Posan *et al.* 2003).

Partial prothrombin time: The partial prothrombin time (PTT) test measures the time it takes for the blood to clot and is normally 25–35 s. Above 35 s is abnormal. It detects defects in the intrinsic pathway, vWD, and hemophilia A and B.

Prothrombin time: *Prothrombin time* (PT) measures the extrinsic cascade (time it takes to form a clot) and measures the presence or absence of clotting factors I, II, V, VII, and X. The normal PT is 11–13 s. PT >13 s is abnormal. It is used to find defects in the extrinsic pathway, prothrombin deficiency, vitamin K deficiency, liver disease, and antiplatelet drugs. International normalized ratio (INR) is a way of allowing reproducibility or standardization of PT results from different laboratories and different laboratory methods. Today, most labs report INR but not the PT (Kitchen and Preston 1999).

Lab values for common bleeding disorders are summarized in Table 10.1.

Table 10.1 Common bleeding disorders and screening tests.

Bleeding disorders	Platelet count	Bleeding time	International normalized ratio	Partial prothrombin time
Thrombocytopenia	Low	Increased	Normal	Normal
von Willebrand disease	Normal or low	Increased	Normal	Normal or prolonged
End-stage liver disease	Low	Increased	Increased	Prolonged
Anticoagulation drugs (warfarin)	Normal	Normal	Increased	Normal
Heparin factors VIII, IX, and XI deficiency	Normal	Normal	Normal	Prolonged
Intestinal malabsorption/ vitamin K deficiency, factor II, V, and X deficiency	Normal	Normal	Increased	Prolonged

Adapted from Patton (2003).

Bleeding disorders: Vessel wall disorders

Blood vessel wall disorders occur due to increased fragility of the blood vessels resulting in mild, not serious bleeding usually localized to the skin, mucosa, and gingiva (Patton 2003). Extra-/intraoral petechiae and ecchymosis is a common feature (D'Amato-Palumbo 2012). There is usually a normal platelet count, PT, and PTT. Examples of blood vessel wall disorders include Cushing's syndrome, Ehlers–Danlos syndrome, and hereditary hemorrhagic telangiectasia (Lukes 2012).

Bleeding disorders: Platelet function

Platelet disorders are classified as congenital or acquired and thrombocytopenias or thrombocytopathies. Table 10.2 lists the classification of platelet disorders (Patton 2003; Gupta *et al.* 2007).

a.   Thrombocytopenia

Thrombocytopenia is the primary cause of bleeding disorders characterized by low platelet counts. The normal range of platelets is 150,000–400,000 cells/mm^3, but in a patient diagnosed with thrombocytopenia the count is <150,000 cells/mm^3 (Terranova *et al.* 2008; Mann and Grimes 2011). A decrease in platelets is due to a decrease in platelet production in the bone marrow, increased sequestration in the spleen, accelerated destruction of platelets, or decreased platelet survival (Patton 2003; D'Amato-Palumbo 2012). Thrombocytopenia can be caused by a decreased production of platelets as a result of bone marrow suppression from cytotoxic drugs indicated for treatment of rheumatoid

Table 10.2   Classification of platelet disorders.

Congenital platelet conditions (rare conditions)
  Thrombocytopenic
      May–Hegglin anomaly
      Wiskott–Aldrich syndrome
      Neonatal alloimmune thrombocytopenia
  Nonthrombocytopenic
      Glanzmann's thrombasthenia
      Platelet-type von Willebrand disease (vWD)
      Bernard–Soulier syndrome
Acquired platelet conditions
  Thrombocytopenic
      Immune (or idiopathic) thrombocytopenia purpura
      Thrombotic thrombocytopenia purpura
      Cytotoxic chemotherapy
      Drug induced
      Leukemia
      Aplastic anemia
      Systemic lupus erythematosus
      Comorbid infection (HIV, mononucleosis)
  Nonthrombocytopenic
      Drug induced (aspirin, nonsteroidal anti-inflammatory drugs, penicillin, cephalosporins)
      Uremia
      Alcoholism
      Liver disease
      Myeloproliferative diseases
      Acquired platelet-type vWD

arthritis and systemic lupus erythematosus (e.g., azathioprine (Imuran), cyclophosphamide (Cytoxan), methotrexate (Rheumatrex), thiazide diuretics (e.g., hydrochlorothiazide), valproic acid, sulfonamides, gold, methyldopa, quinine, quinidine, heparin, and alcohol). Three weeks after chemotherapy is stopped, dental procedures can be scheduled (Patton and Ship 1994). Clinical oral signs/symptoms of thrombocytopenia include petechiae and ecchymosis.

Immune (or idiopathic) thrombocytopenia purpura is a rare autoimmune disease occurring in approximately 23 of every 100,000 people in the USA (Mann and Grimes 2011). ITP may be more prolonged in adults than in children. Extra- and intraoral signs/symptoms of ITP include dry and wet purpura. Purpura is defined as areas of purple or red spots evident within the skin (dry purpura) or mucous membranes (e.g., oral cavity and eyes; wet purpura) as a result of spontaneous hemorrhages of blood (Mann and Grimes 2011). Clinically, it appears as bruising and petechiae circumferential spots (Mann and Grimes 2011). Some patients with ITP do not show any signs of bleeding. It depends on the severity of the thrombocytopenia. Patients with a platelet count <10,000/mcl may show more bleeding (Provan and Newland 2003; Mann and Grimes 2011).

Irreversible thrombocytopenia is caused by end-stage liver disease, splenomegaly, bone marrow irradiation, autoimmune destruction, hemolytic anemias, leukemia, lymphomas, aplastic anemia, thrombotic thrombocytopenic purpura, HIV, and giant hemangiomas (Patton and Ship 1994; Kujovich 2005; Neunert *et al.* 2011).

b.   Thrombocytopathy

Thrombocytopathy is a platelet disorder resulting from impairment in platelet function even though there are adequate numbers of platelets. There is a defect in platelet adhesion, aggregation, or granule release (Patton 2003). Thrombocytopathies may be congenital or acquired. Conditions resulting in thrombocytopathy include the following (Patton and Ship 1994; D'Amato-Palumbo 2012):

- Inherited (congenital) conditions: vWD, which consists of a platelet dysfunction and a factor VIII deficiency
- Acquired conditions:
  - Drug induced (e.g., aspirin, nonsteroidal anti-inflammatory drugs [NSAIDs], clopidogrel (Plavix), ticlopidine (Ticlid)); alcohol taken with aspirin or NSAIDs; uremia; hemodialysis; liver disease; and myeloproliferative disorders—abnormal growth of platelets and other blood cells in the bone marrow, polycythemia vera, and chronic myelogenous leukemia).

Dental patients with end-stage renal disease undergoing hemodialysis are at a high risk for dental bleeding due to the use of heparin during dialysis, which keeps the shut open, impaired platelet function and thrombocytopenia associated with hemodialysis trauma to the platelets. Dental surgical procedures should be scheduled one day after hemodialysis when the heparin has been eliminated and blood urea nitrogen (BUN) and creatinine levels are at the lowest concentrations (Pattin and Ship 1994).

c.   Antiplatelet medications

Antiplatelet drugs are used to reduce absolute number of platelets or alter platelet function, resulting in increased bleeding during and after dental surgery. Risk factor screening for bleeding due to antiplatelet agents is important in patients that have had cardiovascular procedures. Treatment options for patients on antiplatelet drugs who require emergency surgery (Ferraris *et al.* 2012) are as follows:

1. Delaying the surgery
2. Bridging strategies using short-acting antiplatelet agents

3. Performing platelet transfusions for patients with excessive bleeding

4. Administering recombinant factor VIIa for intractable bleeding.

Aspirin irreversibly binds to and acetylates cyclooxygenase enzyme blocking the synthesis of thromboxane A_2 resulting in inhibition of platelet aggregation and vasoconstriction. Since platelets do not synthesize new proteins, suppression of platelet aggregation occurs for 7–10 days, the life of the platelet. The most common indication for "low-dose" aspirin (50–325 mg/day) is prevention of thrombotic cardiovascular events (Berger *et al.* 2008). Low-dose aspirin does not have any anti-inflammatory effects; much larger doses are required. NSAIDs also have the same mechanism of action on platelets; but they bind reversibly, not irreversibly, so that the antiplatelet action is not prolonged as it is with aspirin, usually lasting about 6–12 h. Once an NSAID is discontinued, platelet inhibition is reversed within 1–5 half-life ($t\frac{1}{2}$) of the drug (D'Amato-Palumbo 2012). This is the reason "low-dose" aspirin is used for prophylaxis of cardiac events. Other antiplatelet drugs include clopidogrel (Plavix), ticlopidine (Ticlid), prasugrel (Effient), abciximab (ReoPro), dipyridamole (Persantine), and aspirin–dipyridamole (Aggrenox). *These antiplatelet drugs also are not recommended to be discontinued for invasive dental procedures.* However, a medical consultis recommended because some physicians want the patients to stop it for up to 7 days. Aspirin taken together with another antiplatelet such as clopidogrel or warfarin increases the risk of bleeding (Ferraris *et al.* 2010). Take precautions with patients with combined antiplatelet agents.

Common herbal products with antiplatelet activity include ginger, ginkgo, green tea, black licorice (glycyrrhizic acid), willow bark, clove, flaxseed oil, and feverfew. These products should be discontinued before dental surgery.

Features: Platelet disorders (Patton and Ship 1994)

- Petechiae in skin and oral mucosa (<100,000 platelets)
- Ecchymosis
- Superficial bleeding from cuts and scratches of skin

B. Bleeding disorders: Coagulation disorders

a. *von Willebrand disease*

Clinical synopsis

vWD is an inherited disorder of platelet adhesion, which involves a defect in vWF, which plays an important role in primary hemostasis by binding to both platelets and endothelial components. Also there is a deficiency and/or a qualitative defect in factor VIII. Both characteristics cause a defect in clot formation and fibrin formation. vWD is estimated to occur in 1% of the general population and is one of the most common bleeding disorders in children (Klaassen and Halton 2002).

vWD is usually transmitted as an autosomal dominant disorder. It is classified into four types: Type I, the most common (deficiency in vWF); Type II (qualitative defect in vWF); Type III, a rare event (both Type I and II defects), from a mild form to a severe form; and Type IV, which is referred to as pseudo-vWD or platelet-type vWD, which is primarily a platelet condition that mimics vWD (Patton 2003; D'Amato-Palumbo 2012).

vWD is diagnosed by a positive family history and clinical features including mucocutaneous bleeding, bruising with minimal or no apparent trauma, recurrent spontaneous epistaxis, and oral cavity bleeding events. Other bleeding symptoms include prolonged bleeding following skin laceration or oral surgery and spontaneous gastrointestinal bleeding. Laboratory tests show prolonged

PTT, abnormal assay showing a decrease in factor VIII level, and prolonged BT and/or abnormal platelet function (Federici 1998; Sadler *et al.* 2000; Mannucci *et al.* 2000; Klaassen and Holton 2002; Patton 2003; D'Amato-Palumbo 2012).

Medications

The choice of treatment for patients with vWD depends on the clinical severity, the type of vWD, and the risk of bleeding. The three main therapeutic modalities used in the treatment of vWD are desmopressin acetate (DDAVP; Ferring Inc, Canada), transfusion with plasma concentrates that contain vWF, and antifibrinolytic agents (Klaassen and Holton 2002).

Orofacial findings: Coagulation disorders (Adeyemo *et al.* 2011)

- Orofacial petechiae
- Conjunctival hemorrhage
- Spontaneous nose bleeding
- Posttraumatic gingival bleeding
- Prolonged post-extraction bleeding

Dental notes

The key to treating patients with bleeding disorders is to prevent excessive bleeding during a dental procedure. A thorough medical history, a hematologist consult, a review of lab values, and an assessment of bleeding tendencies are essential. Part of the medical history should include family members with bleeding disorders, past history of prolonged bleeding after an extraction and use of anticoagulation drugs. DDAVP is a synthetic analogue of the antidiuretic hormone L-arginine vasopressin. The mechanism of action of DDAVP is to increase blood levels of factor VIII coagulant activity and vWF and shorten the prolonged BT (Mannucci 1988; Leissinger *et al.* 2013). DDAVP is indicated in the treatment of mild and moderate hemophilia A, vWD, and thrombocytopenia. In addition, DDAVP has also been indicated to help shortening the prolonged skin BTs that occur with uremia, cirrhosis, and platelet dysfunctions of various etiologies (Mannucci 1988). DDAVP is supplied as a nasal inhalant, an intravenous solution, or an oral or sublingual tablet. DDAVP should be administered 30 min before invasive dental procedures to achieve maximum effectiveness. For infusions, blood pressure should be monitored at the start and end of the infusion.

b. Hemophilias

Clinical synopsis

Hemophilias are a group of bleeding disorders caused by an inherited sex-linked recessive trait and are seen only in men; however, women may be carriers. Hemophilia is characterized by a deficiency or an absence of a coagulation factor (antihemophilic factor) (White *et al.* 2001). There are two forms of hemophilia: hemophilia A, a deficiency of factor VIII, and hemophilia B (Christmas disease), a deficiency of factor IX. The missing factor in both forms is a protein that the hemophiliac cannot synthesize.

The clinical hallmark of hemophilia A and B is bleeding into joints and muscles (called hemarthroses). Patients with mild hemophilia usually do not have extensive bleeding until there is trauma or they undergo surgery. The severity of bleeding in hemophilia is generally correlated with the clotting factor level (Srivastava *et al.* 2013). Other bleeding features include skin bruising/purpurae, nose bleeds, and genitourinary and gastrointestinal bleeding. Dentally, the patient may experience gingival bleeding and bullous hemorrhages on the buccal mucosa. Bleeding in a hemophiliac is different from the "superficial" mucosal and skin bleeding seen in platelet disorders or vWD. The INR is not reported since it does not measure the reduction of factors VIII or IX, which is a feature of hemophilia.

Medications

There is no known cure for hemophilia. Hemophiliacs must be careful to prevent or minimize the risk of external and internal bleeding. Since factor VIII cannot be stored in a blood bank for a prolonged period of time, for hemophilia A, fresh blood transfusions must be given.

Dental notes: Hemophilia

There are no contraindications to dental treatment for hemophiliacs; however, caution should be used when administering local and general anesthesia. Hemophiliacs can be treated in a nonhospital setting (Table 10.5). To control bleeding, patient should be administered an antifibrinolytic drug such as tranexamic acid or desmopressin (DDAVP) and a single infusion of deficient factor VIII for hemophilia A and factor IX for hemophilia B every 8–12 h for 1–2 days (Zanon *et al.* 2000; Frachon *et al.* 2005; Gupta *et al.* 2007; Peisker *et al.* 2013). Adverse effects after factor VIII include hemarthrosis, oropharyngeal and dental bleeding, epistaxis, and hematuria (Gupta *et al.* 2007).

There are no restrictions or contraindications concerning the type of local anesthetic agent administered. Epinephrine is not contraindicated and will provide additional hemostasis.

Replacement therapy is required for an inferior alveolar block and lingual infiltration. An inferior alveolar block should be given only after raising clotting factor levels with replacement therapy; this will reduce the risk of bleeding into the muscles and development of a hematoma in the retromolar or pterygoid space, which could compromise the airway. An intraligamentary or intraosseous injection is preferred over a mandibular block. Likewise, hemostatic coverage is requi red for lingual infiltration due to the plexus of blood vessels in the lingual area. Infiltration, intrapapillary, and intraligamentary injections are often done under factor cover although it may be possible for those with adequate experience to administer these injections without it (Brewer and Correa 2006; Srivastava *et al.* 2013). Tranexamic acid or epsilon aminocaproic acid is often used after dental procedures to reduce the need for replacement therapy (Srivastava *et al.* 2013).

During the dental procedure, if the patient experiences prolonged bleeding or difficulty in swallowing, speaking, or breathing, the hematologist/surgeon should be notified immediately. Following extractions, smoking should be avoided and the patient should rinse with warm salt water (1 teaspoon of salt in an 8 oz. glass of warm water) starting the day after the extraction for 5–7 days (Srivastava *et al.* 2013).

Avoid prescribing/recommending NSAIDs and any aspirin-containing drug. Acetaminophen is a good acceptable analgesic (Srivastava *et al.* 2013).

c. End-stage liver disease

Depending upon the severity of liver damage, patients with liver disease most likely will have bleeding problems due to inability of the liver to synthesize all clotting factors except factor VII and vWF (Gupta *et al.* 2007). In addition, patients with severe liver disease may also have thrombocytopenia. Common etiology of liver disease includes hepatitis B and C, alcohol cirrhosis, and hepatocellular carcinoma.

It is common belief that acetaminophen is contraindicated in patients with liver disease; however, even though the half-life of acetaminophen may be prolonged, cytochrome P450 enzyme activity is not increased and glutathione stores are not depleted to critical levels in patients taking recommended doses. In addition, studies using acetaminophen in different liver diseases have not shown an increased risk of hepatotoxicity at currently recommended doses (Benson *et al.* 2005).

For more detail, review Chapter 7.

d. Anticoagulation medications

In order to have a more reproducible value from different laboratories, the PT is reported with its INR or just INR alone, which is a more reproducible valve. This test evaluates the extrinsic coagulation system to form a fibrin clot and measures the presence or absence of clotting factors I, II, V, VII, and X (Patton 2003). Normal values are a PT of 11–13 s or an INR of 1.0 (Patton 2003).

The INR is used to monitor warfarin therapy. Warfarin has a narrow therapeutic range, and even slight changes in dose can lead to either thrombosis or hemorrhage (Eisenstein 2012). Warfarin works on vitamin K–dependent factors, II, VII, IX, and X, which are formed in the liver. Most patients should get an INR within 24 h but not more than 72 h of the dental procedure; however, if the patient has been on warfarin for a while and once the INR becomes stable at <3.0, the frequency of testing can be reduced to within 2 weeks or up to 4 weeks for routine dental treatment (Hirsh *et al.* 2003). It should be noted that some patients on anticoagulant therapy may also have other medical conditions including liver or kidney impairment that could increase the incidence of bleeding during or after dental procedures.

An INR is required for the following dental procedures (Morimoto *et al.* 2009):

- Periodontal probing
- Periodontal subgingival scaling/root planing
- Mandibular blocks
- Periodontal surgery
- Implant surgery
- Extractions
- Biopsies

Table 10.3 lists the acceptable INR for treating patients. Some patients may be on low-intensity warfarin or high-intensity warfarin therapy depending on the indication. Table 10.3 lists the acceptable INR range for different patients on warfarin.

Table 10.3   International normalized ratio (INR) guidelines for dental treatment (Mori *et al.* 2002; Goldhaber 2006).

All patients should have an INR below 4
Acceptable range: INR 2.0–3.0 in patients with low-intensity warfarin therapy:
Pulmonary embolus
Deep vein thrombosis
Atrial fibrillation
Bileaflet mitral value
Acceptable range: INR 3.0–4.0 in patients with high-intensity warfarin therapy:
Mechanical heart valves
Recurrence of embolism while on warfarin
Prevention of recurrent myocardial infarction (MI)

The American College of Chest Physicians (ACCP) recommends that clinicians keep patients on warfarin for minor dental procedures (Douketis *et al.* 2008; Eisenstein 2012). Many minimally invasive dental procedures can be performed on patients taking warfarin as these procedures are not likely to cause bleeding that cannot be managed with local hemostatic measures.

Recommendations for treating patients on anticoagulant drugs are as follows (http://standfordhospital. org/PDF/anticoagulation/dentalProcedure.pdf; Scully and Wolff 2002; Jeske and Suchko 2003; Sandor 2004):

- Literature has documented that warfarin does not have to be discontinued but an INR is still required for procedures that are considered "low risk" for bleeding including examination (periodontal probing), study models, and orthodontic procedures. If the INR >3.5, the procedure can be performed; however, be prepared for administering local hemostatic measures.
- Low-intensity warfarin therapy (INR 2.0–3.0):
  ◦ Procedures that are considered to be "low–moderate" risk for bleeding nonsurgical or simple surgical procedures: oral prophylaxis, periodontal scaling/root planing, restorative procedures, and endodontics. For an INR > 3, it is recommended not to perform these procedures.
  ◦ Procedures that are considered to be "moderate" risk for bleeding: simple tooth extractions, subgingival periodontal debridement with severe inflammation, non-flap periodontal surgery, and prosthetics. For an INR >2.5, it is recommended not to perform these procedures (Douketis *et al.* 2008). It is recommended to consult with the patient's cardiologist.
  ◦ If the risk of bleeding is severe (e.g., a patient at high risk for thrombus formation), it is recommended to contact the physician. Warfarin dose may need to be discontinued or reduced, which should be done at least 5 days before the surgery, and the patients may be treated with bridging therapy to reduce the risk of thromboembolic events and even death (Garcia *et al.* 2008; Eisenstein 2012). Anticoagulant should be started again as soon as possible after the surgery once there are no further bleeding episodes (Douketis *et al.* 2008; Eisenstein 2012). Consultation with the patient's cardiologist is recommended.
- High-intensity warfarin therapy (INR 2.5–3.5):
  ◦ Nonsurgical or simple surgical procedures: INR 2.5–3.5
  ◦ Complex surgical procedures: INR 2.5–3.0
  ◦ Consult with physician

In summary, most literature guidelines recommend that anticoagulated patients can undergo minor invasive dental procedures provided their INR is therapeutic ($\leq$3.0–3.5) (see Table 10.3) (Sonis *et al.* 2003; Douketis *et al.* 2008; Balevi 2010; D'Amato-Palumbo 2012). No alteration in dosing is needed if the INR is within the therapeutic range. If the INR >4, then alteration of anticoagulation is required (Herman *et al.* 1997; Pototski and Amenabar 2007).

The Institute for Safe Medication Practices states that there may be a misunderstanding by the patient regarding previous instructions to discontinue or not discontinue a medication before the dental procedure. Thus, it is advisable to have good communication between the cardiologist and patients (Eisenstein 2012).

The following list shows warfarin–dental drug interactions (Dean and Talbert 1980; Glasheen *et al.* 2005; Hughes *et al.* 2011):

Aspirin, NSAIDs—avoid concurrent use; additive effect of bleeding.
Acetaminophen alone or in combination with a narcotic—increases bleeding; need a dose adjustment based on the PT or INR. Consult with physician.
Amoxicillin—overcoagulation; need a dose adjustment based on the PT or INR. Consult with physician.

Azithromycin (Zithromax)—overcoagulation; need a dose adjustment based on the PT or INR. Consult with physician.

Erythromycin—overcoagulation; need a dose adjustment based on the PT or INR. Consult with physician.

Quinolones: ciprofloxacin (Cipro), levofloxacin (Levaquin)—overcoagulation; need a dose adjustment based on the PT or INR. Consult with physician.

Tetracycline—overcoagulation; need a dose adjustment based on the PT or INR. Consult with physician.

Doxycycline—overcoagulation; need a dose adjustment based on the PT or INR. Consult with physician.

Metronidazole—overcoagulation; need a dose adjustment based on the PT or INR. Consult with physician.

Azole antifungals (ketoconazole)—overcoagulation; need a dose adjustment based on the PT or INR. Consult with physician.

Herbals (ginseng, garlic)—increased bleeding.

Since 2011, alternatives to warfarin have been available that do not require an INR; however, excessive bleeding cannot be reversed with these drugs, physicians cannot check how well the anticoagulant is working, and they are expensive (Huff 2012). Examples of these newer anticoagulants include apixaban (Eliquis), dabigatran (Pradaxa), and rivaroxaban (Xarelto). These drugs are indicated for the prevention of venous thromboembolic events in patients who have had total hip or knee replacement and the prevention of stroke and systemic embolism with non-valvular atrial fibrillation and one or more cardiovascular risk factors.

Heparin is used for short-term anticoagulation in the treatment of thromboembolic disorders and in hemodialysis so that blood does not clot in the machine. Heparin has a relatively short duration of action of 3–4 h with a half-life of approximately 1.5 h (range 1–6 h) and is administered parenterally. On the other hand, warfarin is used for chronic anticoagulation because the maximum effect of a dose occurs up to 48 h after administration, and the effect remains for the next 5 days (Horton and Buswick 1999). Heparin is administered intravenously as an inpatient procedure, so they will most likely not be seen in the dental office.

Low-molecular-weight heparin preparations are administered subcutaneously on an outpatient need and cause less thrombocytopenia and bleeding complications than warfarin (Patton 2003). These agents are used as bridging therapy in high-risk patients that need to stop oral anticoagulants before surgery (Pengo *et al.* 2009). In these cases, warfarin is stopped and the patient is started on heparin, which is usually stopped 4 hours before the dental procedure and then reinstated right after the procedure. Warfarin is started again while heparin is slowly discontinued. With bridging therapy, it is difficult to get INR values back to a therapeutic range. Consultation with the patient's cardiologist is necessary before a dental procedure.

Certain herbal/vitamin products that act as anticoagulants and cause bleeding include black licorice (glycyrrhizic acid), garlic, ginseng, dong quai, vitamin E, chamomile, and alfalfa. Before surgery, question the patient regarding the use of these products and instruct the patient to discontinue until after surgery (Fong Liu *et al.* 2010).

Management of intraoral "visible" bleeding

Intraoral bleeding can be managed with medications or products (Table 10.4). To manage intraoral bleeding after extractions, an antifibrinolytic agent is recommended. Antifibrinolytics work by preventing fibrinolysis by reducing the activity of plasmin, which is responsible for breaking up

Table 10.4 Medications and products used in preventing oral bleeding events (www.rxlist.com; Patton 2003; McBee and Koerner 2005; www.medicalhemostat.blogspot.com/2009/06/hemostasis-market-review-of-gelfoam.html).

Drug/product	Indication	Dose/administration	Adverse effects/precautions
Platelet transfusion	Platelets <50,000 cells/mm^3	Transfusion center: one pack = 50 ml and increase platelet count by 6000. Performed on the morning of the dental procedure	
Fresh frozen plasma	Severe liver disease, immune globulin deficiency, blood transfusion >10 units of blood	1 unit = 150–125 ml	
Epsilon aminocaproic acid (Amicar)	Antifibrinolytic drug: to assist in clot formation after a dental procedure that causes a bleeding event in patients with a bleeding disorder	Requires a prescription: Supplied: 25% oral solution (250 mg/ml), 20 ml administered during the first hour of treatment, followed by a continuing rate of one 1000 mg tablet or two, 500 mg tablets or 5 ml of oral solution per hour. This is continued for 8 h or until the bleeding has been controlled and the patient is clotting OR 5–10 ml qid for 7 days (bite on soaked gauze/rinsing). OR Tablets, dose: 75 mg/kg every 4–6 h for 7–10 days (maximum 24 g/24 h) (For example: 5/1000 mg tablets or 10/500 mg) Call pharmacy ahead of the surgery to make sure they will carry it. Most pharmacies do not have it in stock and will have to order it	Common adverse effects: generally well tolerated Warning: upper urinary tract bleeding
Tranexamic acid (Cyklokapron)	Antifibrinolytic drug: to assist in clot formation after a dental procedure that causes a bleeding event in patients with a bleeding disorder (hemophilia)	Requires a prescription: Supplied: Tablet: 25 mg/kg is given 2 h before surgery, followed by every 8 h for 6–8 days. Factor VIII and factor IX as well as tranexamic acid (injectable) should be given	Common adverse effect: gastrointestinal discomfort occurs in more than 30% of patients after oral administration of 6 g/day. The discomfort disappears when the dose is reduced Thrombosis, deep vein thrombosis, pulmonary embolism, subarachnoid hemorrhage Dosage adjustment for patients with renal insufficiency

Desmopressin acetate (DDAVP)	A synthetic derivative of the antidiuretic hormone L-arginine vasopressin. Administer before treatment in patients with congenital and acquired bleeding disorder including von Willebrand disease and hemophilia		Can develop hypersensitivity with repeated use; topical use only
Tisseel	Fibrin sealant; human fibrinogen combined with bovine thrombin; to control bleeding during surgery that cannot be controlled by conventional methods including sutures, pressure, and electrocautery; very expensive	Thaw prefilled syringe and warm between 91.4 (33°C) and 98.6 (37°C) in a sterile water bath (pouches removed) or nonsterile water bath (in pouches) or incubator (in pouches). Apply as a thin layer by dripping. Absorbed in 10–14 days	
Electrocautery	Soft-tissue bleeding	Apply to soft tissue	Causes necrosis if applied to bone and can cause tissue necrosis
Gauze	Moist cold 2 × 2 gauze with finger pressure. Apply pressure for as long as necessary to control the bleeding, usually 30–60 min		
Gelfoam (Pfizer)	Introduced in 1940s; absorbable gelatin (purified pork skin) sponge material; acts in the intrinsic pathway causing contact activation and platelet aggregation allowing for clot formation; use directly out of box; expensive	Should be placed on top of extraction socket; it swells a lot, so it is difficult to use in small spaces	Do not place inside of flap

(continued)

Table 10.4 *(cont'd)*

Drug/product	Indication	Dose/administration	Adverse effects/precautions
Surgicel (Ethicon)	Plant-based oxidized regenerated cellulose; control bleeding after extractions/oral surgery; expensive; use directly out of box	Absorbs in 7–14 days; remove unabsorbed material	Nidus for infection
ActCel (Coreva Health Science)	Topical hemostatic agent; controls bleeding from oral open wounds	Absorbable in 1–2 weeks	
Collagen (CollaPlug, CollaTape, CollaCote) (Zimmer Dental)	Bovine collagen; indicated for wound protection control of bleeding from open oral wounds including socket preservation; causes platelet aggregation, which bind to collagen fibrils	Can be removed after 2–5 min; however, they are resorbed within 14–56 days	
Ativene (Bard Davol, Inc), Helitene (Integra LifeSciences Corporation), Collagene (Sabra Dental Products), INSTAT MCH (Ethicon)	Microfibrillar collagen (bovine skin); use directly out of box	Binds tightly to blood surfaces, so a dry area is not necessary. Causes minimal swelling compared with Gelfoam; absorbable in 3 months	Causes a foreign body reaction and granulation formation
Sutures	Closing a flap with evidence of bleeding	Any suture material	If there is no open flap

the fibers in blood clots. The most commonly used antifibrinolytic that is easier to obtain from a pharmacy is aminocaproic acid (Amicar). Tranexamic acid (Cyklokapron) is also available but more difficult to obtain. Since these agents are usually not part of the normal stock, it is advisable to notify the pharmacy to have these agents on hand ahead of time. Tranexamic acid can be used along with DDAVP or factor concentrates for oral surgery or mouth bleeding events. A dose of 25 mg/kg orally, every 8 h for 10 days, is required to prevent fibrinolysis and allow wound healing. A 5% solution of tranexamic acid mouthwash made from the intravenous preparation can effectively prevent local bleeding in minor oral cavity bleeding. Aminocaproic acid is another antifibrinolytic agent currently in use. The dose is 50–100 mg/kg every 4–6 h for 7–10 days (maximum 24 g/24 h).

Dental notes: Bleeding disorders (Gupta *et al.* 2007)

1. Always obtain a medical consult and recent blood count and clotting profiles. Consultation with the patient's physician is recommended.
2. Obtain a thorough medical/family history and ask the patient about previous nose bleeding events, spontaneous gingival bleeding, prolonged bleeding after extractions, and family members with bleeding disorders.
3. A complete medication history is important noting the use of aspirin (low dose) and anticoagulants.
4. Patients with petechiae, ecchymoses, hematomas, or excessive/spontaneous gingival bleeding should be suspected of having a bleeding disorder, and referral to a physician is recommended.
5. It must be decided whether the dental procedure will be done in private office or hospital setting with general anesthesia.
6. Table 10.5 reviews the protocol for the medical management of bleeding disorders.
7. Table 10.6 reviews the dental management of patients with bleeding disorders.
8. Coagulation disorders: Bleeding management options depend on the clinical condition of the patient and the type of vWD that is diagnosed (Type I, II, or III) and hemophilia.
9. Platelet disorders: Surgical bleeding will usually not occur with >50,000 cells/mm³ platelets. Spontaneous bleeding usually occurs at <10,000–20,000 circulating platelets (Patton and Ship 1994).
10. A platelet transfusion is necessary when platelet counts are <50,000 (Radmand *et al.* 2013).
11. Patients with reversible, transient thrombocytopenia should have elective dental treatment postponed until there is a platelet count of >50,000 cells/mm³.
12. Patients with irreversible thrombocytopenia require platelet transfusions with counts of <50,000 cells/mm³. One unit of platelets increases the count by 6,000 cells/mm³; usually, a six-unit pack is transfused (Patton and Ship 1994).
13. Recommend to start with an antifibrinolytic agent such as E-aminocaproic acid (Amicar) immediately after dental surgery in patients with thrombocytopenia. Call the pharmacy ahead of time because most pharmacies do not normally stock Amicar. The patient should come for the surgery with Amicar.
14. Post-extraction instructions: Avoid spitting and sucking on a straw for 24 h.
15. Avoid recommending or prescribing analgesics with antiplatelet effects including aspirin and NSAIDs (e.g., naproxen and ibuprofen).

(*continued*)

16. Local anesthesia: Use infiltration and intraligamentary injections rather than nerve blocks; use of epinephrine is not contraindicated unless for other medical reasons.

17. Patients may have poor oral hygiene because they are afraid of trauma to and bleeding of the oral tissues from toothbrushing and flossing. Reinforcement of oral hygiene as well as periodontal disease monitoring are important (Urdaneta *et al*. 2008). Oral hygiene methods may need to be modified in patients with <20,000 cells/mm^3 due to increased risk of gingival bleeding (Patton and Ship 1994). Adjunctive chlorhexidine rinse may be helpful.

Summary of dental management of patients taking antiplatelet/anticoagulant drugs
(Rada 2006)

1. Bleeding should be suspected in patients that have thrombocytopenia, hemophilia, vWD, and end-stage liver disease. In addition, bleeding is anticipated in patients taking anticoagulants and antiplatelet drugs. Be prepared because these patients will bleed and you might not know if the bleeding could be controlled or not. Use local medicinal products/drugs to assist in controlling surgical and postsurgical bleeding.

2. Patients taking "low-dose" aspirin or other antiplatelet drugs [(e.g., clopidogrel (Plavix) and ticlopidine (Ticlid)]: Although there may be an increased chance of bleeding during dental procedures, most studies show there is no significant difference in perioperative or postoperative bleeding in patients taking aspirin (Ardekian *et al*. 2000). As such, many articles have *recommended that it is not advisable to discontinue taking these medications* 7–10 days before surgery as this could result in a more serious medical event (Lockhart *et al*. 2003; Brennan *et al*. 2008). The decision on the dental management of antiplatelet drug–receiving patients needs to be individualized distinguishing between local bleeding in low-risk patients and patients at high risk with associated comorbidities (Konstantinos *et al*. 2012). In fact, most patients with bleeding problems may have a comorbidity that is overlooked by the dentist (Lockhart *et al*. 2003).

3. Dual antiplatelet drugs: Aspirin plus another antiplatelet drug have been shown to reduce cardiac events after coronary stenting. The hazards of premature discontinuation must be stressed, and it is recommended to postpone elective surgery for 1 year; and if surgery cannot be deferred, consider the continuation of aspirin during the perioperative period in high-risk patients (Grines *et al*. 2007).

4. If the patient is taking warfarin, the decision whether to keep them on warfarin depends on the overall risk of bleeding and the general welfare of the patient. The question to ask is what is the risk vs. the benefit? Patients with deep vein thrombosis have a lower risk of bleeding than patients with a prosthetic heart valve or previous heart attack. Consult with the physician.
   - Obtain INR value within 24 h of invasive dental procedure. If patient has been on warfarin for a long time and has a stable INR, then a value from 2 to 4 weeks is acceptable.
   - The ACCP does not recommend discontinuing warfarin for minor dental procedures due to increased risk of developing a thromboembolic event. Consult with the patient's cardiologist.
      1. A 70 kg adult man has a 7%/5 l blood volume. The severity of hemorrhaging may help the practitioner to decide if the patient needs to go to the hospital to control bleeding. The severity of bleeding is divided into four classes (Gutierrez *et al*. 2004; Mehran *et al*. 2011; http://www.fpnotebook.com/mobile/ER/Exam/HmrhgClsfctn.htm):
   - Class I hemorrhage (minimal blood loss): <750 ml (<15%); vital signs are not changed.
   - Class II hemorrhage (mild blood loss): 750–1500 ml (15–30%); BP not elevated; mild tachycardia.

- Class III hemorrhage (moderate blood loss): 1500–2000 ml (30–40%); hypotension/tachycardia.
- Class IV hemorrhage (severe blood loss): >2000 ml (>40%); severe hypotension, tachycardia, and coma.

2. The decision whether to activate emergency services in a patient who is bleeding depends on whether the bleeding is significant. For example, if bleeding has been occurring for several hours after the dental procedure but still blood clots or bleeding stops after pressure is applied in 15 min intervals, there is little concern.

Table 10.5   Medical/drug management of patients with bleeding disorders (Patton 2003; Gupta *et al.* 2007).

Bleeding disorder	Management
Thrombocytopenia	Medical consult with hematologist Review platelet count at least 2 days before dental treatment If platelet count is <50,000, platelet transfusion is necessary for invasive (bleeding) dental procedures (e.g., extractions); transfusion is done the morning of the day of the extraction Other aids for bleeding control: pressure packs and hemostatic and antifibrinolytic agents such as E-aminocaproic acid rinse (see Table 10.4) Avoid aspirin and nonsteroidal anti-inflammatory drugs (NSAIDs)
von Willebrand disease	Consult with hematologist. DDAVP before surgery/factor VIII replacement Local measures to control bleeding. Use of hemostatic agents to control bleeding Avoid aspirin and NSAIDs
Hemophilia	Consult with hematologist Hemophilia A: increase factor VIII levels; replace recombinant (genetically manufactured not from human or animal) and plasma-derived factor VIII DDAVP for a transient increase in factor VIII Antifibrinolytic (inhibits fibrinolysis) (e.g., E-aminocaproic acid rinse), postoperative (3 days) to protect the formed blood clot Good/less tissue trauma surgical technique Use of hemostatic agents Avoid aspirin and NSAIDs
Severe liver disease	Consult with hepatologist Platelet counts; may require platelet transfusion the morning of the dental procedure (e.g., extractions) Careful recommending/prescribing acetaminophen products
Antiplatelet drugs: Aspirin Clopidogrel (Plavix)	Prepare for bleeding during surgery; use pressure until hemostasis is achieved

(continued)

Table 10.5   *(cont'd)*

Bleeding disorder	Management
Ticlopidine (Ticlid) Prasugrel (Effient) Abciximab (ReoPro) Dipyridamole (Persantine) Aspirin–dipyridamole (Aggrenox).	International normalized ratio (INR) does not measure antiplatelet drug bleeding Do not prescribe any medication containing aspirin or NSAIDs
Anticoagulant drugs: Warfarin (Coumadin) Apixaban (Eliquis) Dabigatran (Pradaxa) Rivaroxaban (Xarelto)	Get an INR within 24 h, but not more than 72 h, of the invasive dental procedure (e.g., scaling/root planing, extractions, implant and periodontal surgery). Obtain primary closure No INR is required for Eliquis, Pradaxa, or Xarelto Use postsurgery hemostatic measures including pressure with gauze Do not prescribe any medication containing aspirin or NSAIDs

Table 10.6   Dental discipline management of the patient with bleeding disorders (Gupta *et al.* 2007).

Dental procedure	Management
Local anesthesia	Patients with bleeding disorders should not be administered local anesthesia nerve block injection unless there is no other alternative for anesthesia and antibiotic prophylaxis is given. There is a high risk for hematoma when the anesthetic solution is deposited into a highly vascularized area (Nazif 1970; Gupta *et al.* 2007). Recommend infiltration anesthesia An inferior alveolar nerve block can cause major swelling, pain, dysphasia, respiratory obstruction, and even asphyxia (Bogdan *et al.* 1994; Gupta *et al.* 2007) Use infiltration and intraligamentary injections rather than nerve blocks Use of epinephrine is not contraindicated unless for other medical reasons General anesthesia in a hospital setting is an option
Periodontics	Optimum oral hygiene is of utmost importance. Bleeding may occur during toothbrushing and use of interdental devices. Reassure patient about bleeding that they will experience. Recommend chlorhexidine rinses starting one week before periodontal debridement No factor replacement or platelet transfusion is needed for periodontal probing and oral prophylaxis (supragingival scaling) and polishing Subgingival scaling/root planing also usually does not require factor replacement if procedure is done carefully (Gupta *et al.* 2007) A preprocedural rinse using chlorhexidine gluconate is helpful to reduce gingival inflammation (Gupta *et al.* 2007) Periodontal and implant surgery will require factor replacement Use local and hemostatic agents to control bleeding (Table 10.4)

Table 10.6   *(cont'd)*

Dental procedure	Management
Oral surgery	The greatest potential for bleeding Pre-operative factor levels should be at least 40–50% of normal activity to reduce bleeding but best to get 50–100% (Patton 2003) In some cases, postoperative factor replacement may be necessary Postoperative bleeding due to fibrinolysis usually occurs 3–5 days after surgery and can be controlled by local methods or antifibrinolytic agents (Table 10.4). Consult with hematologist before surgery
Endodontics	Intraligamentary injections are acceptable If a choice to extract or do endodontics, do endodontics Care with placement of clamp for rubber dam and use of saliva ejectors on floor of mouth Some endodontic procedures may require factor replacement; consult with hematologist
Operative/restorative/ prosthodontics	Restorative procedures will not usually cause any significant bleeding; careful with clamp placement and use of saliva ejector Make sure dental prosthesis is not irritating or traumatizing gingiva or mucosa
Orthodontics	No factor replacement is necessary Avoid tissue trauma from wires

References

Adeyemo, T.A., Adeyemo, W.L., Adediran, A., *et al.* (2011) Orofacial manifestations of hematological disorders: anemia and hemostatic disorders. *Indian Journal of Dental Research*, **22**, 454–461.

Ardekian, L., Gaspar, R., Peled, M., *et al.* (2000) Does low-dose aspirin therapy complicate oral surgical procedures? *Journal of the American Dental Association*, **131** (**3**), 331–335.

Balevi, B. (2010) Should warfarin be discontinued before a dental extraction? A decision-tree analysis. *Oral Surgery Oral Medicine Oral Pathology Oral Radiology Endodontology*, **110**, 691–697.

Benson, G.D., Koff, R.S., & Tolman, K.G. (2005) The therapeutic use of acetaminophen in patients with liver disease. *American Journal of Therapeutics*, **12** (**2**), 133–141.

Berger, J.S., Brown, D.L., & Becker, R.C. (2008) Low-dose aspirin in patients with stable cardiovascular disease: a meta-analysis. *American Journal of Medicine*, **121** (**1**), 43–49.

Bogan, C.J., Strauss, M., & Ratnoff, O.D. (1994) Airway obstruction in hemophilia (factor VIII deficiency): a 28-year institutional review. *Laryngoscope*, **104**, 789–794.

Brennan, M.T., Valerin, M.A., Noll, J.L., *et al.* (2008) Aspirin use and post-operative bleeding from dental extractions. *Journal of Dental Research*, **87**, 740–744.

Brewer, A. & Correa, M.E. (2006) The World Federation of Hemophila Guidelines for dental treatment of patients with inherited bleeding disorders. *Haemophilia*, **40**, 1–13.

D'Amato-Palumbo (2012) www. dental care.com Continuing education course. http://media.dentalcare.com/media/en-us/education/ce319/ce319.pdf [accessed February 2, 2014].

Dean, R.P. & Talbert, R.L. (1980) Bleeding associated with concurrent warfarin and metronidazole therapy. *Drug Intelligence & Clinical Pharmacy*, **14**, 864–866.

Douketis, J.D., Berger, P.B., Dunn, A.S., *et al.* (2008) The perioperative management of antithrombotic therapy: American College of Chest Physicians Evidence-Based Clinical Practice Guidelines (8th edition). *Chest*, **133** (**6 Suppl.**), 299S–339S.

Eisenstein, D.H. (2012) Anticoagulation management in the ambulatory surgical setting. *Association of Perioperative Registered Nurses*, **95** (**4**), 510–521.

Federici, A.B. (1998) Diagnosis of von Willebrand disease. *Haemophilia*, **4**, 654–660.

Ferraris, V.A., Saha, S.P., Oestreich, J.H., *et al*. (2012) Update to the Society of Thoracic Surgeons guideline on use of antiplatelet drugs in patients having cardiac and noncardiac operations. *Annuals of Thoracic Surgery*, **94** (**5**), 1761–1781.

Fong Liu, J., Srivastsa, A., & Kaul, V. (2010) Black licorice ingestion: yet another confounding agent in patients with melena. *World Journal of Gastrointestinal Surgery*, **272** (**10**), 30–31.

Frachon, X., Pommereuil, M., Berthier, A.M., *et al*. (2005) Management options for dental extraction in hemophiliacs: a study of 55 extractions (2000-2002). *Oral Surgery Oral Medicine Oral Pathology Oral Radiology Endodontics*, **99** (**3**), 270–275.

Garcia, D.A., Regan, S., Henault, L.E., *et al*. (2008) Risk of thromboembolism with short-term interruption of warfarin therapy. *Archive of Internal Medicine*, **168** (**1**), 63–69.

Glasheen, J.J., Fugit, R.V., & Prochazka, A.V. (2005) The risk of overanticoagulation with antibiotic use in outpatients on stable warfarin regimens. *Journal of General Internal Medicine*, **20**, 653–656.

Goldhaber, S.Z. (2006) "Bridging" and mechanical heart valves. Perils, promises, and predictions. *Circulation*, **113**, 470–472.

Grines, C.L., Bonow, R.O., Casey, D.E. Jr., *et al*. (2007) Prevention of premature discontinuation of dual antiplatelet therapy in patients with coronary artery stents: a science advisory from the American Heart Association, American College of Cardiology, Society for Cardiovascular Angiography and Interventions, American College of Surgeons, and American Dental Association, with representation from the American College of Physicians. *Circulation*, **115**, 813–818.

Gupta, A, Epstein, J.B., & Cabay, R.J. (2007) Bleeding disorders of importance in dental care and related patient management. *Journal of the Canadian Dental Association*, **73**, 77–83.

Gutierrez, G., Reines, H.D., & Wulf-Gutierrez, M.E. (2004) Clinical review: hemorrhagic shock. *Critical Care*, **8**, 373–381.

Herman, W., Konzelman, Jr., J., & Sutley, S. (1997) Current perspectives on dental patients receiving coumarin anticoagulant therapy. *Journal of the American Dental Association*, **128**, 327–335.

Hirsh, J., Fuster, V., Ansell, J., *et al*. (2003) American Heart Association/American College of Cardiology Foundation Guide to Warfarin Therapy. *Circulation*, **107**, 1692–1711.

Horton, J.D. & Buswick, B.M. (1999) Warfarin therapy: evolving strategies in anticoagulation. *American Family Physician*, **59**, 365–646.

Huff, C. (2012) New drugs could improve anticoagulation rates. *American College of Physicians*, April. www.acpinternist.org/archieves/2012/04/anticoagulation.htm (accessed on July 17, 2014).

Hughes, G.J., Patel, P.N., & Saxena, N. (2011) Effect of acetaminophen on international normalized ratio in patients receiving warfarin therapy. *Pharmacotherapy*, **31**, 591–597.

Israels, S., Schwetz, N., Boyar, R., *et al*. (2006) Bleeding disorders: characterization, dental considerations and management. *Journal of the Canadian Dental Association*, **72**, 827–840.

Jeske, A. & Suchko, G. (2003) Lack of a scientific basis for routine discontinuation of oral anticoagulation therapy before dental treatment. *Journal of the American Dental Association*, **134**, 1492–1497.

Kitchen, S. & Preston, F.E. (1999) Standardization of prothrombin time for laboratory control of oral anticoagulant therapy. *Seminars in Thrombosis and Hemostasis*, **25**, 17–25.

Klaassen, R.J. & Halton, J.M. (2002) The diagnosis and treatment of von Willebrand disease in children. *Paediatrics & Children Health*, **7** (**4**), 245–249.

Konstantinos, K.C, Lillis, T., Tsirlis, A., *et al*. (2012) Dental management of antiplatelet-receiving patients: is uninterrupted antiplatelet therapy safe? *Angiology*, **63**, 245–247.

Kujovich, J.L. (2005) Hemostatic effects in end stage liver disease. *Critical Care Clinic*, **21**, 563–587.

Lockhart, P.B., Gibson, J., Pond, H., *et al*. (2003) Dental management considerations for the patient with an acquired coagulopathy (from drugs). *British Dental Journal*, **195**, 123–130.

Lukes, S.M. (2012) Detecting hereditary hemorrhagic telangiectasia. *Dimensions of Dental Hygiene*, April. p 48–51. http://www.dimensionsofdentalhygiene.com/ddhright.aspx?id=13035 [accessed on July 26, 2014].

Mann, M. & Grimes, E.B. (2011) Treating patients with immune thrombocytopenia purpura. *Dimensions of Dental Hygiene*, **9** (**8**), 20–23.

Mannucci, P.M. (1988) Desmopressin: a nontransfusional form of treatment for congenital and acquired bleeding disorders. *Blood*, **72** (**5**), 1449–1455.

McBee, W.L. & Koerner, K.R. (2005) Review of hemostatic agents used in dentistry. *Dentistry Today*, **24**, 62–65.

Mehran, R., Rao, S.V., & Bhatt, D.L. (2011) Standardized bleeding definitions for cardiovascular clinical trials. A consensus report from the Bleeding Academic Research Consortium. *Circulation*, **123**, 2736–2747.

Mori, T., Asano, M., Ohtake, H., *et al.* (2002) Anticoagulant therapy after prosthetic valve replacement-optimal PT-INR in Japanese patients. *Annals of Thoracic and Cardiovascular Surgery*, **8** (**2**), 83–87.

Morimoto, Y., Niwa, H., & Minematsu, K. (2009) Hemostatic management for periodontal treatments in patients on oral antithrombotic therapy: a retrospective study. *Oral Surgery Oral Medicine Oral Pathology Oral Radiology Endodontology*, **108**, 889–896.

Nazif, M. (1970) Local anesthesia for patients with hemophilia. *ASDC Journal of Dentistry for Children*, **37**, 79–84.

Neunert, C., Lim, W., Crowther, M., *et al.* (2011) American Society of Hematology. The American Society of Hematology 2011 evidence-based practice guideline for immune thrombocytopenia. *Blood*, **117** (**16**), 4190–4207.

Patton, L.L. (2003) Bleeding and clotting disorders. In: *Burket's Oral Medicine: Diagnosis and Treatment*, 10th ed., pp. 454–477. BC Decker, Hamilton, ON.

Patton, L.L. & Ship, J.A. (1994) Treatment of patients with bleeding disorders. *Dental Clinics of North America*, **38**, 465–482.

Peisker, A., Raschke, G.F., & Schultze-Mosgau, S. (2013) Management of dental extractions in patients with haemophilia A and B: a report of 58 extractions. *Medicina Oral Patologia Oral y Cirugia Bucal*, **19**, e55–e60.

Pengo, V., Cucchini, U., Denas, G., *et al.* (1999) Standardized low-molecular-weight heparin bridging regimen in outpatients on oral anticoagulants undergoing invasive procedure or surgery. *Circulation*, **119**, 2920–2927.

Posan, E., McBane, R.D., Grill, D.E., *et al.* (2003) Comparison of PFA-100 testing and bleeding time for detecting platelet hypofunction and von Willebrand disease in clinical practice. *Thrombosis & Haemostsis*, **90** (**3**), 483–490.

Pototski, M. & Amenabar, J.M. (2007) Dental management of patients receiving anticoagulation or antiplatelet treatment. *Journal of Oral Sciences*, **49**, 253–258.

Provan, D. & Newland, A.C. (2003) Acquired disorders affecting megakaryocytes and platelets. In: Wickramasingher, S.N. & McCullough, J., eds. *Blood and Bone Marrow Pathology*, pp. 525–555. Elsevier Science Limited, London.

Rada, R.E. (2006) Management of the dental patient on anticoagulant medication. *Dentistry Today*, **125** (**8**), 58–63.

Radmand, R., Schilsky, M., Jakab, S., *et al.* (2013) Pre-liver transplant protocols in dentistry. *Oral Surgery Oral Medicine Oral Pathology Oral Radiology, Endodontology*, **115**, 426–430.

Sadler, J.E., Mannucci, P.M., Berntorp, E., *et al.* (2000) Impact, diagnosis and treatment of von Willebrand disease. *Thrombosis and Haemostasis*, **84**, 160–174.

Sandor, G. (2004) Do patients taking oral anticoagulants need to discontinue their medication before surgical procedures? *Journal of the Canadian Dental Association*, **70**, 482–483.

Scully, C. & Wolff, A. (2002) Oral surgery in patients on anticoagulant therapy. *Oral Surgery, Oral Medicine, Oral Pathology, Oral Radiology, Endodontology*, **94**, 57–64.

Sonis, S., Fazio, R., & Fang, L. (2003) *Oral Medicine Secrets*, pp 113–128. Henley and Belfus Inc., Philadelphia.

Srivastava, A., Brewer, A.K., Mauser-Bunschoten, E.P., *et al.* (2013) Guidelines for the management of hemophila. *Haemophilia*, **19**, e1–e47.

Terranova, L., Gerli, G., & Cattaneo, M. (2008) Platelet disorders in the elderly. In: Balducci, L., Ershler, W., & de Gaetano, G., eds. *Blood Disorders in the Elderly*, pp. 420–433. Cambridge University Press, Cambridge.

Urdaneta, M.B., Urdaneta, M.B., Mendez, V.F., *et al.* (2008) Evaluating periodontal conditions in patients with von Willebrand's disease in Hospital Universitario de Maracaibo (University Hospital, Maracaibo)–Venezuela. *Medicina Oral Patologia Oral y Cirugia Bucal*, **13** (**5**), E303–E306.

White, G.C. 2nd, Rosendaal, F., Aledort, L.M., *et al.* (2001) Definitions in hemophilia. Recommendation of the scientific subcommittee on factor VIII and factor IX of the scientific and standardization committee of the International Society on Thrombosis and Haemostasis. *Thrombosis & Haemostasis*, **85**, 560.

Zanon, E., Martinelli, F., Bacci, C., *et al.* (2000) Proposal of a standard approach to dental extraction in haemophilia patients. A case-control study with good results. *Haemophilia*, **6** (**5**), 533–536.

Chapter 11

Blood dyscrasias

A. Red blood cell disorders	174
a. Anemia	174
b. Myeloproliferative disorders	181
B. White blood cell disorders	182
a. Leukemia	182
b. Lymphoma	186
c. Multiple myeloma	187
References	189

Introduction

Blood is composed of cells and plasma, an interstitial fluid. Blood plasma is a pale yellowish liquid containing inorganic salts, carbohydrates such as glucose, fats, minerals, hormones, vitamins, waste matter, proteins (albumin), and fibrinogen (clotting). The majority of blood cells are red blood cells (RBCs; erythrocytes), and the remainder is white blood cells (WBCs; leukocytes) and platelets (thrombocytes).

Blood cells make up about 45% of the volume of blood with the remainder being plasma (Table 11.1). The average Hct is 45% (lower in women). The *hematocrit* measures the volume or percentage of RBCs in total blood volume (RBCs and plasma) (Billett 1990). *Hemoglobin (Hgb) is the molecule in the RBC that carries oxygen.* The life span of an RBC is about 120 days, and the number averages about 5 million/mm^3 (lower in women). The number of RBCs is kept constant, and if the number is increased or decreased for any reason, a compensatory adjustment occurs. Erythropoiesis is the process by which new red cells are formed in the bone marrow to make up for losses and normal destruction. Table 11.1 reviews normal complete blood count (CBC) with differential, which measures the percentage of each type of WBC.

The following list shows the conditions and diseases related to the different percentages of WBCs (http://www.nlm.nih.gov/medlineplus/ency/article/003657.htm; http://www.nlm.nih.gov/medlineplus/ency/article/003644.htm).

Neutrophils:
Increased percentage:

- Acute infection
- Acute stress

The Dentist's Quick Guide to Medical Conditions, First Edition. Mea A. Weinberg, Stuart L. Segelnick, Joseph S. Insler, with Samuel Kramer.
© 2015 John Wiley & Sons, Inc. Published 2015 by John Wiley & Sons, Inc.

Table 11.1   CBC with differential (Beutler and Waalen 2006; Goldman and Schafer 2011).

Blood test	Male	Female	Notes
RBCs	4.7–6.1 million cells/mm^3	4.2–5.4 million cells/mm^3	*Low RBC:* anemia; bone marrow failure (from radiation, tumor); erythropoietin deficiency (secondary to kidney disease); hemolysis (due to transfusion, blood vessel injury); hemorrhage; leukemia; malnutrition; multiple myeloma; deficiencies of iron, folate, and vitamin B$_{12}$ and B$_6$; pregnancy *High RBC:* cigarette smoking, congenital heart disease, dehydration from diarrhea, renal cell carcinoma, hypoxia, PV
Hematocrit (Hct)	40.7–50.3%	36.1–44.3%	*Low Hct:* anemia; bleeding; leukemia; deficiencies of iron, folate, vitamin B$_{12}$, and vitamin B$_6$ *High Hct:* congenital heart disease, dehydration, PV, hypoxia
Hemoglobin (Hgb)	13.8–17.2 g/dl (or about 130 g/dl) (1–2 g less in African–Americans)	12.1–15.1 g/dl (or about 120 g/dl) (1–2 g less in African–Americans)	*Low Hgb*: anemia, kidney disease, cancer *High Hgb*: PV, dehydration, hypoxia
WBCs Neutrophils: 40–60% Lymphocytes: 20–40% Monocytes: 2–8% Eosinophils: 1–4% Basophils: 0.5–1% Band (young neutrophils): 0–3%	4 500–10,000 cells/mcl	4 500–10,000 cells/mcl	*Low WBCs:* bone marrow deficiency or failure, systemic lupus erythematosus, liver disease, disease of the spleen, radiation therapy or exposure *High WBCs*: anemia, burns, bone marrow tumors, rheumatoid arthritis, infectious diseases, leukemia

- Gout
- Myelocytic leukemia
- Rheumatoid arthritis
- Rheumatic fever
- Thyroiditis
- Trauma

Decreased percentage:

- Aplastic anemia
- Chemotherapy
- Influenza or other viral infection
- Widespread bacterial infection
- Radiation therapy or exposure

Lymphocytes:

Increased percentage:

- Chronic bacterial infection
- Infectious hepatitis
- Infectious mononucleosis
- Lymphocytic leukemia
- Multiple myeloma
- Viral infection (such as infectious mononucleosis, mumps, and measles)

Decreased percentage:

- Chemotherapy
- HIV infection
- Leukemia
- Radiation therapy or exposure
- Sepsis

Monocytes:

Increased percentage:

- Chronic inflammatory disease
- Parasitic infection
- Tuberculosis
- Viral infection (e.g., infectious mononucleosis, mumps, and measles)

Eosinophils:

Increased percentage:

- Allergic reaction
- Cancer
- Collagen vascular disease
- Parasitic infection

Basophils:

Decreased percentage:

- Acute allergic reaction

A. Red blood cell disorders

a. Anemia

Anemia literally means "lack of blood" and is usually classified according to its etiology such as a decrease in the number, size, or function of RBCs; excessive blood loss; a deficiency of Hgb or Hct; a deficiency in absorption of iron, vitamin B_{12}, or folic acid; destruction of red cells; or structurally abnormal Hgb. With a shortage of Hgb, there is less oxygen delivered from lungs to capillaries, resulting in hypoxia and many classic signs and symptoms.

Hgb estimates the erythrocyte function and is more stable to plasma volume changes such as dehydration, which makes it more reliable for the assessment of anemia; however, in many settings, automated methods for Hgb determination are not available and rough values are estimated using observed Hct levels, which is a simpler and cheaper approach. So, both Hgb and Hct work together and both levels must be evaluated for the diagnosis of anemia (Quinto *et al.* 2006).

Diagnosing anemia

Though anemia of chronic disease (ACD) is the most common cause of anemias, there are still many more etiologies to account for the various anemias (Brill and Baumgardner 2000).

There are two general methodologies to recognizing the causes of anemia: identifying the mechanisms responsible for a decrease in Hgb concentration and classifying anemia according to the variation in size of the RBC (e.g., the mean corpuscular volume [MCV]). MCV is the average volume of RBC in a specimen (Schrier 2013).

The first method utilizes the approach that the cause of anemia is a result of one or more of the three mechanisms: excessive blood loss, a decreased RBC production, and an increased RBC destruction (Tefferi 2003; Schrier 2013). Mature RBCs circulate for about 110–120 days and are then removed from the circulation by macrophages. A decreased production of RBCs may be due to the body failing to make enough new RBCs or a lack of nutrients including iron, vitamin B_{12}, or folate. Increased RBC destruction due to hemolysis occurs when the life span of an RBC is <100 days (Schrier 2013). This can be due to an inherited hemolytic anemia (e.g., thalassemia major and sickle cell disease (SCD)) or acquired hemolytic anemia (e.g., malaria and thrombotic thrombocytopenia purpura) (Schrier 2013).

The second approach to recognize the causes of anemia focuses on the variation in size of the RBC. Anemia is classified according to the MCV measurement as microcytic anemia (MCV is below normal; small average RBC size), macrocytic anemia (MCV is above normal; large average RBC size), or normocytic anemia (MCV is within normal). Table 11.2 describes the most common causes of the different types of anemia. The three most common causes of microcytosis in clinical practice are iron deficiency, alpha or beta thalassemia minor, and (less often) the anemia of inflammation (ACD).

Anemia and its symptoms can also be classified as mild, moderate, or severe. Symptoms, when they occur, are usually due to the underlying etiology of blood loss, destruction, or underproduction of RBCs (Carley 2003). Mild anemia, Hgb 9.5–11 g/dl, is often asymptomatic. Moderate anemia, Hgb 8–9.5 g/dl, may present with other symptoms and usually requires treatment to prevent long-term complications. Severe anemia, Hgb <8 g/dl, will require further workup and immediate treatment and could be life-threatening (http://www.medscape.com/viewarticle/457482; Abshire 2001; Lesperance *et al.* 2002; Segel *et al.* 2002; Tender and Cheng 2002).

Many individuals may be functionally anemic despite having Hct and Hgb levels within the acceptable range. For example, chronic pulmonary or cardiac disease may create increased oxygen demands due to increased need for oxygen or impaired oxygen utilization and symptoms traditionally suggestive of anemia (Segel *et al.* 2002; Carley 2003).

Table 11.2 Common causes of anemia (Tefferi *et al.* 2005; Chulilla *et al.* 2009; Schrier 2013).

RBC indices (size and shape of RBCs):	Normal values:	
		Low MCV (<80 fl) (microcytosis or microcytic anemia): iron deficiency, hereditary thalassemia, lead poisoning, anemia of chronic disorders
MCV: determines the classification of anemia as microcytic, macrocytic, or normocytic	MCV: 80–100 fl	*High MCV (>100 fl) (macrocytosis or macrocytic anemia)*: alcohol abuse, folate and vitamin B_{12} deficiency (pernicious anemia), acute myeloid leukemias, reticulocytosis (hemolytic anemia, response to blood loss), liver failure, drug-induced anemia (e.g., chemotherapeutics and hydroxyurea)
		Normal MCV (80–100 fl) (normocytosis or normocytic anemia): excessive, acute blood loss; bone marrow suppression; early iron deficiency; chronic renal failure; sickle cell anemia; anemia due to inflammation, infection, or malignancy; hemolytic anemia
MCH	MCH: 26–33 picograms/cell	*High >33*: Macrocytic anemia *Low <26*: Microcytic anemia
MCV	82–98 fl	*High >98:* Macrocytic anemia *Low <80:* Microcytic anemia

Laboratory evaluation

When evaluating for anemia, a CBC with WBC differential and RBC indices including Hgb, Hct, MCV, mean corpuscular hemoglobin (MCH), and mean corpuscular hemoglobin concentration (MCHC) should be ordered.

The MCV measures the average RBC volume and the MCH determines the mean Hgb per erythrocyte. So, MCV and MCH increase (macrocytic) and decrease (microcytic) equally (Chulilla *et al.* 2009). The MCHC measures the concentration of Hgb in a volume of packed RBCs and increases in only a few rare diseases (Chulilla *et al.* 2009).

The reticulocyte count measures how fast immature RBCs or reticulocytes are synthesized in the bone marrow and helps to distinguish among the different types of anemia. For example, anemia with a high reticulocyte count indicates blood loss and the one with a low reticulocyte count is indicative of a decreased production of RBCs (Schrier 2013).

Summary of anemia

Microcytic anemia

Iron-deficiency anemia (IDA): It is more common in women than men and the most common cause of microcytosis in the USA (Van Vranken 2010). A number of factors contribute to developing IDA including a reduction in RBC production due to a deficiency in iron intake or absorption, pregnancy, or most frequently overt or occult chronic slow bleeding. Microcytosis is often an incidental finding when a blood test is taken (Van Vranken 2010).

The required daily intake of iron in menstruating women is 2–3 mg and in men is 0.5–1.0 mg (http://www.uptodate.com/contents/causes-and-diagnosis-of-iron-deficiency-anemia-in-the-adult/abstract/5). The regulation of normal iron levels in the body is through absorption, not excretion of iron (Killip *et al.* 2007). This absorption is regulated by the production of new RBCs and the degree of saturation of the spleen, liver, and bone marrow, which are the iron-storage centers in the body. Ferritin is a protein that reflects iron stores in the body. A definitive diagnosis of iron-deficiency anemia is made when serum ferritin levels are decreased and MVC <80 fl (Chulilla *et al.* 2009). In the blood plasma, iron is bound to transferrin, a protein carrier. Total iron-binding capacity (TIBC), a test that measures the blood's capacity to bind iron with transferrin, can be used in differentiating iron-deficiency anemia and ACD when the serum iron level is decreased (Van Vranken 2009).

Anemia is usually detected by routine laboratory screening performed before the patient is symptomatic. Symptoms usually do not appear until the anemia worsens with an Hct <20% and Hgb <7 g/dl. Few symptoms are seen early in the condition. The first sign and symptom a patient usually has is weakness or fatigue, due to low Hgb levels, which causes hypoxia and triggers compensating mechanisms (Chulilla *et al.* 2009). Clinically evident may be pallor of the face, nail beds and conjunctivae; spooning of the nail beds (koilonychias); and glossitis (inflamed/red tongue) (Billett 1990). Additionally, there is altered taste sensation, angular cheilitis, gingival bleeding, post-extraction bleeding, and a few reported cases of periodontal disease (Hutter *et al.* 2001; Adeyemo *et al.* 2011; http://www.ncbi.nlm.nih.gov/pubmed/?term=Hatipoglu%20H%5Bauth%5D, H., http://www.ncbi.nlm.nih.gov/pubmed/?term=Hatipoglu%20MG%5Bauth%5D,M.G., http://www.ncbi.nlm.nih.gov/pubmed/?term=Cagirankaya%20LB%5Bauth%5D 2012). Other non-oral signs/symptoms include resting tachycardia, angina, and orthostatic hypotension.

Treatment begins with eliminating the cause. In children IDA is usually related to a nutritional deficiency and in menstruating women to menstrual blood loss. In men and nonmenstruating women, iron loss can be due to occult bleeding in the gastrointestinal (GI) tract (e.g., malignancy and ulcers) (Hershko and Skikne 2009; Van Vranken 2013). Drug-induced IDA is common with NSAIDs, aspirin, and corticosteroids. The next phase is iron replacement, specifically ferrous sulfate tablets (dose for adults: 300 mg bid–qid). A common adverse side effect of ferrous sulfate is black-colored feces.

Plummer–Vinson syndrome

Plummer–Vinson syndrome is a symptom complex caused by iron deficiency (Hoffman and Jaffe 1995). It presents as a classic triad of chronic iron deficiency, dysphagia, and esophageal web (due to mucous membrane formation) (Novacek 2006). There is also a predisposition to develop oropharyngeal cancer, which comes from the degenerative changes in the oral mucosa of the oral cavity, pharynx, and esophagus (Lawoyin *et al.* 2006). Clinically, all features of iron-deficiency anemia are present in Plummer–Vinson syndrome including glossitis (sore, red/fiery tongue), tongue ulcers, and depapillated atrophic tongue (Lawoyin *et al.* 2006).

Thalassemia

Microcytic anemia associated with normal serum levels is most likely hereditary thalassemia. In this anemia, the body synthesizes a defective form of Hgb. Thalassemia includes a variety of diseases characterized by decreased or absent production of alpha and/or beta globin chains of Hgb A, the major Hgb in adults (Adams and Coleman 1990). Thalassemia is classified as minor, intermedia, and major. Most adults with alpha or beta thalassemia minor are asymptomatic and may be diagnosed because of the presence of microcytic, hypochromic red cells, with or without minor degrees of anemia (Benz 2013). Beta thalassemia major (Cooley's anemia) is more common in African–Americans and the people of Mediterranean ancestry and is best diagnosed as increased levels of HgbA2 on hemoglobin electrophoresis or liquid chromatography (HPLC), while molecular methods are usually required for the diagnosis of the alpha thalassemia variants (Henderson *et al.* 2009; Van Vranken 2010). These individuals show the most soft and hard orofacial deformities starting at birth and the worst prognosis (Van Vranken 2010; Amini *et al.* 2013). Alpha thalassemia is caused by an underproduction of alpha globin chains and is usually seen in people of African or Southeast Asian ancestry (Van Vranken 2010).

Macrocytic anemia

Macrocytosis or macrocytic anemia is diagnosed with a MCV >100 fl. Macrocytic anemias are classified as megaloblastic anemias, which are those resulting from disorders of DNA synthesis of erythrocyte precursors in bone marrow, and nonmegaloblastic anemias, which are caused primarily by alcoholism, liver disease, and hypothyroidism. A blood smear should be performed to differentiate the two anemias (Davenport 1996). The most common causes of macrocytosis include alcohol abuse, vitamin B_{12} and folate deficiencies, and medications (e.g., HIV antiretroviral drugs, isoniazid, methotrexate, Dilantin, metformin, nitrous oxide, and NSAIDs) (Savage *et al.* 2000; Aslinia *et al.* 2006; Kaferle and Strzoda 2009).

Vitamin B_{12} deficiency
Hemoglobin is produced in the bone marrow from amino acids and iron, which requires vitamin B_{12} found in various foods such as eggs, milk, cheese, and liver. Once ingested, vitamin B_{12} is absorbed in the small intestine with the help of intrinsic factor, a protein formed in the lining of the stomach. Once absorbed, it is stored in the liver and then released as needed. Vitamin B_{12} is required for RBC formation and nuclear growth and division of cells. In order for this to happen, there must be adequate supply of vitamin B_{12} and adequate secretion of intrinsic factor. Vitamin B_{12} deficiency occurs when the mucous membrane of the stomach is defective and unable to produce intrinsic factor.

Causes of vitamin B_{12} deficiency include the following: (i) inadequately supplied in the diet especially in strict vegetarians; (ii) pernicious anemia; (iii) Addison's disease; (iv) lowered production of intrinsic factor causing a reduced absorption of the vitamin; (v) surgical resection of the stomach, ileum, or small intestine; (vi) Celiac disease; (vii) Crohn's disease; (viii) chronic intake of H_2-receptor antagonists and proton pump inhibitors (antiulcer medications); and (ix) parasitic infection (e.g., tapeworm), causing the breakdown of the vitamin in the intestine (Davenport 1996; Adeyemo *et al.* 2011).

Oral signs and symptoms
Vitamin B_{12} deficiency shows in the oral cavity as part of megaloblastic changes occurring in the GI (Adeyemo *et al.* 2011). Oral signs and symptoms of vitamin B_{12} deficiency may be clinically seen in asymptomatic anemic patients (Table 11.2). Other non-oral signs and symptoms include fatigue, shortness of breath, and neurological problems (Pontes *et al.* 2009). There are no dental drug–vitamin B_{12} interactions.

Lab tests/values
A CBC, a peripheral blood smear, and a reticulocyte count are ordered. There will be an elevated HCV, decreased vitamin B_{12} levels, presence of intrinsic antibody levels in the serum, and elevated homocyteine and methylmalonic acid (MMA) blood levels (Ward 2002; Oh and Brown 2003).

Treatment of vitamin B_{12} deficiency involves monthly vitamin B_{12} subcutaneous or intramuscular injections or oral tablets for a lifetime (Oh and Brown 2003). Oral lesions are the first initial signs/symptoms that appear in these patients. It is important to recognize these various oral and non-oral signs and symptoms and refer to a physician before neurologic signs evolve because early recognition and treatment could prevent or reverse the neurologic problems (Pontes *et al.* 2009).

Folic acid deficiency

Folate deficiency is rarely seen today because many food products are fortified with folic acid. Folic acid deficiency does not cause tissue problems the way vitamin B_{12} deficiency does.

Normocytic anemia

In normocytic anemia, Hgb levels are decreased but the MCV is within the reference range between 80 and 100 fl (RBC size is normal) and reticulocytes are <4%. Normocytic anemia is relatively common. Although normocytic anemia commonly results from early iron deficiency or chronic disease, hemoglobinopathies, enzyme defects, RBC membrane defects, G6PD deficiency, and other hemolytic anemias also result in normocytic anemia (Schrier 2013).

The first step in the evaluation of normocytic anemia is determination of the reticulocyte count to distinguish cases of increased RBC turnover, such as hemolysis, from bone marrow disorders. Hemolytic anemias and anemias due to blood loss have elevated reticulocyte counts in the days following an episode but RBC production is not impaired. On the other hand, low reticulocyte count suggests bone marrow hypofunction. Leukemia and aplastic anemia reduce RBC production. A peripheral blood smear is also essential in the evaluation for normocytic anemia because it will determine if there is a subpopulation of RBCs with distinctive size or shape abnormalities (Harrington 2007).

Hemolytic anemia

G6PD: Many of the hemolytic anemias have distinctive peripheral blood features, such as sickle cells in SCD, spherocytes in hereditary spherocytosis and autoimmune hemolytic anemia, schistocytes in microangiopathic hemolytic anemia, and bite cells in glucose-6-phosphate dehydrogenase (G6PD) deficiency (Harrington 2007).

In hemolytic anemia, there is a defect in the RBCs so the body removes them from circulation by hemolysis. The RBCs can no longer carry oxygen through the body so that during a hemolytic crisis the individual will feel fatigue and out of breath. Hemolytic anemia can be inherited or acquired. Intrinsic hemolytic anemia is usually inherited and develops when the RBCs produced by the body are defective. Patients with G6PD deficiency have intrinsic hemolytic anemia. Extrinsic or acquired hemolytic anemia occurs when healthy RBCs are destroyed by the spleen, infection, tumors, or autoimmune diseases (e.g., HIV, hepatitis, and leukemia) (Dhaliwal *et al.* 2004).

G6PD deficiency is the most common human enzyme defect. G6PD deficiency is a genetic disorder characterized by hemolysis of normal RBCs. G6PD is an enzyme that is required for RBCs to function properly. G6PD helps to convert nicotinamide adenine dinucleotide phosphate (NADP) to its reduced form, NADPH, which protects cells from oxidative damage (Frank 2005). It is more common in black than white males and the people of Mediterranean and Middle East (Sephardic Jewish) descent. Acute hemolysis is caused by infection, ingestion of fava beans, or exposure to an oxidative drug (Frank 2005). Drug-induced hemolysis is considered the most common adverse clinical consequence of G6PD deficiency (Youngster *et al.* 2010). Patients most likely already know they have G6PD deficiency and what drugs will trigger a crisis. Hemolytic anemia will only develop in these patients if the individual is exposed to the triggering chemical or drug. The conversion of nicotinamide adenine dinucleotide phosphate to its reduced form in erythrocytes is the basis of diagnostic testing for the deficiency (Frank 2005).

The key to treating a patient with G6PD deficiency is to prevent a hemolytic crisis by avoiding the triggers including infection, certain drugs, and fava beans (Frank 2005). Acute hemolysis is usually self-limiting and requires a blood transfusion in rare severe episodes (Frank 2005). It is controversial which drugs are contraindicated or should be used with precaution. A 2010 evidenced-based review of PubMed articles wrongly classified drugs as contraindicated to give to patients with G6PD deficiency

(Youngster *et al.* 2010). In reality, there are only a few drugs that are contraindicated in these patients (Youngster *et al.* 2010). NSAIDs or aspirin can trigger a hemolytic episode and should not be recommended or prescribed to a patient with G6PD deficiency. Since dental infections can trigger an episode, it is imperative to aggressively treat any dental infection (Sams *et al.* 1990). Penicillins, cephalosporins, and quinolone antibiotics (e.g., ciprofloxacin) should be avoided (Youngster *et al.* 2010). Bisulfites used as a preservative in epinephrine (Dhaliwal *et al.* 2004) should be avoided. It is safest to use a local anesthetic without epinephrine. Acetaminophen in high doses should be avoided but in normal recommended doses is not contraindicated (http://www.g6pd.org/en/g6pddeficiency/SafeUnsafe/LowRisk.aspx).

Sickle cell disease

Sickle cell anemia or SCD is a disease of the erythrocytes caused by an autosomal recessive single-gene defect in the β-globin chain of HbA that produces HbS. The RBCs become hard and sticky and take a "C" or "sickle" shape, which "clogs" the flow, and some cells will die early. Deoxygenation occurs because of the reduced affinity of oxygen to the defective Hgb. This can cause severe pain, infection, and stroke. When an individual inherits one sickle cell gene ("S") from one parent and one normal gene ("A") from the other parent, it is the sickle cell trait. These individuals usually do not have any of the signs of the disease and live a normal life, but they can pass the trait on to their children. Clinical features of the disease are first evident between 6 months and 3 years of age (Ramakrishna 2007). Triggers of vaso-occlusive crisis include hypoxia, dehydration, changes in body temperature, and infections including endodontic and periodontal abscesses (Sun and Xia 2013; Rada *et al.* 1987; Sams *et al.* 1990). There is no treatment for SCD other than symptomatic treatment.

Dental management

The most common clinical manifestation of SCD is vaso-occlusive crisis, where pain arises almost in any part of the body. When a patient is in crisis, dental treatment should be postponed. A diagnosis of SCD includes the clinical features of chronic hemolytic anemia and vaso-occlusive crisis, and electrophoresis confirms the diagnosis with the presence of homozygous HbS (Charache 1990).

A patient should only receive dental treatment when they are not in vaso-occlusive crisis. Elective dental procedures should not be performed in patients who are poorly controlled unless absolutely essential since there is an increased risk of chronic anemia and delayed wound healing (Ramakrisha 2007). Reducing stress during the dental appointment is helpful. Preventive dental care is important to prevent infections. Management of caries is extremely important as non-treated caries leading to periapical infection can precipitate a crisis. Infections have to be managed aggressively with local and systemic measures including appropriate dental treatment, antibiotics, and surgical procedures if necessary (i.e., incision and drainage and extraction) (Mello *et al.* 2012; Sams *et al.* 1990; Bryant and Boyle 2011). Table 11.3 summarizes dental care of the patient with sickle cell anemia.

One complication of SCD is nephropathy, which can be worsened by NSAIDs, so NSAIDs should only be used up to 1 week at most; however, NSAIDs can accelerate renal injury from the disease itself and thus should be avoided. Narcotics can be used for moderate to severe pain (http://sickle.bwh.harvard.edu/scdmanage.html; Okpala and Tawil 2002; Yale *et al.* 2000).

ACD/*inflammation*

The features of anemia due to chronic disease/inflammation include a low serum iron, low TIBC (transferrin), and a normal to increased serum ferritin concentration (Schrier 2013). The anemia is usually mild and not progressive (Van Vranken 2010). A low MCV is usually seen in patients with hepatoma or renal cell carcinoma.

Table 11.3   Oral signs and symptoms and the dental management of anemia (Sams *et al.* 1990; Soriano *et al.* 2002; Lawoyin *et al.* 2006; Adeyemo *et al.* 2011; Mello *et al.* 2012).

Anemia	Oral tissue changes	Dental notes
Iron-deficiency anemia	Glossitis, burning tongue, depapillated tongue, angular cheilitis, pallor lips and oral mucosa	Most likely the patient will be taking ferrous sulfate tablets Tetracycline/doxycycline/minocycline + iron supplement (ferrous sulfate): do not give the two drugs together, space apart about 2 h
Plummer–Vinson syndrome	Increased incidence to develop oral squamous cell carcinoma—screening of the tongue during recare appointments; painless oral swellings, gingival bleeding, recurrent herpes simplex virus infections, candidiasis, lymphadenopathy	Recommend medical consultation before dental treatment.
Anemia of chronic disorders		
Vitamin B_{12} deficiency	Glossitis, stomatitis, angular cheilitis; sore, burning mouth; gingival bleeding; ulcerative gingivitis; depapillated tongue; "beefy" red/smooth/glossy tongue referred to as magenta tongue; aphthous ulcers; alteration of taste; paresthesia; bone loss	Be aware of oral lesions and refer to a physician if vitamin B_{12} deficiency is suspected especially in vegetarians
Sickle cell disease (SCD) Sickle cell trait	Sickle cell crisis: orofacial (nonspecific) pain, dental caries, gingival overgrowth, pallor of mucosa, smooth tongue, "step ladder" of alveolar bone, decreased trabeculation, paresthesia of mental nerve, maxilla overdevelopment, malocclusion, delayed tooth eruption, enamel hypomineralization, pulpal necrosis Sickle cell trait: no symptoms	Medical consult is recommended Patient with sickle cell trait can be treated normally without any precautions Majority of patients are already aware of their disease When a patient is in crisis, dental treatment should be postponed. Only palliative treatment can be given. Anesthesia: epinephrine should be avoided to prevent further vasoconstriction and tissue ischemia. Nitrous oxide and oral sedation are not contraindicated. Since patients with SCD have a higher oxygen demand, 70% N/30% O_2 is acceptable. Adequate hemoglobin levels must be reached for general anesthesia

Table 11.3   *(cont'd)*

Anemia	Oral tissue changes	Dental notes
		Recommend antibiotics after surgery Meticulous oral home care and maintain periodontal health Caries control using fluoride supplementation For oral surgery procedures, patients must have adequate hemoglobin levels and maintain adequate oxygenation, body temperature, and hydration Pain medications: NSAIDs should be avoided. Acetaminophen and narcotics for moderate to severe pain are adequate Antibiotics: all are recommended

Summary: Dental management of anemia

In any anemic patient, it is recommended to avoid aspirin and NSAIDs, which can cause bleeding. In addition, aspirin, NSAIDs, and corticosteroids can cause GI problems. Acetaminophen is the analgesic of choice in anemic patients except for patients with G6PD deficiency. Benzodiazepines for anxiety and oral sedation can cause respiratory depression. Epinephrine should be avoided in G6PD-deficient anemia but can be used in patients with mild anemia.

Besides oral signs and symptoms, there are non-oral features of anemia including spooning of nail beds, brittle nails, tachycardia, and heart failure in severe anemia.

Table 11.3 reviews various oral signs and symptoms and the dental management of different types of anemia.

b.   Myeloproliferative disorders

Myeloproliferative disorders are a group of conditions that cause any blood cell including platelets, RBCs, and WBCs to develop abnormally in the bone marrow. Myeloproliferative disorders are divided into polycythemia vera (PV), essential thrombocythemia, and primary myelofibrosis. Since PV is more common than the other conditions, it will only be discussed.

Primary PV is a rare disorder wherein the bone marrow produces excessive erythrocytes, although the number of platelets and WBCs are also increased. Sometimes, it is called erythrocytosis if only the RBCs are increased. It is considered to be a cancer of mesenchymal tissues with a moderately good prognosis. The prothrombotic mechanisms of an elevated Hct are evident in PV (Barbui *et al.* 2013). The predominant increase of red cell count characterizes the PV hematologic phenotype, and the consequent blood hyperviscosity is a chief cause of vascular disturbances that severely influence morbidity and mortality. The incidence of PV is approximately five per million and occurs more frequently in middle-aged, Caucasians, and males (Bander *et al.* 1991).

Secondary PV can be acquired or congenital and is often linked with a history of cardiovascular occlusive lesions (e.g., stroke and transient ischemic attacks) or other conditions such as lung disease that lead to oxygen shortage (Hoffman *et al.* 2008; Besa 2012).

Signs/symptoms

The following are signs/symptoms of PV: bleeding (oral and GI); reddish purple tongue, cheeks, gingiva, oral mucosa, and lips; spontaneous gingival bleeding (no deep bleeding as seen in other hereditary coagulation disorders); easy bruising and bleeding after minor trauma; nose bleeds; difficulty in lying down in dental chair; peptic ulcers; gout; and bluish red and itchy skin, face, ears, and palms of hands. The most frequently observed sign is splenomegaly, which is the enlargement of the spleen (Bander *et al.* 1991).

Diagnosis/lab values/management

Diagnosis of PV is based on blood counts: RBC mass (RCM)—male: 2.36 ml/kg; female: 2.32 ml/kg and/or platelet count >4,000 µl; WBC 12,000 µl; and elevated leukocyte alkaline phosphatase score >100. Blood oxygen levels are below reference range. The primary treatment of PV is phlebotomy (bloodletting), which keeps Hct <45% and reduces packed cell volume and low-dose aspirin (antiplatelet effect) (Landolfi *et al.* 2006). Hydroxyurea (Hydrea) or analgrelide (Agrylin) is taken to suppress the production of platelets. There are no known drug interactions with dental drugs.

Dental management

It is important to collaborate with the patient's hematologist during dental treatment. There may be comorbidities that will be determined from the medical history and medical consultation. A copy of the patient's blood test results should be obtained and recorded in the chart. The patient's Hgb should be >16 g/dl; HCH 45–52%; and platelets <600 × 10^3/mm^3 (Bander *et al.* 1991).

There are a few criteria necessary for a patient with PV to be treated in the dental office. Since the patient may be taking low-dose aspirin, there may be an increased risk of bleeding. Patients that are controlled will not have as much problems as if they were not controlled; however, using the most conservative treatment is always advisable. Areas to observe in the patient include the following:

• Spontaneous gingival bleeding.
• Purple/reddish color of oral tissues.
• Periodontal condition.
• Excessive bleeding during and after dental procedures. Bleeding could occur up to 10 days after surgery. Monitor postoperative visits frequently and carefully.

B.   White blood cell disorders

In contrast to RBCs, WBCs are nucleated and move spontaneously along close to the walls of the blood vessels. There are three types of WBCs that vary in kind, shape, function, and origin. Granulocytes make up about 70% of the total WBCs.

WBC disorders include lymphoma, leukemia, multiple myeloma, and myelodysplastic syndrome.

a.   Leukemia

Clinical synopsis

Leukemia is a blood cancer wherein a WBC (leukocyte) becomes malignant and multiplies inside bone marrow, which causes an excessive number to be released into the blood. This affects the centers where WBCs are formed including the bone marrow, spleen, and lymph nodes. Leukemic cells can also invade the gingiva especially in AML subtype acute monocytic leukemia (M5) (Cooper *et al.* 2000). In the different forms of leukemia, there is an abnormal increase in the granulocytes, lymphocytes, or monocytes. Leukemia may be acute (rapid and severe) or chronic (slowly progressing). Other factors that classify leukemia include the type of cell involved (myeloid, lymphoid, or monocytic) and increase or non-increase in the number of abnormal cells in the blood (Genc *et al.* 1998; Mathur *et al.* 2012).

Different types of leukemia include the following (Vardiman *et al.* 2009):

- Chronic lymphocytic leukemia (CLL): common in adults over 55 years of age
- Chronic myelogenous (myeloid) leukemia (CML): primarily seen in adults
- Acute lymphocytic leukemia (ALL): the most common type of leukemia in children
- Acute myelogenous (myeloid) leukemia (AML)—subtype acute monocytic leukemia: most common acute leukemia in adults; average age 65.

Treatment/diagnostics/lab values

For a definitive diagnosis, a specimen of marrow or tissue from lymph nodes is examined. Initial dental diagnostic workup of a patient includes knowing the CBC and differential. Patients with CLL have increased number of lymphocytes (lymphocytosis) (lymphocytes >10,000 mm^3) and may have low RBCs and platelets. A peripheral blood smear will show abnormal lymphocytes called smudge cells (Schiffer and Anastasi 2013). In AML, there is bone marrow failure resulting in symptoms related to anemia, neutropenia, and thrombocytopenia. Although there is a decrease in neutrophils (neutropenia), there is usually an increase in the number of WBCs to 100,000–200,000 mm^3; however, sometimes there is no increase. These WBCs are immature and do not function properly resulting in an increased incidence of bacterial infections. The patients become anemic because the bone marrow contains abnormally large numbers of immature WBCs which obstruct the formation of normal RBCs and platelets. In acute myeloid leukemia, the increase in monocytes causes hemorrhages and gingival enlargement.

There is no cure for leukemia (AML). Treatment consists of remission induction and consolidation. Initially in the induction phase, there is radiation of the spleen and lymph nodes or the entire body and chemotherapeutic drugs that suppress the growth and proliferation of abnormal cells. Afterward, the patient continues on remission therapy with long-term chemotherapy. A patient in the induction phase should not be treated in the dental office. Once the patient is in the consolidation phase, then dental treatment can be rendered. Leukapheresis, a procedure often done before chemotherapy, passes the patient's blood through a machine to remove WBCs and leukemic cells and returns the remaining blood cells and plasma to the patient (Ranganathan *et al.* 2008). Blood transfusions are done to treat the anemia.

Oral and general implications

Signs and symptoms of leukemia are often not specific and may appear to be that of the flu. Oral adverse effects in patients with leukemia become evident depending upon the age of the patient, nutritional status, type of malignancy, pretreatment oral status, oral care (dental office and home care) during treatment, and pretreatment neutrophil counts (Mathur *et al.* 2012).

The dentist should be aware of certain signs and symptoms that could be suggestive of AML including gingival (spontaneous) bleeding, diffuse hemorrhagic gingival enlargement, petechiae, and ulcerations that develop rapidly (Chi *et al.* 2010). Children with leukemia often develop gingivitis; this is one of the initial signs of the disease.

Treatment phases of AML include remission induction and consolidation phases. In the remission induction phase, treatment is done immediately with chemotherapy, irradiation, or bone marrow transplantation, which results in immunosuppression. Consolidation phase prevents relapse. Oral adverse effects of these treatments include gingival bleeding, ecchymoses, ulcerations, oral mucositis, taste alteration, skin desquamation, xerostomia, anemia, and infections (e.g., bacterial, fungal, and viral) (Blum *et al.* 2004; Mathur *et al.* 2012). On the other hand, chronic leukemia is not treated immediately and may be monitored with treatment beginning with the first signs/symptoms appearing. The prognosis for acute leukemia with treatment is much better than in patients with chronic leukemia.

Besides oral signs/symptoms, the patient may feel fatigue, which may be evident many months before clinical manifestations appear due to anemia (Schiffer and Anastasi 2013).

A common classification of oral complications in children with acute leukemia is as follows (Emidio *et al.* 2010):

1. **First-degree complications:** Infiltration of leukemic cells into the oral structures such as gingiva (gingival enlargement) and bone.
2. **Second-degree complications:** Due to effects of radiation or chemotherapy. Examples include increased tendency to bleeding, susceptibility to infections, and ulcers. Vomiting is often seen, which may cause erosion of the palatal surface of maxillary anterior teeth.
3. **Third-degree complications:** Due to adverse effect of therapy including a systemic condition. Examples include ulcerations, oral mucositis, taste alteration, skin desquamation, candidiasis, herpetic lesions, gingival bleeding, xerostomia, dysphasia, and fungal infections. Adverse effects seen later in therapy include tissue atrophy, permanent taste loss or change, fibrosis, edema, soft-tissue necrosis, loss of teeth, decrease in salivary flow, caries, and osteoradionecrosis. In the presence of severe mucositis following chemotherapy or irradiation, the diagnosis of oropharyngeal HSV disease is difficult (Hirsch *et al.*, 2013).

Dental notes: Acute leukemia

Table 11.4 lists common oral complications seen in leukemic patients. Early and radical dental intervention reduces the frequency of complications, reducing the risk for oral and accompanying systemic problems (Xavier and Hedge 2010). Care must be taken when patients are actively receiving treatment because there is impaired clotting and even brushing and flossing can cause excessive bleeding. A medical consultation is required for patients undergoing active treatment. Patients that are suspected of having leukemia should visit their physician immediately.

There are no special precautions or contraindication to using epinephrine in local anesthetics or any non-narcotic or narcotic analgesic prescribed in dentistry.

Since all types of blood cells are affected, there most likely will be complications of bleeding due to thrombocytopenia (platelet count), delayed healing due to granulocytosis, infection due to neutropenia, and general fatigue and shortness of breath due to normocytic anemia.

An oncologist consultation is strongly recommended before dental treatment is started. Any dental procedures should be completed before leukemia treatment starts to help avoid subsequent oral complications pre- and post-therapy. Oral hygiene is of utmost importance. Oral hygiene instructions should be emphasized. Any endodontic treatment or extractions should be completed before treatment is started. The child should rinse as often as possible with water. Topical fluoride treatment should be administered when possible (Xavier and Hedge 2010).

Death may occur in patients with AML as a consequence of uncontrolled infection or hemorrhage (Seiter 2012; http://emedicine.medscape.com/article/197802-clinical).

Table 11.4 Acute leukemia: common oral complications and their management (Wu *et al.* 2002; Vissink *et al.* 2003; Demirer *et al.* 2007; Xavier and Edge 2010; Seiter 2012; Schiffer and Anastasi 2013).

Oral complications	Management
Gingival enlargement: develops very quickly without signs of extensive oral biofilm	Early sign in acute leukemia (AML); no treatment until medical (oncologist) consult. Due to invasion in the gingiva of leukemic cells. If patient is actively undergoing treatment, then only oral hygiene instruction including prescribing a non alcoholic rinse (e.g., Crest Pro-Health, ACT, Biotene, Listerine Total Care Zero, and Tom's of Maine) should be given and no invasive periodontal therapy initiated. It is best to avoid brushing and flossing and to wipe the teeth gently with gauze. Therapy for the leukemia may resolve the gingival condition
Gingival bleeding: develops very quickly without signs of extensive oral biofilm	Early sign in acute leukemia (AML); no treatment until medical (oncologist) consult. Due to thrombocytopenia, coagulopathy, or both. If patient is actively undergoing treatment, then only oral hygiene instruction including non alcoholic oral rinse should be given and no invasive periodontal therapy initiated. It is best to avoid brushing and flossing and to wipe the teeth gently with gauze. Therapy for the leukemia may resolve the gingival condition
Bacterial infections	Incidence of bacterial infection is directly related to the number of neutrophils. Neutropenia: <500 cells/µl. Highest risk of infection when <100 cells/µl
Opportunistic infections: fungal/viral	Fungal infection: can cause alteration in taste, a burning feeling, and dysphagia. Treatment with fluconazole. Clotrimazole troches or topical nystatin for oral lesions but these products contain sugar (Buchner and Roos 1992). Other alternatives for non–sugar-containing topical agents include a mixture of diphenhydramine/Maalox or oral sucralfate suspension (Shenep *et al.* 1988) Herpes infection: Especially reactivation of a previous herpes simplex I viral infection. Pain is the main symptom. Hydration is important. HSV-seropositive patients treated for acute leukemia by chemotherapy alone should be considered for antiviral prophylaxis (Hirsch *et al.*, 2013). Drugs: acyclovir or valaciclovir
Oral mucositis	Redness of mucous membrane; loss of the epithelial barrier; loss of taste; sore mouth; and ulceration on lips, tongue, and gingiva. With this comes reduced food intake and poor nutrition. Mucositis cannot be prevented; however, make sure dentures fit properly, restore any faculty restorations, and do any surgical procedures including extractions at least one month before treatment starts. It usually resolves about 7–14 days after the first signs appear. Regular toothbrushing with extra-soft brush, rinsing with 1 tsp baking soda in 1 cup of water, non alcoholic rinse, and no flossing if platelets are <40,000. Suck on ice cubes or sugar-free ice pops or candies

b. Lymphoma

Clinical synopsis

Lymphoma is a type of blood cancer that develops in the lymph nodes. Its primary feature is WBCs become malignant, multiplying and spreading abnormally to other parts in the body. The two major conditions of lymphoma are Hodgkin disease and non-Hodgkin lymphoma. Non-Hodgkin lymphoma is more common than Hodgkin lymphoma and thus will only be discussed, and dental management is the same for Hodgkin and non-Hodgkin lymphoma. Approximately 55,000–60,000 new cases of non-Hodgkin lymphoma are diagnosed yearly in the USA and have been increasing in number in the past years. Non-Hodgkin lymphoma has been implicated with chronic inflammatory diseases such as Sjögren's syndrome, celiac disease, and rheumatoid arthritis (Ansell and Armitage 2005). Clinical presentation of non-Hodgkin lymphoma is either aggressive or indolent with lymphadenopathy for many years (Ansell and Armitage 2005).

Non-Hodgkin lymphoma is classified according to microscopic features and the presence of specific proteins on the surface of the cells. There is B-cell or T-cell lymphoma and numerous types of both of these. Burkitt's lymphoma is a type of B-cell lymphoma (Jaffe *et al.* 2001). MALT lymphoma is a B-cell lymphoma usually affecting people in their 60s. Staging determines if cells have spread within the lymph nodes or to other parts of the body:

In stage I, cells are in only one lymph node area, and in stages II, III, and IV, cells spread from lymph nodes to other parts of the body (Carbone *et al.* 1971; Moormeier *et al.* 1990). The outcome of patients with lymphoma is highly variable. The primary factors that affect outcome and prognosis of a case are the histology and morphology of the lymphoma (Ansell and Armitage 2005; Cheson 2008). Certain viral and bacterial infections (e.g., HIV, hepatitis C virus, and Epstein–Barr virus), pesticides, and chemicals increase the risk of non-Hodgkin lymphoma.

Diagnosis/lab values

Diagnosis of non-Hodgkin and Hodgkin lymphoma is established from many tests; all or some can be used: a physical exam; a CBC with WBC differential and platelet count and an examination of the peripheral smear for the presence of atypical cells; chest X ray; CT scan; endoscopy; MRI; and bone marrow and lymph node biopsies are examples of some of the tests. Other tests include renal and hepatic function, including lactate dehydrogenase; testing for HIV, hepatitis B, and hepatitis C; electrolytes; uric acid; and contrast-enhanced computed tomography scan of the chest, abdomen, and pelvis (Freedman and Friedberg 2013).

Part of the clinical dental examination should include palpation and observation of the Waldeyer's ring (tonsils, base of the tongue, and nasopharynx) and standard lymph node sites (e.g., cervical and supraclavicular).

Oral and general signs/symptoms

There are no oral signs or symptoms. Other symptoms include painless palpable neck lymph nodes, fatigue, night sweats, abdominal pain, fever, weight loss, and flu-like symptoms.

Treatment

Treatment of non-Hodgkin lymphoma with chemotherapy, radiation, radioimmunotherapy (e.g., ibritumomab (Zevalin) and tositumomab (Bexxar)), monoclonal antibodies (e.g., rituximab (Rituxan)), and stem cell transplant usually in combination can extend life with lymphoma, and sometimes cure it. Chemotherapy is the most important therapeutic treatment, especially for lymphomas with an aggressive phenotype (Ansell and Armitage 2005).

Dental notes

See Chapter 12 regarding head and neck cancer.

c. Multiple myeloma

Clinical synopsis

Multiple myeloma is a blood cancer in which plasma cells, which are WBCs from the bone marrow, become malignant and multiply and produce and release monoclonal immunoglobulin that eventually causes organ damage. Multiple myeloma has no cure, but stem cell transplant and/ or chemotherapy can allow people to live for years with the condition. It usually affects people with a mean age of 66 years (Kyle *et al.* 2003).

Diagnostics/lab values

Initially, serum or urine protein electrophoresis or immunofixation and bone marrow aspirate analysis are ordered (Nau and Lewis 2008). In addition, CBC, imaging tests, metastatic bone survey, and serum creatinine may be required.

Oral and general signs/symptoms

Signs and symptoms are related to the infiltration of plasma cells into the bone or other organs or to kidney damage. Early on in the disease there may not be any symptoms. As the plasma cells invade the bone, more symptoms appear. Some common signs/symptoms are bone pain (in back, hips, and ribs); bone fractures; fatigue and weakness (due to anemia); excessive thirst; thickening of the blood (hyperviscosity); weight loss, nausea, and constipation (due to hypercalcemia); and renal disease. In about 14% of dental patients presenting with mandibular pain, swelling, bleeding mobile teeth, and soft-tissue masses from amyloid and plasma cell deposits, a diagnosis of multiple myeloma is made (Junquera *et al.* 2011). Impaired antibodies and leukopenia cause recurrent infections (Nau and Lewis 2008). Amyloidosis presents with amyloid deposits in oral tissues as plaques, nodules, and papules. Radiographic osteolytic lesions are more common in the mandibular posterior areas (Shah *et al.* 2012).

Treatment

The initial therapy to treat symptomatic multiple myeloma is known as induction therapy, using many different drugs. Radiation, chemotherapy, and autologous stem cell transplantation (ASCT) is the standard treatment for patients with symptomatic multiple myeloma. The purpose of a stem cell transplant is to restore stem cells destroyed by radiation, chemotherapy, and the disease itself. Pamidronate (Acredia) and Zoledronic (Zometa) are two intravenous bisphosphonates approved for bone pain resulting from hypercalcemia. Patients who can get an ASCT usually are placed on melphalan (Alkeran) and prednisone, which reduces the adverse effects of the chemotherapeutic drug.

Bisphosphonates (antiresorptive therapy)

A detailed description of bisphosphonates is found in Chapter 13. Bisphosphonates or antiresorptive agents are indicated in multiple myeloma for bone pain and hypercalcemia. In these cancer cases, bisphosphonates are prescribed intravenously. The risk of developing antiresorptive osteonecrosis of the jaw (ARONJ), the most current nomenclature, is an adverse effect of bisphosphonates or antiresorptive drugs especially in multiple myeloma patients. In addition, smoking and obesity were considered risk factors for ARONJ in cancer patients taking intravenous zoledronic acid (Wessel *et al.* 2008; Edwards *et al.* 2009; Hellstein *et al.* 2011).

Dental notes

1. Dental treatment is allowed only if the patient is in long-term remission. Patients in relapse should only have urgent dental care (Shah *et al.* 2012).
2. Osteonecrosis of the jaw (ONJ), bisphosphonate-associated osteonecrosis of the jaw, or antiresorptive agent–induced ONJ (ARONJ), which is the most current nomenclature, is an adverse effect of bisphosphonates, especially intravenous (Edwards *et al.* 2009). Any invasive dental

Table 11.5   Dental management of WBC disorders (Nau and Lewis 2008; Brunetti *et al.* 2010; Xavier and Hedge 2010; Shah *et al.* 2012).

Leukemia	Oncologist consultation required
	Antibiotic prophylaxis may be required for dental procedures that cause bleeding; WBC <2,000 mm^3 or absolute neutrophil count <1000 mm^3
	Best time to treat patients is when all blood counts are at the highest
	Best time to treat patients is when they are in remission and not taking any treatment; still acceptable if they are in remission and on long-term chemotherapy
	Oral hygiene is important but stopped if platelet counts are <20,000 mm^3 and neutrophil count is <500 mm^3
	Consider fluoride therapy
	Be aware of development of opportunistic infections (bacterial, fungal, and herpetic)
	Treat dental caries and other infections including endodontic and periodontal
	Bleeding concerns; check on platelet counts
Lymphoma	Oncologist consultation
	No precautions with using epinephrine
	Follow dental notes in Chapter 12 (Head and Neck Radiation and Chemotherapy)
Multiple myeloma	Oncologist consultation
	Obtain blood test report and evaluate WBCs with differential and platelet counts
	Only treat patients in long-term remission
	May require antibiotic prophylaxis
	Caution used if taking antiresorptive therapy; risk for ARONJ
	May have bleeding problems
	Adjust dentures so there are no rough or irritating edges
	Analgesics: if anemia is present, avoid prescribing NSAIDs and aspirin; if kidney insufficiency is present, avoid NSAIDs
	Evaluate patient's kidney function (serum creatinine) because some dental drugs may require dosing interval adjustment (refer to Chapter 3) (Shah *et al.* 2012)
	Opiates are the recommended analgesics

procedure involving bone trauma could potentially result in ARONJ. These procedures include extractions, periodontal surgery, scaling/root planing, and implant surgery. Endodontic therapy, orthodontic therapy, and restorative dentistry and prosthodontics have the least risk for developing ONJ (Edwards *et al.* 2009; Hellstein *et al.* 2011). If a patient requires an extraction, it is recommended, if possible, to do endodontic treatment and reduce the occlusal height of the tooth instead of the extraction. Dentures should not have any irritating edges (Shah *et al.* 2012).

3. Increased risk for infection due to a decreased lymphocyte function.
4. Increased risk for bleeding due to impaired platelet function or thrombocytopenia (Shah *et al.* 2012).
5. Recommended to do dental treatment to eliminate inflammation and infections before chemotherapy, radiation, or antiresorptive drugs are started. If the patient will be getting a stem cell transplant, then the patient must wait at least 3 days after the procedure to have dental treatment (Shah *et al.* 2012).

For summary on dental management of WBC disorders see Table 11.5.

References

Abshire, T.C. (2001). Sense and sensibility: approaching anemia in children. *Contemporary Pediatrics*, **18** (**9**), 104–113. [accessed on July 19, 2014].

Adams, J.G. III & Coleman, M.B. (1990) Structural hemoglobin variants that produce the phenotype of thalassemia. *Seminars in Hematology*, **27**, 229–238.

Adeyemo, T.A., Adeyemo, W.L., Adediran, A., *et al.* (2011) Orofacial manifestations of hematological disorders: anemia and hemostatic disorders. *Indian Journal of Dental Research*, **22**, 454–461.

Amini, F., Borzabadi-Farahni, A., Mashayekhi, Z., *et al.* (2013) Soft-tissue profile characteristics in children with beta thalassemia major. *Acta Odontologica Scandinavica*, **71**, 1071–1076.

Ansell, S.M. & Armitage, J. (2005) Non-Hodgkin's lymphoma: diagnosis and treatment. *Mayo Clinic Proceedings*, **80**, 1087–1097.

Aslinia, F., Mazza, J.J., & Yale, S.H. (2006) Megaloblastic anemia and other causes of macrocytosis. *Clinical Medicine & Research*, **4**, 236–241.

Bander, V.M., Lawrence, C., & Mehler, S. (1991) Polycythemia vera: dental management considerations. *Special Care in Dentistry*, **11**, 227–230.

Barbui, T., Finazzi, G., & Flanaga, A. (2013) Myleoproliferative neoplasms and thrombosis. *Blood*, **122**, 2176–2184.

Benz, E.J. (2013) Clinical manifestations and diagnosis of the thalassemias. Topic 7116 Version 39.0. http://www.uptodate.com/contents/clinical-manifestations-and-diagnosis-of-the-thalassemias?source=see_link [accessed on July 19, 2014].

Besa, E.C. (2012) Secondary polycythemia. www.emedicine.medscape.com/article/205039-overview#a0104 [accessed on July 19, 2014].

Beutler, E. & Waalen, J. (2006) The definition of anemia: what is the lower limit of normal of the blood hemoglobin concentration? *Blood*, **107**, 1747–1750.

Billett, H.H. (1990) Hemoglobin and hematocrit. In: H.K. Walker, W.D. Hall, & J.W. Hurst (eds), *Clinical Methods: The History, Physical, and Laboratory Examinations*, 3rd ed, Chapter 151. Butterworths, Boston.

Blum, W., Mrózek, K., Ruppert, A.S., *et al.* (2004) Adult de novo acute myeloid leukemia with t(6;11) (q27;q23): results from Cancer and Leukemia Group B Study 8461 and review of the literature. *Cancer*, **101** (**6**), 1420–1427.

Brill, J.R. & Baumgardner, D.J. (2000) Normocytic anemia. *American Family Physician,* **62** (**10**), 2255–2264.

Brunetti, G, Caravita, T., Cartoni, C., *et al.* (2010) Pain management in multiple myeloma. *Expert Review of Anticancer Therapy*, **10**, 415–425.

Bryant, C. & Boyle, C. (2011) Sickle cell disease, dentistry and conscious sedation. *Dental Update*, **38** (**7**), 486–488, 491–492.

Buchner, T. & Roos, N. (1992) Antifungal treatment strategy in leukemia patients. *Annals of Hematology*, **65**, 153–161.

Carbone, P.P., Kaplan, H.S., & Musshoff, K. (1971) Report of the Committee on Hodgkin's Disease Staging Classification. *Cancer Research,* **31**, 1860–1861.

Carley, A. (2003) Anemia, when is it not iron deficiency? *Journal of Pediatric Nursing*, **29**, 205–211.

Charache, S. (1990) Fetal hemoglobin, sickling and sickle cell disease. *Advances in Pediatrics*, **37**, 1–31.

Cheson, B.D. (2008) Staging and evaluation of the patient with lymphoma. *Hematology/Oncology Clinics of North America*, **22 (5)**, 825–837, vii–viii.

Chi, A.C., Neville, B.W., Krayer, J.W., *et al.* (2010) Oral manifestations of systemic disease. *American Family Physician*, **82 (11)**, 1381–1388.

Chulilla, J.A.M., Colas, M.S.R., & Martin, M.G. (2009) Classification of anemia for gastroenterologists. *World Journal of Gastroenterology*, **15 (37)**, 4627–4637.

Cooper, C.L., Loewen, R., & Shore, T. (2000) Gingival hyperplasia complication acute myelomonocytic leukemia. *Journal of the Canadian Dental Association*, **66**, 78–79.

Davenport, J. (1996) Macrocytic anemia. *American Family Physician*, **53**, 155–162.

Demirer, S., Ozdemir, H., Sencan, M., *et al.* (2007) Gingival hyperplasia as an early diagnostic oral manifestation in acute monocytic leukemia: a case report. *European Journal of Dentistry*, **1**, 11–114.

Dhaliwal, G., Cornett, P.A., & Tierney, L.M. (2004) Hemolytic anemia. *American Family Physicians*, **69**, 2599–2607.

Edwards, B.J., Hellstein, J.W., Jacobsen, P.L., *et al.* (2009) Updated recommendations for managing the care of patients receiving oral bisphosphonate therapy: an advisory state from the American Dental Association Council on Scientific Affairs. *Journal of the American Dental Association*, **139 (12)**, 1674–1677.

Emidio, T.C., Maeda, Y.C., Caldo-Teixeira, A.S., *et al.* (2010) Oral manifestations of leukemia and antineoplastic treatment—a literature review (part II). *Brazilian Journal of Health*, **1**, 136–149.

Frank, J.E. (2005) Diagnosis and management of G6PD deficiency. *American Family Physician*, **72**, 1277–1282.

Freedman, A.S. & Friedberg, J.W. (2013) Evaluation and staging of non-Hodgkin lymphoma. http://www.uptodate.com/contents/evaluation-and-staging-of-non-hodgkin-lymphoma [accessed on July 27, 2014].

Genc, A., Atalay, T., Gedikoglu, G., *et al.* (1998) Leukemic children: clinical and histopathological gingival lesions. *Journal of Clinical Pediatric Dentistry*, **22**, 253–256.

Goldman, L., & Schafer, A.I., eds. (2011) *Cecil Medicine*, 24th ed, Chapter 161. Saunders Elsevier, Philadelphia, PA.

Harrington, A. (2007) Laboratory evaluation of normocytic anemia. *Newspath*, http://www.cap.org/apps/cap.portaL?_nfpb=true&cntvwrPtlt_actionOverride=%2Fportlets%2FcontentViewer%2Fshow&_windowLabel=cntvwrPtlt&cntvwrPtlt%7BactionForm.contentReference%7D=newspath%2F0707%2Flaboratory_evaluation_normocytic_anemia.html&_state=maximized&_pageLabel=cntvwr [accessed on July 19, 2014].

Hellstein, J.W., Adler, R.A., Edwards, B., *et al.* (2011) Managing the care of patients receiving antiresorptive therapy for prevention and treatment of osteoporosis. *Journal of the American Dental Association*, **142**, 1243–1251.

Henderson, S., Timbs, A., McCarthy, J., *et al.* (2009) Incidence of haemoglobinopathies in various populations-the impact of immigration. *Clinical Biochemistry*, **42 (18)**, 1745–1756.

Severe periodontal destruction in a patient with advanced anemia: a case report

Hershko, C. & Skikne, B. (2009) Pathogenesis and management of iron deficiency anemia: emerging role of celiac disease, *helicobacter pylori*, and autoimmune gastritis. *Seminars in Hematology*, **46 (4)**, 339–350.

Hoffman, R., Xu, M., Finazzi, G., *et al.* (2008) The polycythemias. In: R. Hoffman, E.J. Benz, Jr., & S.J. Shattil, S.J., *et al.* (eds). *Hoffman Hematology: Basic Principles and Practice*, 5th ed, Chapter 68. Churchill Livingstone Elsevier, Philadelphia, PA.

Hoffman, R.M. & Jaffe, P.E. (1995) Plummer-Vinson syndrome: a case report and literature review. *Archives of Internal Medicine*, **155**, 2008–2011.

Hutter, J.W., Van der Velden, U., Varoufaki, A., *et al.* (2001) Lower numbers of erythrocytes and lower levels of hemoglobin in periodontitis patients compared to control subjects. *Journal Clinical Periodontology*, **28**, 930–936.

Jaffe, E.S., Harris, N.L., Stein, H., *et al.* (eds). (2001) *World Health Organization Classification of Tumours: Pathology and Genetics of Tumours of Haematopoietic and Lymphoid Tissues.* World Health Organization, Geneva.

Junquera, L., Gallego, L., & Pelaz, A. (2011) Multiple myeloma and bisphosphonate-related osteonecrosis of the mandible associated with dental implants. *Case Reports in Dentistry*, **2011**, 568246.

Kaferle, J. & Strzoda, C.E. (2009) Evaluation of macrocytosis. *American Family Physician*, **79 (3)**, 203–208.

Killip, S., Bennett, J.M., & Chambers, M.D.(2007) Iron deficiency anemia. *American Family Physicians*, **75**, 671–678.

Kyle, R.A., Gertz, M.A., Witzig, T.E., *et al.* (2003) Review of 1027 patients with newly diagnosed multiple myeloma. *Mayo Clinical Proceedings*, **78 (1)**, 21–33.

Landolfi, R., Cipriani, M.C., & Novarese, L. (2006) Thrombosis and bleeding in polycythemia vera and essential thrombocythemia: pathogenetic mechanisms and prevention. *Best Practice & Research Clinical Haematology*, **19 (3)**, 617–633.

Lawoyin, D, Reid, E., Obayomi, T., *et al.* (2006) Plummer Vinson syndrome: a case report and literature review. *The Internet Journal of Dental Science*, **5 (2)**. http://ispub.com/IJDS/5/2/10116 [accessed on July 27, 2014].

Lesperance, L., Wu, A.C., & Bernstein, H. (2002). Putting a dent in iron deficiency. *Contemporary Pediatrics*, **19 (7)**, 60–79.

Mathur, V.P., Dhillon, J.K., & Kalra, G. (2012) Oral health in children with leukemia. *Indian Journal of Palliative Care*, **18**, 12–18.

Mello, S.M., Paulo, C., Araujo, R., *et al.* (2012) Oral considerations in the management of sickle cell disease: a case report. *Oral Health Dental Management*, **11 (3)**, 125–128.

Moormeier, J.A., Williams, S.F., & Golomb, H.M. (1990) The staging of non-Hodgkin's lymphomas. *Seminars in Oncology*, **17**, 43–50.

Nau, O.C. & Lewis, W.D. (2008) Multiple myeloma: diagnosis and treatment. *American Family Physician*, **78**, 853–859.

Novacek, G. (2006) Plummer-Vinson syndrome. *Orphanet Journal of Rare Diseases*, **1**, 36–40.

Oh, R. & Brown, D.L. (2003) Vitamin B$_{12}$ deficiency. *American Family Physicians*, **67 (5)**, 979–986.

Okpala, I. &Tawil, A. (2002) Management of pain in sickle cell disease. *Journal of the Royal Society of Medicine*, **95 (9)**, 456–458.

Management of pain in sickle-cell disease

Pontes, H.A.R., Neto, N.C., Ferreira, K.B., *et al.* (2009) Oral manifestations of vitamin B$_{12}$ deficiency: a case report. *Journal of the Canadian Dental Association*, **75**, 533–537.

Quinto, L., Aponte, J.J., Menende, C., *et al.* (2006) Relationship between haemoglobin and haematocrit in the definition of anemia. *Tropical Medicine and International Health*, **11**, 1.

Rada, R.E., Bronny, A.T., Hasiakos, P.S. (1987) Sickle cell crisis precipitated by periodontal infection: report of two cases. *Journal of the American Dental Association*, **114**, 799–801.

Ramakrishna, Y. (2007) Dental considerations in the management of children suffering from sickle cell disease: a case report. *Journal of Indian Society of Pedodontics and Preventive Dentistry*, **25**, 140–143.

Ranganathan, S., Sesikeran, S., Gupta, V., *et al.* (2008) Emergency therapeutic leukaphereis in a case of acute myeloid leukemia M5. *Asian Journal of Transfusion Science*, **2**, 18–19.

Hirsch, H.H., Martino, R., Ward, K.N., Boeckh, M., Einsele, H., Ljungman, P. (2013) Fourth European Conference on Infections in Leukaemia (ECIL-4): guidelines for diagnosis and treatment of human respiratory syncytial virus, parainfluenza virus, metapneumovirus, rhinovirus, and coronavirus. *Clinical Infectious Disease*, **56 (2)**, 258–266

Sams, D.R., Thornton, J.B., & Amamoo, P.A. (1990) Managing the dental patient with sickle cell anemia: a review of the literature. *Pediatric Dentistry*, **12**, 316–320.

Savage, D.G., Ogundipe, A., Allen, R.H., *et al.* (2000) Etiology and diagnostic evaluation of macrocytosis. *The American Journal of the Medical Sciences*, **319 (6)**, 343–352.

Schiffer, C.A. & Anastasi J (2013) Clinical manifestations, pathologic features, and diagnosis of acute myeloid leukemia. *UptoDate,* Topic 4497 Version 21.0. http://www.uptodate.com/contents/clinical-manifestations-pathologic-features-and-diagnosis-of-acute-myeloid-leukemia [accessed on July 27, 2014].

Schrier, S.L. (2013) Approach to the adult patient with anemia. *UpToDate,* Topic 71331, Version 20.0. http://www.uptodate.com/contents/approach-to-the-adult-patient-with-anemia [accessed on July 27, 2014].

Segel, G.B., Hirsh, M.G., & Feig, S.A. (2002). Managing anemia in pediatric office practice: Part 1. *Pediatrics in Review,* **23** (**3**), 75–83.

Seiter, K. (2012) Acute myelogenous leukemia clinical presentation. http://emedicine.medscape.com/article/197802-clinical [accessed on July 19, 2014].

Shah, A., Latoo, S., & Ahmad, I. (2012) Multiple myeloma in dentistry. In: A. Gupta (ed). *Multiple Myeloma— An Overview.* http://www.intechopen.com/books/multiple-myeloma-an-overview/multiple-myeloma-and-dentistry [accessed on July 19, 2014].

Shenep, J.L., Kalwinsky, D.K., Hutson, P.R., *et al.* (1988) Efficacy of oral sucralfate suspension in prevention and treatment of chemotherapy-induced mucositis. *Journal of Pediatrics,* **113**, 758–763.

Soriano, C.A., Montoya, G.J.A., & Garrido, L.G.D. (2002) Thalassemias and their dental implications. *Medicina Oral,* **7**, **36–40**, 41–45.

Sun, K. & Xia, Y. (2013) New insights into sickle cell disease: a disease of hypoxia. *Current Opinions in Hematology,* **20** (**3**), 215–221.

Tefferi, A. (2003) Anemia in adults: a contemporary approach to diagnosis. *Mayo Clinic Proceedings,* **78** (**10**), 1274–1280.

Tefferi, A., Hanson, C.A., & Inwards, D.J. (2005) How to interpret and pursue an abnormal complete blood cell count in adults. *Mayo Clinic Proceedings,* **80**, 923–936.

Tender, J. & Cheng, T.L. (2002). Iron deficiency anemia. In: F.D. Burg, J.R. Ingelfinger, R.A. Polin, & A.A. Gershon (Eds.). *Gellis & Kagan's Current Pediatric Therapy,* 17th ed, pp. 633–637. W.B. Saunders, Philadelphia. http://www.uptodate.com/contents/causes-and-diagnosis-of-iron-deficiency-anemia-in-the-adult/abstract/5 [accessed on July 19, 2014].

Van Vranken, M. (2010) Evaluation of microcytosis. *American Family Physician,* **82**, 1117–1122.

Vardiman, J.W., Thiele, J., Arber, D.A., *et al.* (2009) The 2008 revision of the World Health Organization (WHO) classification of myeloid neoplasms and acute leukemia: rationale and important changes. *Blood,* **114**, 937–951.

Vissink, A., Burlage, F.R., & Spijkervet, F.K.L. (2003) Prevention and treatment of the consequences of head and neck radiotherapy. *Critical Reviews of Oral Biology and Medicine,* **3**, 213–225.

Ward, P.C. (2002) Modern approaches to the investigation of vitamin B12 deficiency. *Clinics in Laboratory Medicine,* **22** (**2**), 435–445.

Wessel, J.H., Dodson, T.B., & Zavras, A.L. (2008) Zoledronate, smoking, and obesity are strong risk factors for osteonecrosis of the jaw: a case-control study. *Journal of Oral and Maxillofacial Surgery,* **66**, 625–631.

Wu, J., Fantasia, J.E., & Kaplan, R. (2002) Oral manifestations of acute myelomonocytic leukemia: a case report and review of the classification of leukemias. *Journal of Periodontology,* **73**, 664–668.

Xavier, A.M. & Hedge, A.M. (2010) Preventive protocols and oral management in childhood—leukemia—the pediatric specialist's role. *Asian Pacific Journal of Cancer Prevention,* **11**, 39–43.

Yale, S.H., Nagib, N., & Guthrie, T. (2000) Approach to the vaso-occlusive crisis in adults with sickle cell disease. *American Family Physician,* **61** (**5**), 1349–1356.

Youngster, I., Arcavi, L., Schechmaster, R., *et al.* (2010) Medications and glucose-6-phosphate dehydrogenase deficiency: an evidence-based review. *Drug Safety,* **33** (**9**), 713–726.

Chapter 12

Musculoskeletal and connective tissue disorders

A. Osteoporosis	193
B. Osteoarthritis	197
C. Rheumatoid arthritis	198
D. Gout	201
E. Fibromyalgia syndrome	203
F. Systemic lupus erythematosus	205
G. Sjögren's syndrome	208
References	210

Musculoskeletal disorders comprise diseases of the muscles, joints and bones, autoimmune disorders, and non-autoimmune disorders. In the USA, musculoskeletal disorders account for approximately 131 million patient visits to a physician per year (Millett *et al.* 2008).

A. Osteoporosis

Clinical synopsis

About 8 million women and 2 million men in the USA have been diagnosed with osteoporosis and 34 million people with osteopenia (Sweet *et al.* 2009). Osteoporosis is characterized as low bone mass and structural deterioration of bone tissue, which increases the risk for fractures (Wellbery 2007). According to the World Health Organization, osteoporosis is subjectively defined as a bone mineral density (BMD) that is 2.5 standard deviations (SDs) or more below the mean in younger women, as measured at the femoral neck. Osteopenia is defined as a BMD that is 1 SD or more below the younger women's mean (U.S. Preventive Services Task Force 2010, http://www.uspreventive servicestaskforce.org/3rduspstf/osteoporosis/osteorr.htm).

Diagnostics/lab values

BMD is the amount of bone in a given area in the body and is measured at these different parts, usually the lumbar spine, total hip, or femoral neck. Dual-energy X-ray absorptiometry is currently the recommended test to measure BMD.

The Dentist's Quick Guide to Medical Conditions, First Edition. Mea A. Weinberg, Stuart L. Segelnick, Joseph S. Insler, with Samuel Kramer.
© 2015 John Wiley & Sons, Inc. Published 2015 by John Wiley & Sons, Inc.

Treatment

Treatments for osteopenia include weight-bearing exercises and possible calcium and vitamin D supplementation. Decisions about pharmacologic treatment for fracture prevention depend on fracture risk and patient preference (Wellbery 2007).

In the mid-1990s **bisphosphonates** were first introduced and prescribed as alternates to hormone replacement therapies for osteoporosis and to treat osteolytic tumors and possibly slow tumor development. In 1996, alendronate (Fosamax®) was the first bisphosphonate drug approved for osteoporosis in postmenopausal women.

The most current nomenclature for these drugs is antiresorptive therapy. One of the more important adverse effects of these drugs relating to dentistry is *antiresorptive osteonecrosis of the jaw (ARONJ)*. Developing ARONJ is at lowest risk in patients taking oral antiresorptives for low bone mass (Hellstein *et al.* 2011). Besides bisphosphonates, other antiresorptive agents taken for osteopenia/osteoporosis include the following:

- Denosumab (Prolia®, Xgeva®), administered subcutaneously, is a monoclonal antibody that binds to receptor activator of nuclear factor kappa-B ligand (RANKL).
- Denosumab works by inhibiting the maturation of osteoclasts by binding to RANKL.
- Antiangiogenic medications such as bevacizumab (Avastin®), cetuximab (Erbitux®), panitumumab (Vectibix®), and trastuzumab (Herceptin®) inhibit the growth of blood vessels.

Bisphosphonates: There are two subclasses of bisphosphonates: non-nitrogenous and nitrogenous bisphosphonates. The non-nitrogenous or first-generation bisphosphonates are not as potent as the nitrogenous, second- and third-generation bisphosphonates, which contain nitrogen and appear to be implicated in causing ARONJ.

Bisphosphonates are prescribed in the treatment and prevention of the following (Table 12.1):

1. Corticosteroid-induced osteoporosis
2. Postmenopausal osteoporosis
3. Hypercalcemia with metastatic cancer to help decrease bone pain and fracture by reducing blood calcium levels
4. Paget's disease
5. Chronic renal disease in patients undergoing dialysis (precipitates bone fragility)

Mechanism of action

Bisphosphonates, which are potent antiresorptive agents, inhibit bone removal or resorption by osteoclasts, thereby allowing the buildup of new bone. This will then help to prevent fractures of

Table 12.1 Bisphosphonates (Weinberg *et al.* 2014).

Generic name	Trade name	Route of administration	Indication	Potency factor
Etidronate	Didronel	Oral	Paget's disease	1
Tiludronate	Skelid	Oral	Paget's disease	10
Clodronate	Bonefos, Loron, Ostac	Oral	Hypercalcemia (bone metastases)	10
Alendronate	Fosamax	Oral	Osteoporosis	500
Risedronate	Actonel	Oral	Osteoporosis	2,000
Ibandronate	Boniva	Oral/IV	Osteoporosis	1,000
Pamidronate	Aredia	IV	Bone metastases	100
Zoledronate	Zometa	IV	Bone metastases	10,000

the hip and spine. Normally, an equilibrium exists between osteoblasts and osteoclasts. In patients taking bisphosphonates, there are no more osteoclasts to get rid of necrotic bone allowing new bone that is formed to lay down on diseased bone. If necrotic bone cannot be resorbed during normal healing, then the necrotic bone will inhibit healing and affect blood supply to the area, resulting in antiresorptive-associated osteonecrosis of the jaw (ARONJ) (Ruggiero 2008; Hellstein *et al.* 2011). In addition, bisphosphonates inhibit the increased osteoclastic activity and skeletal calcium release into the bloodstream induced by various stimulatory factors released by tumors.

Adverse effects of bisphosphonates

Although first observed in 2004 in patients taking intravenous bisphosphonates, cases of ARONJ are being seen in patients taking oral bisphosphonates. Patients are considered to be at risk for ARONJ if they are currently taking or previously were taking a bisphosphonate. Bisphosphonates, once taken into the body, bind to bone and stay there for long periods of time, even if discontinued. This long half-life of about 10 years or more is of concern because even if the drug is discontinued before dental procedures, it is still in the body. In some patients at lower risk a 5-year break from the drug after 5 years of use is recommended (Wellbery 2008).

Risk factors for the development of ARONJ include the following (Marx 2007):

- History of or currently taking bisphosphonates (especially IV formulations but also oral)
- History of cancer (breast, lung, prostate, multiple myeloma, or metastatic disease to the bone), osteoporosis, Paget's disease, chronic renal disease on dialysis
- Corticosteroid therapy
- Diabetes
- Smoking
- Alcohol use
- Poor oral hygiene
- Chemotherapeutic drugs.

Osteonecrosis of the jaw (ONJ) occurs after precipitating causes such as extractions or periodontal and implant procedures where there is poor or delayed wound healing in the mouth (Migliorati *et al.* 2013). The following are local dental risk factors for ARONJ in patients taking intravenous or oral bisphosphonates (Otomo-Corgel 2007):

- Extractions
- Periodontal surgery
- Dental implant surgery
- Ill-fitting dentures that are irritating to the tissues
- Less likely with endodontic therapy, orthodontics, scaling and root planing; still patients should be advised about the complication of developing ARONJ.
- ARONJ can also occur spontaneously without any prior dental procedure.

Clinical signs:
The following are signs and symptoms of ARONJ:

- Irregular mucosal ulcer with exposed bone in the maxillofacial area
- Pain or swelling in the area
- Infection
- Pain
- Mobility of teeth
- Numbness or heavy sensation

Table 12.2　Staging criteria for ARONJ.

Grade	Symptom severity
1	Asymptotic
2	Mild
3	Moderate
4	Severe

Novartis (East Hanover, NJ), a drug company that manufactures Aredia and Zometa developed a staging criterion for ARONJ (Table 12.2).

Treatment of ONJ depends on the severity of the case. Regardless of the severity, any necrotic bone should be removed. Conservative treatment of ONJ is recommended, including antibiotics, oral rinses (chlorhexidine), pain control, and periodontal debridement where needed. Some situations may require antibiotic prophylaxis starting 1 day before and extending 3–7 days after the dental procedure (Hellstein *et al.* 2011). During endodontic treatment, it has been suggested not to instrument beyond the apex (Hellstein *et al.* 2011).

Dental management

If a patient has been taking an oral bisphosphonate for more than 3 years, the risk of developing ARONJ increases (Zak *et al.* 2007). *Although the risk of developing ARONJ is low in patients taking oral bisphosphonates* (Migliorati *et al.* 2005; Edwards *et al.* 2008), dental treatment may need to be altered. There are currently no data from clinical trials evaluating dental management of patients on oral bisphosphonate therapy. Preventive care is extremely important to reduce the incidence of ARONJ. Recommendations focus on conservative surgical procedures, proper sterile technique, appropriate use of oral disinfectants, and the dentist's clinical and professional judgment (American Dental Association of Scientific Affairs 2006). Consultation with the patient's physician is necessary.

Patients taking oral bisphosphonates for less than 3 years can have invasive dental treatment, but if the patient has been taking bisphosphonates for more than 3 years, the C-terminal cross-linked telopeptide (CTx) blood test can be performed to determine the amount of bone resorption. Its use is controversial; some clinicians do not think that this test is useful. Fleisher *et al.* (2010) have suggested that radiographic PDL widening may be a more sensitive indicator for predicting the risk of developing ARONJ than using the CTx test (Fleisher *et al.* 2010). The CTx test is performed by Quest Diagnostics and sent to its lab in California (http://www.questdiagnostic.com). If the results of the CTx blood test are >150 pg/ml, then dental procedures can be performed. Values <100 pg/ml are associated with a high risk of developing ARONJ (Fugazzotto *et al.* 2007; Marx 2007; Grant *et al.* 2008). It is recommended to discontinue the drug for 3 months prior to the planned procedure and send for CTx testing. Once treatment is done, extend the "drug holiday" for an additional 3 months (Marx *et al.* 2005; Cartsos *et al.* 2008; Marx 2007). Thus, patients on long-term oral bisphosphonates should be treated with caution (Wang *et al.* 2007). In 2011, a panel (American Dental Association Council on Scientific Affairs) reported there was insufficient evidence to recommend a drug holiday from antiresorptive drugs (Hellstein *et al.* 2011).

On the other hand, in patients taking IV bisphosphonates, usually for cancer, any invasive dental procedures should be avoided; however, dentists need to exercise their professional judgment, perhaps after consultation with the patient's physician, in deciding whether invasive treatment is needed under the particular clinical situations (American Dental Association Council on Scientific Affairs 2006).

Summary: Dental notes

There are concerns regarding the dental management of patients currently taking or having a history of taking bisphosphonates because of the development of ARONJ. Although the majority of reports of bisphosphonate-associated ONJ are in patients taking IV bisphosphonates, more reports are being documented in patients taking oral bisphosphonates. Thus, patients undergoing long-term IV or oral bisphosphonate therapy should be treated with caution and close observation after dental procedures. It is important to discuss the patients' dental needs with their physician.

The Food and Drug Administration (FDA), drug companies, and dental societies/associations (e.g., American Academy of Periodontology, American Association of Endodontists, American Academy of Oral Medicine, and American Association of Oral and Maxillofacial Surgeons) have issued precautions and recommendations for dentists to follow regarding prevention, diagnosis, and treatment guidelines for ARONJ.

It is advised that patients have a dental examination and all dental procedures be completed prior to the start of bisphosphonate therapy; careful medical history is needed to determine if a patient will require or is currently on bisphosphonates. Patients should go for routine dental maintenance visits at least every 6 months and maintain good oral hygiene. Routine restorative and dental hygiene procedures may be performed. An elective dental procedure is not advised in patients on IV bisphosphonates (Weinberg *et al.* 2014).

B. Osteoarthritis

Clinical synopsis

Osteoarthritis is a degenerative articular disease of the cartilage and bone of a joint (knee, hand, shoulder, and hip). The deterioration of the bone and cartilage results in the development of joint pain, stiffness, and limitation of motion. In contrast to rheumatoid arthritis (RA) and gout, osteoarthritis affects men and women equally (Sinusas 2012). Pain is due to inflammation of the articular capsule, synovitis, or in some cases muscle spasm. Sometimes, the pain and swelling may mimic acute gouty arthritis.

The temporomandibular joint (TMJ) is also affected by osteoarthritis.

Heberden's nodes characteristically involve the distal interphalangeal joints of the fingers. They can develop quickly or slowly and can severely limit motion and interfere with proper oral home care.

Diagnostics/lab values

There are no specific lab tests to diagnose osteoarthritis. Diagnosis is based on physical exam, patient's symptoms, and X rays. The goal of testing is to properly diagnose osteoarthritis. Differential diagnoses are other forms of arthritis such as RA and other disorders of pain. Some commonly found features of osteoarthritis are Bouchard's nodes and Heberden's nodes (Rees *et al.* 2012). Bouchard's nodes are bony enlargements at the middle joint or proximal interphalangeal joint of the finger. Heberden's nodes, which are more common than Bouchard's nodes, are bony enlargements involving the distal interphalangeal joints.

Treatment

Many patients take analgesics such as acetaminophen or aspirin or nonsteroidal anti-inflammatory drugs (NSAIDs). Be cautious if prescribing additional analgesics for postoperative pain. Prescription combination opioid analgesic containing acetaminophen should not be prescribed to a patient already taking OTC acetaminophen. This may increase the dose to >3 g/day, which could increase the risk for developing hepatotoxicity (Khandelwal *et al.* 2011; Krenzelok and Royal 2012). It should be noted that in 2011, McNeil, manufacturers of Tylenol, voluntarily reduced the maximum daily dose to 3000 mg/day for the 500 mg tablets. Generic manufacturers have not to date changed the recommendations. Other regimens include supplemental glucosamine and chondroitin and corticosteroid injections (triamcinolone acetonide and lidocaine 1%). These injections are helpful only for a short term, lasting about 4–8 weeks (Sinusas 2012). Surgical or joint preservation surgery/total or partial joint replacement is reserved when pharmacologic treatment has failed (Sinusas 2012).

Dental notes

1. A medical consultation is usually not required.
2. No antibiotic prophylaxis is required.
3. Keep short appointments due to pain in joints.
4. Semi-supine position in the dental chair may be more comfortable than supine. Patients may require help getting in and out of the chair. Many patients may be using a cane, walker, or a wheelchair.
5. For osteoarthritis of the hand, oral home care devices may need changes: electric toothbrush, bigger handles for toothbrush, and electric flosser (Sonicare, WaterPik).
6. Patients may be taking aspirin or NSAIDs. No contraindications for treatment. May experience slightly more bleeding during a dental procedure (e.g., scaling/root planing, periodontal and implant surgery, and extractions). Symptom management is considered the first-level therapeutic approach (Patel and Manfredini 2013).

C. Rheumatoid arthritis

Clinical synopsis

Whereas osteoarthritis is caused by "wear and tear" or degeneration of the joints (three or more joints), RA is caused by an inflammatory and an autoimmune reaction wherein the host's body produces antibodies that target T lymphocytes with an increase in interleukin and tumor necrosis factor (TNF) and chronic inflammation of the joints (O'Dell 2012). This destroys connective (synovial) tissue, joints, and cartilage. There is a tendency toward symmetrical distribution of joint involvement and the most involved joint is the toe, followed by the wrist, knee, elbow, shoulder, hip, and tarsometatarsal joints. Duration of morning stiffness usually lasts past an hour, which serves as an index of activity.

RA is a multisystem disease involving one or more extra-articular symptoms including rheumatoid (subcutaneous) nodules of the finger joints, pulmonary fibrosis, obesity, pericarditis, myocarditis, valvulitis of the heart, splenomegaly, and normocytic anemia (Sayah and English 2005; Scrivo *et al.* 2013).

Diagnostics/lab values

Whereas osteoarthritis is diagnosed based on physical findings, RA is diagnosed based on a positive/ elevated rheumatoid factor (RF), anti-cyclic citrullinated peptide antibodies, synovial fluid analysis (to detect crystals in the joint and to look for signs of joint infection), C-reactive protein levels, and erythrocyte sedimentation rate (Klareskog *et al.* 2009; Goldman *et al.* 2013). Other testing done including antinuclear antibody (ANA) testing helps to rule out systemic lupus erythematosus (SLE) and complete blood count with differential and platelet count and liver and kidney function test help to rule out other disorders.

Treatment

There is no cure for RA, but some medications can help to reduce symptoms of pain, inflammation, and swelling and prevent further joint damage. Table 12.1 lists common nonbiologic or biologic disease-modifying antirheumatic drugs (DMARDs), TNF-α inhibitors, and the appropriate dental management of patients taking these medications (Li *et al.* 2013) (Table 12.3). Biologic agents are drugs similar to a naturally occurring substance. For example, rituximab is a biologic agent because it is a manufactured antibody similar to a naturally occurring antibody. The earlier the patient is placed on DMARDs, the lesser subsequent joint damage may occur (Lard *et al.* 2010). For mild active RA, the initial rapid relief drug of choice is either an NSAID or a corticosteroid and then start on DMARD treatment with hydroxychloroquine or sulfasalazine. For moderate to severe active RA, an NSAID is started followed by a DMARD (e.g., methotrexate). If the patient is resistant to this

Table 12.3 Drugs used to treat rheumatoid arthritis (RA) and dental management (Weinblatt 2003; Kalantzis *et al.* 2005; Mucke 2012; Li *et al.* 2013; Schur and Moreland 2013; www.nytimes.com/health/guides/disase/rheumatoid-arthritis/medications.html).

Antirheumatic drug	Dental implications
Rapidly acting anti-inflammatory drugs for mild active RA: Nonsteroidal anti-inflammatory drugs (NSAIDs)	Antiplatelet effect—bleeding
Rapidly acting anti-inflammatory drugs for mild active RA: Corticosteroids Administered orally or via intra-articular injections into the joints to reduce inflammation	Consult with physician regarding steroid supplementation for dental surgeries. This depends on whether the patient is on everyday or alternate-day steroid, which causes less inhibition of endogenous steroids. If supplemental steroids are require in a patient taking everyday steroids, usually, the patient takes double the usual dose.
Nonbiologic disease-modifying antirheumatic drugs (DMARDs) or host-modulating drugs and chemotherapy drugs (to minimize or prevent joint damage): Hydroxychloroquine (Plaquenil) Methotrexate (Rheumatrex) Leflunomide (Arava) Sulfasalazine	Methotrexate: stomatitis (mouth sores and ulcerations) is dose dependent, and folic acid supplementation with tablets or diet may relieve the stomatitis but this is controversial. OTC analgesics and chlorhexidine oral rinse may be helpful (Kalantzis *et al.* 2005); liver disease in patients with comorbidities, increased incidence of bacterial infections. Methotrexate may increase the risk for bacterial infections, which could compromise the periodontal condition as well as dental implants. It is safe to keep the patient on methotrexate for dental surgery (Pieringer *et al.* 2007; Sakai *et al.* 2011); consult with patient's physician. Hydroxychloroquine (Plaquenil) may cause a lichenoid-like reaction or rash intraorally. Patients taking DMARDs/immunosuppressant drugs are monitored monthly or in 1–3 months with a complete blood count; liver function tests; fasting lipids; eye exam; and electrolytes, urea, creatinine, and fasting glucose (Hsu and Katelaris 2009). Drug–drug interaction: Methotrexate + NSAID = increased toxicity of methotrexate

(continued)

Table 12.3   *(cont'd)*

Antirheumatic drug	Dental implications
Biologic (DMARDs) (synthesized from living cells): targets cytokines and tumor necrosis factor (TNF) Adalimumab (Humira) Etanercept (Enbrel) Infliximab (Remicade) Abatacept (Orencia) Rituximab (Rituxan) Anakinra (Kineret)	Risk for developing infections with TNF-blocking drugs (adalimumab, etanercept, infliximab). It has been recommended to discontinue these drugs before surgery and restart them only after wound healing is complete (Pieringer *et al.* 2007). Rituximab (infusions) causes severe mouth reactions including: painful perioral and intraoral sores and ulcers and low WBC, RBC, and platelets, which may result in bacterial infections, delayed healing, and bleeding problems. It is recommended to perform all necessary dental procedures before the patient starts rituximab therapy. While on rituximab, it may be necessary to place the patient on antibiotic prophylaxis for routine dental care including restorative and periodontal scaling. Consult with patient's rheumatologist. *Caution should be used when scheduling dental surgery in patients taking rituximab. This decision depends greatly on the indication for administering rituximab in the patient. Some references state at least 6 months between the last rituximab infusion and the scheduled invasive dental surgery. Consult with patient's treating physician regarding scheduling dental surgery*
Immunosuppressant drugs; also used for other medical conditions including after organ transplantation and ulcerative gastrointestinal disorders: Azathioprine (Imuran) Cyclosporine (Sandimmune, Neoral) Tacrolimus (Prograf)	Cyclosporine and tacrolimus: gingival enlargement (Ellis *et al.* 2004). Difficult for patient to perform home care. Maintain oral health with frequent recare appointments; high blood pressure and kidney function problems. Drug–drug interaction: Cyclosporine + NSAIDs = increased nephrotoxicity
Immunomodulator: (reduces immunoglobulin production, decreases matrix metalloproteinases (MMP-1 and MMP-3) Iguratimod (developed and approved in Japan and China)	Elevation of liver enzymes and thrombocytopenia
Janus kinase inhibitors: Tofacitinib (Xeljanz)	FDA-approved in 2013 for RA, inflammatory bowel disease, psoriasis, organ transplant rejection. Opportunistic infections, decreased neutrophils, increased liver enzyme test, nasopharyngitis

therapy, then a combination of DMARDs is initiated (e.g., methotrexate with either a TNF inhibitor or sulfasalazine) or prescribe leflunomide with NSAID or corticosteroid (Schur and Moreland 2013). Methotrexate is the current standard-of-care drug for RA, especially severe and resistant forms; however, there are numerous adverse effects which make it difficult to take for a long term. Combination DMARDs are usually necessary because a single DMARD loses effectiveness over time (Weinblatt 2003).

For many years, gold compounds have been indicated for active RA to inhibit macrophage activity in joints; however, since the use of DMARDs, including methotrexate, which is much better tolerated and orally administered, gold compounds have been used less frequently.

Dental notes (Treister and Glick 1999; Browning 2001; Grover *et al.* 2011; Mayer *et al.* 2009)

1. Obtain a medical consultation to determine if the patient has active RA.
2. Morning and early afternoon appointments are ideal.
3. RA should be suspected if the patient complains of polyarthritis with morning stiffness and pain lasting at least 30 min. SLE is a differential diagnosis (Klareskog *et al.* 2009; Venables and Maini 2013).
4. Patients on DMARD therapy will routinely be monitored by their physician for drug toxicity and disease activity; ask your patients about their schedule.
5. In patients taking rituximab, serious infections with delayed wound healing can occur after invasive dental surgery. Consult with patient's rheumatologist.
6. Monitor home care and caries and periodontal disease; patients with RA may exhibit periodontal disease (Mercardo *et al.* 2001).
7. Smoking cessation; tobacco use is a risk factor for RA.
8. Patients on corticosteroids may have to have additional supplementation for more invasive dental procedures; consult with patient's physician.
9. Be aware of adverse effects of DMARDs (refer to Table 12.3)
   a. Decreased coagulation—decreased platelets; bleeding problems
   b. Decreased WBCs; infection problems
10. Some patients may require antibiotic prophylaxis; consult with physician.
11. Be aware of altered liver function tests when prescribing antibiotics; dosing interval may need to be changed.
12. Evaluation of TMJ in the RA patient is required; anterior open bite may develop (Sasaguri *et al.* 2009).
13. Dental drug interaction: amoxicillin + methotrexate = especially high amoxicillin doses can cause increased serum methotrexate levels with nausea, vomiting, mouth ulcers and low blood cell counts, which can lead to anemia, bleeding problems, and infections (www.drugs.com).

D. Gout

Clinical synopsis

Gout, a type of arthritis, is a hereditary disease characterized by a sudden-onset acute attack usually of the first metatarsophalangeal joint, although it can occur in the finger, ankle, foot, knee, or wrist. It is primarily a condition with monarticular rather than polyarticular involvement; however, RA must be ruled out when there is polyarticular involvement. The duration of an acute attack is a few days while the next attack can be up to a year. If the primary acute attack is not treated, the condition becomes chronic wherein the pain and inflammation are more severe at each attack.

Gout usually affects adults >20 years of age and rarely is seen in children and young adults. It primarily affects men between 40 and 50 years (Helmick *et al.* 2008).

Gout is due to an overproduction of uric acid in the blood without compensatory overexcretion by the kidneys resulting in the accumulation of monosodium urate in the joints, bones, and soft tissue, which causes inflammation in the joints. The rate of monosodium urate deposition at affected joints is slow and insidious, and the appearance of tophi is related to the duration of gout and the degree of hyperuricemia and is a definitive sign of gouty arthritis (Harris *et al.* 1999).

Many patients with gout are hypertensive with vascular complications. Some of these patients have proteinuria due to intrinsic renal disease. As the kidney function fails, hyperuricemia becomes worse.

There are four stages of gout, which are based on the progression of the disease (Harris *et al.* 1999):

1st stage: Hyperuricemia is confirmed but the patient does not show symptoms. No treatment is required.
2nd stage: Acute gouty arthritis: Hyperuricemia results in the deposition of uric acid crystals in joint spaces leading to pain and inflammation of the joints. After this first attack, which can last up to 10 days, it may not be for months or years till the next attack even if treated.
3rd stage: Intercritical gout refers to the time interval when the patient does not experience any attack or symptoms
4th stage: chronic tophaceous gout: This stage occurs over a long time and is characterized by damage to joints and kidneys. This is a severely disabling stage of the disease.

Diagnostics/lab values

Gouty arthritis is not always definitively diagnosed by hyperuricemia (saturation of serum for urate). Having high uric acid blood levels is important but for a definitive diagnosis, synovial joint fluid from the inflamed joint positive for uric acid crystals is required.

Treatment

There are drugs to treat acute attacks of gout and for long-term control of gout. An NSAID is the first drug for the treatment of an acute attack. Corticosteroid administered orally or injected into the joint space is also indicated for an acute attack.

Allopurinol and febuxostat decrease the production of uric acid. Probenecid increases uric acid elimination via the kidneys (Stamp 2013). Colchicine, one of the oldest treatments for gout, inhibits tyrosine phosphorylation in neutrophils in response to crystals.

In addition to pharmacologic therapy, patients are instructed to avoid high-purine foods, limit alcohol, and reduce weight. Table 12.4 lists common interactions with dental drugs that the dentist should be aware.

Dental notes

1. Note drug interactions in Table 12.2.
2. There are no contraindications to dental procedures, even if the patient is having an acute attack.
3. Avoid prescribing aspirin or any combination drug with aspirin since it could decrease urate excretion.

Table 12.4 Dental drug–drug interactions with medications for gout (Harris *et al.* 1999; Stamp 2013).

Antigout drug	Dental drug	Recommendations
Colchicine	Clarithromycin	May increase blood levels of colchicine to dangerously high levels affecting liver and kidney, muscles, blood cells and nervous system. Consult with physician
Colchicine	Erythromycin	May increase blood levels of colchicine to dangerously high levels affecting liver and kidney, muscles, blood cells and nervous system. Consult with physician
Probenecid	Penicillin V Amoxicillin	Reduces excretion of probenecid resulting in elevated blood levels of probenecid. This is not a noticeable interaction and in some cases is used to increase the efficacy of the penicillin in certain infections
Ketorolac (Toradol)	Probenecid	Not recommended to take both concomitantly. If taken together, adverse effects include drowsiness, dizziness, and blood in urine

E. Fibromyalgia syndrome

Clinical synopsis

Fibromyalgia is a common chronic multisystem syndrome characterized by generalized long-term, total-body, diffuse pain with tenderness in the joints, muscles, tendons, and other soft tissue. There is a greater incidence in middle-aged women (Chakrabarty and Zoorob 2007). Other symptoms include disturbed sleep, stress, depression, stiffness, chronic fatigue, flu-like symptoms, and aching (Blumenthal 2002; Balasubramaniam *et al.* 2007). Fibromyalgia is common, effecting primarily white women over 59 years of age (Wolfe *et al.* 1995).

Oral signs/symptoms

Oral symptoms include xerostomia, temporomandibular disorder (TMD), glossodynia, dysgeusia, dysphagia, fatigue complaints in the orofacial area, pain on mandibular movement, and painful areas in the head and neck region (Rhodus *et al.* 2003; Sollecito *et al.* 2003; De Silva *et al.* 2012).

Diagnostics/lab values

There are no specific laboratory tests used to diagnose fibromyalgia. Fibromyalgia is usually diagnosed on clinical characteristics while sometimes excluding autoimmune disease such as SLE (Blumenthal 2002). The American College of Rheumatology (ACR) has set up criteria as follows: (i) widespread pain involving both sides of the body, above and below the waist and the axial skeletal system, for at least 3 months and (ii) presence of 11 tender points among the nine pairs of specified sites making up 18 points (Wolfe *et al.* 1990; Chakrabarty and Zoorob 2007; Wolfe *et al.* 2010). Complete blood count and differential are normal in fibromyalgia (Blumenthal 2002). Patients may also be positive to an ANA test; however, in many cases, there may be false positives (Blumenthal 2002). Thus, diagnosis of fibromyalgia is adequately (or satisfactorily) performed with a thorough history, physical examination, and routine blood testing (Blumenthal 2002).

Treatment (Chakrabarty and Zoorob 2007)

Treatment of fibromyalgia consists of both pharmacologic and nonpharmacologic therapies (exercise, hypnosis, acupuncture). Currently, there are three FDA-approved medications for the treatment of fibromyalgia: an anticonvulsant [pregabalin (Lyrica)] and selective norepinephrine–serotonin reuptake

Table 12.5　Dental drug–fibromyalgia drug interactions (www.drugs.com).

Dental drugs	Fibromyalgia drugs	Notes
Epinephrine	Tricyclic antidepressant (amitriptyline)	Moderate interaction: Limit the amount of 1:100,000 epinephrine to two cartridges (1.7 ml) which is equivalent to 0.034 mg (0.017 mg per cartridge). The reason for this is that tricyclic antidepressants inhibit the norepinephrine/epinephrine (NE/EPI) pump allowing norepinephrine to accumulate in the synapse. So, when epinephrine is injected and the NE/EPI pump is inhibited by the tricyclic antidepressant, the amount of epinephrine elevates resulting in possible cardiac problems. This interaction does not occur with selective serotonin reuptake inhibitors (SSRIs) (e.g., fluoxetine) because it selectively affects serotonin and not norepinephrine.
Epinephrine	Duloxetine (Cymbalta)	Moderate interaction: duloxetine is a selective norepinephrine–serotonin reuptake inhibitor drug that in part inhibits the NE/EPI reuptake pump; could cause increased risk of cardiovascular events when epinephrine is administered. Limit the amount of 1:100,000 epinephrine to two cartridges (1.7 ml), which is equivalent to 0.034 mg (0.017 mg per cartridge)
Acetaminophen/ codeine, oxycodone, hydrocodone, ibuprofen/oxycodone	Tramadol	Major interaction: consult with physician; can increase the risk of seizures and breathing problems
Ciprofloxacin, levofloxacin	Tramadol	Major interaction: Consult with physician; may cause seizures
Lidocaine with epinephrine dental anesthesia	Tramadol	Major interaction: especially in elderly patients or using alcohol or in alcohol withdrawal or with a history of seizures or brain tumor or head trauma. Consult with physician before using lidocaine
Bupropion (Zyban) for smoking cessation	Tramadol	Major interaction: especially in elderly patients or using alcohol or in alcohol withdrawal or with a history of seizures or brain tumor or head trauma. Consult with physician before using lidocaine
Ketoconazole	Tramadol	Minor interaction: can increase nausea, constipation, difficulty concentration, dizziness

inhibitors, [duloxetine (Cymbalta) and milnacipran (Savella)] for neuropathic pain and fatigue and improving function (Arnold *et al.* 2009; Straube *et al.* 2010).

- Tricyclic antidepressants such as amitriptyline and fluoxetine (selective serotonin reuptake inhibitor) have been effective.
- Many patients may require an analgesic such as tramadol (Ultram), which is a central-acting narcotic for moderate to severe pain. NSAIDs are used but generally are not effective (Chakrabarty and Zoorob 2007).
- A muscle relaxant such as cyclobenzaprine (Flexeril) at bedtime.
- Pregabalin (Lyrica), a second-generation anticonvulsant, is indicated for neuropathic pain.

Dental drug–fibromyalgia drug interactions

Table 12.5 reviews more commonly encountered drug–drug interactions in patients taking medications for fibromyalgia.

Dental notes (Rhodus *et al.* 2003; Sollecito *et al.* 2003; Balasubramaniam *et al.* 2007)

1. With a diagnosis of fibromyalgia when all other diseases have been ruled out, there is no need for a medical consultation.
2. Limit 1:100,000 epinephrine to two cartridges if the patient is taking a tricyclic antidepressant (amitriptyline).
3. Xerostomia is an adverse effect of cyclobenzaprine and pregabalin.
4. Patients with fibromyalgia may present with xerostomia and TMD; treat accordingly.
5. Patients may have trouble keeping their mouth open due to fatigue of jaw muscles; use mouth props if necessary.
6. Perform palpation of the head and neck muscular structures.
7. High prevalence of orofacial pain complaints in fibromyalgia patients.

F. Systemic lupus erythematosus

Clinical synopsis

SLE, frequently referred to as lupus, is an autoimmune disease with an unknown etiology. Essentially, it is a type of rheumatoid disease wherein the immune system attacks host cells, tissues, and organs, resulting in chronic inflammation (Trail and Claiborne 2013). SLE is more common in women, particularly African–American (Lawrence *et al.* 1998).

SLE causes much mortality and potentially severe bodily damage, and patients having it are at high risk for neuropsychiatric conditions, renal damage, cardiovascular diseases, digestive tract problems, and respiratory and urinary conditions (Urowitz *et al.* 2008; Fangtham and Petri 2013; Mosca and van Vollenhoven 2013). In addition, there is skin involvement (cutaneous lupus) showing the characteristic malar rash (butterfly rash), which characteristically shows flat or raised erythema over the malar eminence without affecting the nasolabial folds (Sims and Smith 1996), which is included as a criterion for the diagnosis. Discoid rash is evident as raised patches or adherent keratotic scaling.

Jaccoudarthropathy is characteristic of SLE where there are swan-neck deformities of the fingers without synovial or joint involvement (Blumenthal 2002). Approximately 50–60% of SLE patients develop nephritis during the first 10 years of the disease (Dooley *et al.* 2004; Hahn *et al.* 2012).

Approximately 10% of cases are drug-induced lupus (DIL). Common drugs that cause DIL include the following: high risk, hydralazine (muscle relaxant) and procainamide (antiarrhythmic); moderate risk, quinidine (antiarrhythmic); and low risk, acebutolol, carbamazepine, isoniazid (antituberculosis), methyldopa, minocycline, and sulfasalazine. This condition will resolve when the medication is discontinued; however, if that is not possible, an NSAID or low-dose corticosteroid can be prescribed for arthralgia and arthritis. To treat the skin rash, low-dose systemic or topical corticosteroid in combination with hydroxychloroquinecan be prescribed (Marshall 2011). If a drug-induced lupus is suspected, consult with a physician. Drug-induced lupus does not damage major organ systems as does SLE.

Diagnostics/lab values

There is no single diagnostic marker, so it is diagnosed based on clinical and laboratory criteria. ANA titer is obtained from patients with unexplained multiorgan system involvement. Usually, there is no muscle tenderness as in fibromyalgia. An ANA titer of 1:40 or higher is definitive for SLE and the most sensitive test according to the ACR Classification Criteria for SLE (Gill *et al.* 2003). Other conditions characterized with a positive ANA titer are fibromyalgia, Sjögren's syndrome (SS), scleroderma, and RA (Blumenthal 2002). In 2012, the Systemic Lupus International Collaborating Clinics group revised the ACR Classification Criteria to improve the overall understanding of SLE (Petri *et al.* 2012).

Laboratory abnormalities in SLE include the following: WBC—leukopenia; RBC—anemia (hemolytic); and platelets—thrombocytopenia ($<100,000/mm^3$). There is also elevated creatinine, low albumin, and microscopic hematuria (Blumenthal 2002).

Oral signs/symptoms

The oral cavity is affected in about 50% of patients. Painful or painless ulceration is observed usually on the hard palate (but also seen on soft palate), buccal mucosa, gingiva, tongue, vermilion border of lips and nasal tissues. In addition, patients should be monitored for periodontal disease and oral candidiasis.

Treatment

Table 12.6 lists common medications to treat SLE and their dental implications. Remission can happen but usually occurs with flare-ups. The prognosis of patients with SLE has improved significantly (20-year survival is 80%) in the past decade due to more effective treatment (Amissaho-Arthur and Gordon 2010). Besides treating lupus, comorbidities including cardiovascular diseases must also be addressed.

Dental notes (Alibila *et al.* 2007; Toscano *et al.* 2010; Trail and Claiborne 2013; www.ifnc.og/OnlineLibraryHome/Dental-Oral%20Problems/038c.pdf)

1. Rheumatologist consultation is recommended.
2. Antibiotic prophylaxis may or may not be required; check with rheumatologist. The reason for giving antibiotics is that half of the patients with SLE also have Libman–Sacks endocarditis, a heart condition that is usually undetected until death.
3. Frequent recare appointments, meticulous oral home care, and electric toothbrush or ultra-soft bristled tooth brush under hot water may be recommended.
4. Patients with comorbid respiratory problems should not be administered nitrous oxide, which would further depress respiration.

Table 12.6   Common medications for systemic lupus erythematosus (SLE) and their dental implications (Merrill 2012; Postal *et al.* 2012; Mosca and van Vollenhoven 2013).

SLE drugs	Indications	Dental implications
Rituximab	Active disease; non-labeled use; biologic; targets the B-cells. Used in patients with severe organ involvement who are refractory to other drugs or cannot tolerate other drugs; adverse effects include multiple organ involvement including kidney, CNS, and hematological	Causes severe mouth reactions including: painful perioral and intraoral sores and ulcers and low WBC, RBC, and platelets, which may result in bacterial infections and bleeding problems
Belimumab	In 2011, the first FDA-approved biologic (human monoclonal antibody) for SLE; severe disease with organ involvement and refractory cases. Some adverse effects include infections, heart problems, and suicide thoughts	In some patients neutropenia and thrombocytopenia
Nonsteroidal anti-inflammatory drugs (NSAIDs)	Mild disease, non-organ involvement	Bleeding
Corticosteroids	Effective (low dose) in SLE but many adverse effects and toxicities including peptic ulcer disease (do not prescribe NSAIDs for dental pain), osteoporosis, oral candidiasis, and psychiatric problems	Consult with rheumatologist; dosing may need to be increased in certain invasive/stressful dental procedures. Drug–drug interaction: Corticosteroid + NSAID + increased risk of GI bleeding
Hydroxychloroquine (Plaquenil)	Antimalarial drug; used with additional therapy when disease gets worse and steroid doses are increased; in skin and arthritis	Lichenoid reaction (intraoral red lesion or rash).
Mycophenolate Mofetil Methotrexate azathioprine	Immunosuppressants: in severe cases and when not on steroid, dose cannot be reduced to acceptable levels (nonresponding). For renal disease, Mycophenolate Mofetil with steroid. For maintenance therapy, Mycophenolate Mofetil or azathioprine	Azathioprine and Mycophenolate Mofetil: hepatotoxicity; evaluate liver test. Opportunistic bacterial infection with methotrexate (could compromise the periodontal condition as well as dental implants). Avoid prescribing NSAIDs with methotrexate

5. If the undiagnosed patient has red/white lesions on lips and/or mucous membranes that look nonspecific, do a biopsy.
6. Painful oral lesions may limit eating; incorporate nutritional counseling; avoid alcohol-containing mouth rinses; rinse with 1 teaspoonful baking soda in a full glass of water. Avoid citrus and spicy food.
7. During dental surgery, patients that have the "lupus anticoagulant" antibody in the presence of a platelet deficiency, may experience abnormal bleeding.
8. Be aware of comorbid conditions associated with SLE. Kidney damage may require dosing interval of dental drugs including tetracycline and NSAIDs. Doxycycline can be prescribed in patients with kidney insufficiency. Know the GFR/CrCl before prescribing any medications.
9. Painless oral or nasopharyngeal ulcers.
10. Fibromyalgia is more common than in SLE.

G. Sjögren's syndrome

Clinical synopsis

SS is a progressive autoimmune condition characterized by peri-epithelially lymphocytic infiltrates in host tissues with the synthesis of autoantibodies resulting in diminished lacrimal and salivary gland function (Kyriakidis *et al.* 2013). It most commonly occurs in women aged 40–50 years.

Primary SS presents only as SS with the cardinal signs and symptoms of SS, while secondary SS presents with the characteristic signs and symptoms of SS associated with multiple comorbidities such connective tissue diseases including RA, fibromyalgia, and SLE (Carr *et al.* 2012).

Diagnostics/lab values

To assist in the diagnosis, two principal symptoms that comprise the "sicca complex" should be present: xerostomia, often the first symptom experienced, and keratoconjunctivitis sicca (dry eyes) (Ramos-Casals *et al.* 2005). In addition, burning mouth, dysphagia, and taste disturbances have been reported (Pinto 2014). Pinto (2014) describes xerostomia as the patient's subjective perception of dryness in the oral cavity; whereas hyposalivation is the objective confirmation of oral dryness as determined by flow measurement. There are different tests to quantify xerostomia including the salivary gland scintigraphy, parotid sialography, unstimulated production of saliva, and Saxon test (Fox and Creamer 2012). There are different tests to evaluate tear production. One common test is the Schirmer's test, which is performed by placing a tissue paper in the corner of the eye and determining if the eye can produce enough tears (Afonso *et al.* 1999).

Oral signs and symptoms

Prominent signs and symptoms of SS and its management are reviewed in Table 12.7. Other signs/symptoms include hoarseness, oral sores, and loss of taste.

Treatment

The goal of treatment of SS is to relieve symptoms. Besides muscarinic receptor agonists for the management of xerostomia/hyposalivation, other newer agents that have been used in the treatment of primary SS show questionable efficacy (Table 12.8).

Table 12.7 Signs and symptoms of Sjörgren's syndrome (SS) and its management (Ramos-Casals *et al.* 2005; Gupta *et al.* 2006; Wu 2009; Carr *et al.* 2012; Pinto 2014).

Oral signs/symptoms	Dental management
Xerostomia and salivary gland hyposalivation	Highly recommended drugs are systemic sialogogues (muscarinic agonists): pilocarpine 5–10 mg three times a day or cevimeline 30 mg three times a day. These agents may not be as effective in the later stages of SS where there is irreversible salivary gland damage. In clinical trials, the use of salivary lubricants or substitutes in severe cases is not agreed, and topical moisturizers also seemed to be marginally acceptable.
	Remineralizing products (MI paste, MI paste Plus, NovaMin), Oral Biotene products, carboxymethyl or hydroxyethyl solutions (Optimoist, Salix, Salivart, Moi-Stir spray), Prevident, xylitol-containing chewing gum, drinking water frequently, and regular oral home care.
Dysphagia	Clinical studies show promising positive results with an electric stimulator
Oral burning	According to many clinical studies, oral burning is difficult to treat with favorable outcomes; tricyclic antidepressants have been helpful
Oral candidiasis (secondary to oral dryness and/or changes in salivary composition)	Due to high rate of development of resistance to most topical agents, systemic antifungal (fluconazole) treatment is feasible

Table 12.8 Drugs for Sjörgren's syndrome (SS) (Ramos-Casals *et al.* 2005; Kruszka and O'Brian 2009; Carr *et al.* 2012).

Drugs for SS	Notes
Treating systemic involvement of SS: Infliximab Interferon α Rituximab	There is insufficient evidence to prescribe immunomodulators, biologic agents/monoclonal antibody agents, or immunosuppressive drugs for ocular or oral symptoms, but these drugs may be recommended for systemic features of SS including renal, respiratory, hepatic, neurologic, and vascular problems. Adverse effects of rituximab include fatal skin and mouth reactions from Stevens–Johnson syndrome/toxic epidermal necrolysis, increased risk of postoperative infections, and delayed wound healing. Consult with patient's rheumatologist. *Caution should be used when scheduling dental surgery in patients taking rituximab. This decision depends greatly on the indication for administering rituximab in the patient. Some references state at least 6 months between the last rituximab infusion and the scheduled invasive dental surgery. Consult with patient's treating physician regarding scheduling dental surgery.* In addition, it can cause reactivation of hepatitis B infection
Treating the eye problems	Artificial tear substitutes, eye ointments or gels, cyclosporine eye drops (increases tear production)

Dental notes

1. Recommend physician consultation to determine if there is systemic involvement.
2. Review oral symptoms and medications the patient is already taking.
3. Hyposalivation can lead to dental caries, fungal infections, and periodontal disease, besides being annoying to the patient. Encourage the patient to do oral self-exams to report any ulcers or mouth problems. Fluoride supplementation is recommended for high–dental risk patients. Maintaining meticulous home care as well as frequent recare appointments are important (Gupta *et al.* 2006).
4. Encourage patients not to sleep with dentures.

References

Afonso, A.A., Monroy, D., Stern, M.E. *et al.* (1999) Correlation of tear fluorescein clearance and Schirmer test scores with ocular irritation symptoms. *Ophthalmology*, **106**, 803–810.

Alibila, J.B., Clokie, C.M.L., & Sandor, G.K.B. (2007) Systemic lupus erythematosus: a review for dentists. *Journal of the Canadian Dental Association*, **73**, 823–828.

American Dental Association Council on Scientific Affairs (2006) Dental management of patients receiving oral bisphosphonate therapy. *Journal of the American Dental Association*, **137 (8)**, 1144–1150.

Amissaho-Arthur, M.B. & Gordon, C. (2010) Contemporary treatment of systemic lupus erythematosus: an update for clinicians. *Therapeutic Advances in Chronic Disease*, **1**, 163–175.

Arnold, L.M., Clauw, D.J., Wohlreich, M.M., *et al.* (2009) Efficacy of duloxetine in patients with fibromyalgia: pooled analysis of 4 placebo-controlled clinical trials. *Primary Care Companion to the Journal of Clinical Psychiatry*, **11**, 237–244.

Balasubramaniam, R., Laudenbach, J.M., & Stoopler, E.T. (2007) Fibromyalgia: an update for oral health care providers. *Oral Surgery, Oral Medicine, Oral Pathology, Oral Radiology and Endodontology*, **104**, 589–602.

Blumenthal, D.E. (2002) Tired, aching, ANA-positive: does your patient have lupus or fibromyalgia? *Cleveland Clinic Journal of Medicine*, **69 (2)**, 143–152.

Browning, M. (2001) Rheumatoid arthritis: a primary care approach. *Journal of the American Academy of Nurse Practitioners*, **13**, 399–408.

Carr, A.J., Ng, W.F., Figueiredo, F. *et al.* (2012) Sjogren's syndrome—an update for dental practitioners. *British Dental Journal*, **213 (7)**, 353–357.

Cartsos, V.M., Zhu, S., & Zavras, A.I. (2008). Bisphosphonate use and the risk of adverse jaw outcomes: a medical claims study of 714,217 people. *Journal of the American Dental Association*, **139**, 23–30.

Chakrabarty, S. & Zoorob, R. (2007) Fibromyalgia. *American Family Physician*, **76**, 247–254.

De Silva, L.A., Kazyiama, H.H., de Siqueira, J.T., *et al.* (2012) High prevalence of orofacial complains in patients with fibromyalgia: a case-control study. *Oral Surgery, Oral Medicine, Oral Pathology, Oral Radiology and Endodontology*, **113**, e29–e34.

Dooley, M.A., Aranow, C., & Ginzler, E.M. (2004) Review of ACR renal criteria in systemic lupus erythematosus. *Lupus*, **13**, 857–860.

Edwards, B.J., Hellstein, J.W., & Jacobson, P.L. (2008) Updated recommendations for managing the care of patients receiving oral bisphosphonate therapy: an advisory statement from the American Dental Association Council on Scientific Affairs. *Journal of the American Dental Association*, **139**, 1674–1677.

Ellis, J.S., Seymour, R.A., Taylor, J.J., *et al.* (2004) Prevalence of gingival overgrowth in transplant patients immunosuppressed with tacrolimus. *Journal of Clinical Periodontology*, **31 (2)**, 126–131.

Fangtham, M. & Petri, M. (2013) Update: Hopkins Lupus Cohort. *Current Rheumatology Reports*, **15**, 360.

Fleisher, K.E., Welch, G., Kottal, S., *et al.* (2010) Predicting risk for bisphosphonate-related osteonecrosis of the jaws: CTX versus radiographic markers. *Oral Medicine, Oral Pathology, Oral Radiology and Endodontology*, **110 (4)**, 509–516.

Fox, R. & Creamer, P. (2012) Classification and diagnosis of Sjögren's syndrome. *UpToDate,* Topic 5603. Version 9.0. http://www.uptodate.com/contents/classification-and-diagnosis-of-sjogrens-syndrome [accessed on July 27, 2014].

Fugazzotto, P.A., Lightfoot, W.S., Jaffin, R. *et al*. (2007) Implant placement with or without simultaneous tooth extraction in patients taking oral bisphosphonates: postoperative healing, early follow up, and the incidence of complications in two private practices. *Journal of Periodontology*, **7819**, 1664–1669.

Gill, J.M., Quisel, A.M., Rocca, P.V., *et al*. (2003) Diagnosis of systemic lupus erythematosus. *American Family Physician*, **68**, 2179–2187.

Goldman, K., Gertel, S., & Amital, H. (2013) Anti-citrullinated peptide antibodies is more than an accurate tool for diagnosis of rheumatoid arthritis. *Israel Medical Association Journal*, **15 (9)**, 516–519.

Grant, B.T., Amenedo, C., Freeman, K., *et al*. (2008). Outcomes of placing dental implants in patients taking oral bisphosphonates: a review of its cases. *Journal of Oral and Maxillofacial Surgery*, **66**, 223–230.

Grover, H.S., Gaba, N., Gupta, A., *et al*. (2011) Rheumatoid arthritis: a review and dental care considerations. *Nepal Medical College Journal*, **13 (2)**, 74–76.

Gupta, A., Epstein, J.B., & Sroussi, H. (2006) Hyposalivation in elderly patients. *Journal of the Canadian Dental Association*, **72**, 841–846.

Hahn, B.H., McMahon, M.A., Wilkinson, A., *et al*. (2012) American College of Rheumatology Guidelines for Screening, Treatment, and Management of lupus nephritis. *Arthritis Care & Research*, **64**, 797–808.

Harris, M.D., Siegel, L.B., & Alloway, J.A. (1999) Gout and hyperuricemia. *American Family Physician*, **59**, 925–934.

Hellstein, J.W., Adler, R.A., Edwards, B., *et al*. (2011) Managing the care of patients receiving antiresorptive therapy for prevention and treatment of osteoporosis. *Journal of the American Dental Association*, **142**, 1243–1251.

Helmick, C.G., Felson, D.T., Lawrence, R.C., *et al*. (2008) National Arthritis Data Workgroup. Estimates of the prevalence of arthritis and other rheumatic conditions in the United States. Part 1. *Arthritis and Rheumatism*, **1**, 15–25.

Hsu, D.C. & Katelaris, C.H. (2009) Long-term management of patients taking immunosuppressive drugs. *Australian Prescriber*, **32**, 68–71.

Kalantzis, A., Marshman, Z., Falconer, D.T., *et al*. (2005) Oral effects of low-dose methotrexate treatment. *Oral Surgery, Oral Medicine, Oral Pathology, Oral Radiology, and Endodontology*, **100**, 52–62.

Khandelwal, N., James, L.P., Saunders, C., *et al*. (2011) Unrecognized acetaminophen toxicity as a cause of indeterminate acute liver failure. *Hepatology*, **53**, 567–576.

Klareskog, L., Catrina, A.I., & Paget, S. (2009) Rheumatoid arthritis. *Lancet*, **373**, 659–672.

Krenzelok, E.P. & Royal, M.A. (2012) Confusion. Acetaminophen dosing changes based on NO evidence in adults. *Drugs*, **12 (2)**, 45–48.

Kruszka, P. & O'Brian, R.J. (2009) Diagnosis and management of Sjögren syndrome. *American Family Physician*, **79**, 465–470.

Kyriakidis, N.C., Kapsogeorgou, E.K., & Tzioufas, A.G. (2013) A comprehensive review of autoantibodies in primary Sjörgen's syndrome: clinical phenotypes and regulatory mechanisms. *Journal of Autoimmunity*, **51**, 67–74.

Lard, L.R., Visser, H., Speyer, I., *et al*. (2001) Early versus delayed treatment in patients with recent-onset rheumatoid arthritis: comparison of two cohorts who received different treatment strategies. *American Journal of Medicine*, **111**, 446–451.

Lawrence, R.C., Helmick, C.G., Arnett, F.C. *et al*. (1998) Estimates of the prevalence of arthritis and selected musculoskeletal disorders in the United States. *Arthritis & Rheumatism*, **41**, 367–369.

Li, J., Mao, H., Liang, Y. *et al*. (2013) Efficacy and safety of iguratimod for the treatment of rheumatoid arthritis. *Clinical and Developmental Immunology*, 2013, 310628.

Marshall, J.L. (2011) Identifying drug-induced lupus. *U.S. Pharmacist*, **37**, HS6–HS8.

Marx, R.E. 2007. *Oral and Intravenous Bisphosphonate-Induced Osteonecrosis of the Jaws: History, Etiology, Prevention, and Treatment*, p. 15. Quintessence, Chicago, IL.

Marx, R.E., Sawatari, Y., Fortin, M. *et al*. (2005). Bisphosphonate-induced exposed bone (osteonecrosis/osteoporosis) of the jaws: risk factors, recognition, prevention, and treatment. *Journal of Oral and Maxillofacial Surgery*, **63**, 1567–1575.

Mayer, Y., Balbir-Gurman, A., & Machtei, E.E. (2009) Anti-tumor necrosis factor-alpha therapy and periodontal parameters in patients with rheumatoid arthritis. *Journal of Periodontology*, **80**, 141–1420.

Mercardo, R.B., Marshall, R.I., Klestov, A.C., *et al*. (2001) Relationship between rheumatoid arthritis and periodontitis. *Journal of Periodontology*, **72**, 779–787.

Merrill, J.T. (2012) Treatment of systemic lupus erythematosus. A 2012 update. *Bulletin of the NYU Hospital for Joint Diseases*, **70 (3)**, 172–176.

Migliorati, C.A., Casiglia, J., Epstein, J., *et al.* (2005). Managing the care of patients with bisphosphonate-associated osteonecrosis: an American Academy of Oral Medicine position paper. *Journal of the American Dental Association*, **136**, 1658–1668.

Migliorati, C.A., Saunders, D., Conlon, M.S., *et al.* (2013) Assessing the association between bisphosphonate exposure and delayed mucosal healing after tooth extraction. *Journal of the American Dental Association*, **144 (4)**, 406–414.

Millett, E.J., Gobezie, R., & Boykin, R.E. (2008) Shoulder osteoarthritis: diagnosis and management. *American Family Physician*, **78 (5)**, 605–611.

Mosca, M. & van Vollenhoven, R. (2013) New drugs in systemic lupus erythematosus: when to start and when to stop. *Clinical and Experimental Rheumatology*, **31 (Suppl. 78)**, S82–S85.

Mucke, H.A. (2012) Iguratimod: a new disease-modifying antirheumatic drug. *Drugs Today*, **48**, 577–586.

O'Dell, J.R. (2012) Rheumatoid arthritis. In: L. Goldman & A.I. Schafer (eds). *Goldman's Cecil Medicine*, 24th ed., Chapter 272, pp. 1681–1689. Elsevier/Saunders, New York.

Otomo-Corgel, J. (2007) Implants and oral bisphosphonates: risky business? *Journal of Periodontology*, **78**, 373–376.

Patel, D.N. & Manfredini, D. (2013) Two commentaries on interventions for the management of temporomandibular joint osteoarthritis. *Evidenced-Based Dentistry*, **14**, 5–7.

Petri, M., Orbal, A.M., Alarcón, G.S., *et al.* (2012) Derivation and validation of the Systemic Lupus International Collaborating Clinics classification criteria for systemic lupus erythematosus. *Arthritis & Rheumatism*, **64**, 2677–2686.

Pieringer, H., Stuby, U., & Biesenbach, G. (2007) Patients with rheumatoid arthritis undergoing surgery: how should we deal with antirheumatic treatment? *Seminars in Arthritis and Rheumatism*, **36 (5)**, 278–286.

Pinto, A. (2014) Management of xerostomia and other complications of Sjogren's syndrome. *Oral Maxillofacial Surgery Clinics*, **26 (1)**, 63–73.

Postal, M., Costallat, L.T.L., & Appenzeller, S. (2012) Biological therapy in systemic lupus erythematosus. *International Journal of Rheumatology*, **2012**, 578641.

Ramos-Casals, M., Tzioufas, A.G., & Font, J. (2005) Primary Sjorgen's syndrome: new clinical and therapeutic concepts. *Annals of the Rheumatic Diseases*, **64**, 347–354.

Rees, F., Doherty, S., Hui, M., *et al.* (2012) Distribution of finger nodes and their association with underlying radiographic features of osteoarthritis. *Arthritis Care & Research*, **64 (4)**, 533–538.

Rhodus, N.L., Fricton, J., Carlson, P., *et al.* (2003) Oral symptoms associated with fibromyalgia syndrome. *The Journal of Rheumatology* **30**, 1841–1845.

Ruggiero, S.L. (2008). Bisphosphonate-related osteonecrosis of the jaws. *Compendium*, **29 (2)**, 97–105.

Sakai, R., Komano, Y., Tanaka, M., *et al.* (2011) The REAL database reveals no significant risk of serious infection during treatment with a methotrexate dose of more than 8 mg/week in patients with rheumatoid arthritis. *Modern Rheumatology*, **21**, 444–448.

Sasaguri, K., Ishizaki-Takeuchi, R., Kuramae, S., *et al.* (2009) The temporomandibular joint in a rheumatoid arthritis patient after orthodontic treatment. *Angle Orthodontist*, **79 (4)**, 804–811.

Sayah, A. & English, J.C. 3rd. (2005) Rheumatoid arthritis: a review of the cutaneous manifestations. *Journal of the American Academy of Dermatology*, **53**, 191–209.

Schur, P.H. & Moreland, L.W. (2013) General principles of management of rheumatoid arthritis in adults. *UpToDate*, Topic 7516 Version 15.0. http://www.uptodate.com/contents/general-principles-of-management-of-rheumatoid-arthritis-in-adults [accessed on July 27, 2014].

Scrivo, R., Vasile, M., Müller-Ladner, U., *et al.* (2013) Rheumatic diseases and obesity: adipocytokines as potential comorbidity biomarkers for cardiovascular diseases. *Mediators of Inflammation*, **2013**, 808125.

Sims, G.N. & Smith, H.R. (1996) Outpatient management of systemic lupus erythematosus. *Cleveland Clinic Journal of Medicine*, **63**, 94–100.

Sinusas, K. (2012) Osteoarthritis: diagnosis and treatment. *American Family Physician*, **85 (1)**, 45–56.

Sollecito, T.P., Stoopler, E.T., DeRossi, S.S., *et al.* (2003) Temporomandibular disorders and fibromyalgia: comorbid conditions? *General Dentistry*, **51**, 184–187.

Stamp, L.K. (2013) Safety profile of anti-gout agents: an update. *Current Opinions in Rheumatology*, **26 (2)**, 162–168.

Straube, S., Derry, S., Morre, R.A. *et al* (2010) Pregabalin in fibromyalgia: meta-analysis of efficacy and safety from company clinical trial reports. *Rheumatology*, **49**, 706–715.

Sweet, M.G., Sweet, J.M., Jeremiah, M.P., *et al.* (2009) Diagnosis and treatment of osteoporosis. *American Family Physician*, **79 (3)**, 193–200.

Toscano, N.J., Holtzclaw, D.J., Shumaker, N.D., *et al* (2010) Surgical considerations and management of patients with mucocutaneous disorders. *Compendium*, **31**, 344–359.

Trail, A.C. & Claiborne, D.M. (2013) Treating patients with lupus. *Dimension of Dental Hygiene*, 53–57. http://www.dimensionsofdentalhygiene.com/2013/10_October/Features/Treating_Patients_with_Lupus.aspx [accessed on July 27, 2014].

Treister, N. & Glick M. (1999) Rheumatoid arthritis: a review and suggested dental care considerations. *Journal of the American Dental Association*, **130**, 689–698.

U.S. Preventive Services Task Force (2013) Screening for osteoporosis in post-menopausal women: recommendations and rationale. Agency for Healthcare Research and Quality, Rockville, MD; July 2010. http://www.ahrq.gov/clinic/3rduspstf/osteoporosis/osteorr.htm [accessed on December 28, 2013].

Urowitz, M.B., Gladman, D.D., Tom, B.D.M., *et al.* (2008) Changing patterns in mortality and disease outcomes for patients with systemic lupus erythematosus. *The Journal of Rheumatology*, **35**, 2152–2158.

Venables, P.J.W. & Maini, R.N. (2013) Diagnosis and differential diagnosis of rheumatoid arthritis. *UpToDate*, Topic 6504. Version 11.0. http://www.uptodate.com/contents/diagnosis-and-differential-diagnosis-of-rheumatoid-arthritis [accessed on July 27, 2014].

Wang, H. L., Weber, D., & McCauley, L.K. (2007) Effect of long-term oral bisphosphonates on implant wound healing: literature review and a case report. *Journal of Periodontology*, **78**, 584–594.

Weinberg, M.A., Westphal-Thiele, C., & Fine, J.B. (2014) *Oral Pharmacology for the Dental Hygienist*. Pearson Publications, Upper Saddle River, NJ.

Weinblatt, M.E. (2003) Rheumatoid arthritis in 2003: where are we now with treatment. *Annals of the Rheumatic Diseases*, **62 (Suppl, II)**, ii94–ii96.

Wellbery, C. (2007) Pharmacologic treatment of osteopenia not usually indicated. *American Family Physician*, **76 (5)**, 711.

Wolfe, F., Smythe, H.A., Yunus, M.B., *et al.* (1990) The American College of Rheumatology 1990 criteria for the classification of fibromyalgia. Report of the Multicenter Criteria Committee. *Arthritis & Rheumatism*, **33**, 160–172.

Wolfe, F., Ross, K., Anderson, J., *et al.* (1995) The prevalence and characteristics of fibromyalgia in the general population. *Arthritis & Rheumatism* **38**, 19–28.

Wolfe, F., Clauw, D.J., Fitzcharles, M.A., *et al.* (2010) The American College of Rheumatology preliminary diagnostic criteria for fibromyalgia and measurement of symptom severity. *Arthritis Care & Research*, **62**, 600–610.

Wu, A.J. (2008) Optimizing dry mouth treatment for individuals with Sjögren's syndrome. *Rheumatic Disease Clinics of North America*, **34 (4)**, 1001–1010.

Zak, M., Spina, A.N., Spinazze, R.P., *et al.* (2007). Bisphosphonates and the dental patient: Part 1. *Compendium* **28 (9)**, 510–516.

Chapter 13

HIV and oral health care

HIV prevalence	214
Biology of HIV	216
Oral lesions	221
Highly active antiretroviral therapy	223
Fusion/entry inhibitors	225
Impact of medical treatment on PLWHA	227
Dental notes: Dental treatments	227
Dental notes: Clinical ramifications for dental treatment	232
Summary	233
References	234

Clinical synopsis

HIV/AIDS has posed unique problems for the medical and dental health professional over the course of the epidemic. Obstacles faced by the dental practitioner include the lack of standardized procedures for HIV testing, a standardized protocol for counseling and treating HIV patients, payment codes for HIV testing, and standardized laboratory indices to assess the health of HIV patients seeking dental treatment. People living with HIV/AIDS (PLWHA) have their own set of obstacles including fear of dentists, stigma, limited oral health literacy, patient dissatisfaction with their dentists, lack of dental insurance or other means to pay for services, and the severity of pain or discomfort associated with previous dental visits. Consequently, the unmet needs for oral health care among PLWHA are higher than for the general population. It is critical for PLWHA to obtain dental care in spite of the many burdens they face because untreated oral disease can lead to conditions that are more severe to their physical health and quality of life (Benjamin 2012).

Another problem is the limited recognition, among non-dental clinicians, about oral disease and the promotion of good oral health in the immune-compromised individual. New public health strategies, and information on oral health care, are beginning to reach the PLWHA community. These initiatives will help to inform the PLWHA community that good oral health is a vital component of their overall health and well-being.

Dentists should be encouraged to become familiar with the specific difficulties faced by PLWHA to better facilitate access to dental care for those living with the virus as well as those who are not

The Dentist's Quick Guide to Medical Conditions, First Edition. Mea A. Weinberg, Stuart L. Segelnick, Joseph S. Insler, with Samuel Kramer.
© 2015 John Wiley & Sons, Inc. Published 2015 by John Wiley & Sons, Inc.

yet aware of their HIV status. This chapter will attempt to summarize key aspects of HIV/AIDS in the context of diagnosis and treatment, current medical regimens, recent updates in oral health care, and practical suggestions for the dental clinician on how to produce better outcomes for PLWHA.

HIV prevalence

Epidemiologic studies have demonstrated that there are three primary routes of HIV transmission: sexual, parenteral (blood-borne), and perinatal. Laboratory studies have demonstrated that HIV has a short lifespan when exposed to air outside of a host. However, the air does not totally kill the virus. When virus-containing fluid is allowed to dry, the amount of viable virus is reduced by 90–99%. Unlike the common cold, flu, or tuberculosis, HIV specifically targets the immune cells designed to kill it. The fragility of the virus and shortened survival preclude transmission from casual contact such as coughing, hugging, and shaking hands; insect bites; and surface contact from toilet seats or other surfaces.

There are currently more than 1.1 million people in the USA living with HIV infection (Rathbun *et al.* 2013) and almost 1 in 6 (15.8%) are unaware of their infection. Gay/bisexual men, particularly young African–American men having sex with men (MSM), and injection drug users are most seriously affected by the disease. When compared with other racial groups, African–Americans are at the greatest risk of the disease (CDC 2013). In the USA, the estimated incidence rate of HIV has remained overall stable in recent years. In 2011, an estimated 49,273 people were diagnosed with HIV infection in the USA and in that same year, an estimated 32,052 people progressed to AIDS (UNAIDS 2013). An estimated 19,343 people with an AIDS diagnosis died in 2010. Overall, approximately 636,000 people with an AIDS diagnosis have died in the USA (CDC 2011) since the inception of the epidemic. Deaths associated with HIV/AIDS diagnosis are primarily due to opportunistic infections (OIs). AIDS-related mortality rates in the USA have decreased over the past three decades, as treatment for HIV and associated OIs have improved, but there is still a constant steady state of new infections annually.

The global burden of HIV/AIDS is staggering. Worldwide, 33.4 million are currently living with HIV/AIDS; more than 25 million people have died of AIDS since the first cases were reported in 1981 (AIDS.gov 2010). In 2008 alone, 2 million people died due to HIV/AIDS, and another 2.7 million were newly infected (AIDS.gov 2010). Ninety seven percent of people living with HIV reside in low- and middle-income countries, with those living in sub-Saharan Africa being the most affected (UNAIDS 2013). Although the number of HIV-infected individuals receiving treatment in resource-poor countries has increased 10-fold since 2002, the epidemic continues to devastate sub-Saharan Africa. Many of the countries hardest hit by HIV also suffer from problems of food insecurity, paucity of clean water, inadequate sanitation, and other epidemics like malaria and tuberculosis.

Historical perspective

In the summer of 1981, young homosexual men in San Francisco and New York were being seen with flu-like symptoms, unusual malignancies, and infections by healthcare providers. Their immune systems were not able to fend off pathogenic organisms responsible for the OIs resulting in chronic symptoms of diarrhea, anorexia, wasting, alopecia, premature aging, and death. In some, dark purple skin lesions developed on the face and on other parts of the body. This was later diagnosed as a relatively rare and aggressive form of cancer called Kaposi sarcoma (Greene 2007). This chronic disease, referred to as the "gay plague," baffled clinicians and spread fear within the homosexual community. The health of these young men deteriorated rapidly. Most died as their doctors struggled to treat these unusual infections and malignancies. In the early days of the AIDS epidemic, research and epidemiologic data were not available and as a result, many theories about AIDS focused on the lifestyle of homosexual men (Altman 1982) and consequently this set of symptoms was originally called gay-related immune deficiency.

By late 1982, epidemiologic evidence indicated that AIDS was an infectious disease transferred by body fluids and by exposure to contaminated blood or blood products (MMWR 1982a). Reports surfaced indicating that the disease was being identified in patients with hemophilia (MMWR 1982b) and others receiving blood transfusions (MMWR 1982c), intravenous drug abusers (Masur *et al.* 1981), infants born to infected mothers (MMWR 1982b), and sexually active women whose partners were infected (Harris *et al.* 1983). During the period of 1981–1984, more than 50% of hemophilic patients in the USA had become infected and presented with the clinical symptoms of AIDS (MMWR 1982b).

Public outcry demanded more research and implementation of public health measures and policies to prevent the spread of the disease. Researchers in Europe and the USA continued to attempt to isolate and identify the organism responsible for this deadly illness. The first needle-exchange program for intravenous drug abusers was set up in Amsterdam in 1984 (Lane and Stryker 1993). Additional programs were implemented throughout Europe and the USA. Soon thereafter, a heterosexual epidemic of AIDS was reported among immigrants from Central Africa, that preferentially affected women, with none of the previously described risk factors (Klatt 2013). In 1983, Dr. Luc Montagnier and colleagues at the Institute Pasteur identified a new human retrovirus, which they named lymphadenopathy-associated virus (Barré-Sinoussi 2003). However, the causal link between this virus and the chronic disease was forged by Robert Gallo and his colleagues at the National Institutes of Health in 1984 (Popovic *et al.* 1984; Schupbach *et al.* 1984). During this period, Jay Levy at UCSF independently confirmed the virus, which he named AIDS-associated retrovirus (ARV) (Levy 1984). In May, 1986, the International Committee of the Taxonomy of Viruses, chaired by Harold Varmus, recommended that this pathogen with many names be called the human immunodeficiency virus (HIV) (Coffin *et al.* 1986). In 1985, the isolation of the virus and the identification of the genomic sequence enabled scientists to develop laboratory tests for the diagnosis of HIV in patients and in blood products collected for transfusion. Policies were established to protect the quality of the blood supply by HIV testing prior to their use for transfusion.

When compared with other pathogens, the virus appears to have a relatively simple 9 kb RNA genome (Nikolaitchik *et al.* 2013). However, the virus has the ability to bind to and destroy specific cells within the host's immune system, designed to fight viral infection. Confounding the problem is the inherent transcriptional error rate that enables the virus to rapidly mutate, which gives the progeny a different immunologic identity enabling them to invade the host's immune system. The first possibility of treatment came with the identification of three enzymes, reverse transcriptase, protease, and integrase. In 1987, Zidovudine (AZT), a drug originally designed to fight cancer, was found to inhibit HIV transcription (Greene 2007). However, this single drug was not capable of containing the mutated forms, and its effectiveness proved short-lived as the first documented case of AZT-resistant virus was in 1993 (García-Lerma *et al.* 2004; Greene 2007). During this period, researchers identified CD4 as an essential white blood cell surface protein for viral-cell binding. An additional 12 years passed before the cofactors CCR5 and CXCR4 were identified (Yi1 *et al.* 1998).

The mortality rate in developed countries began to decline by the mid-1990s with the introduction of antiretroviral medications and the implementation of highly active antiretroviral therapy (HAART) protocols (Greene 2007; Klatt 2013). The use of these medications in HIV-infected pregnant women also resulted in a substantial decline in mother-to-child transmission (Anderson 2005).Without access to these antiretroviral medications, mother-to-child HIV transmission, as well as infant and maternal mortality rates, continues to increase in lower-income and resource-poor countries.

Biology of HIV

HIV is a member of a class of viruses known as retroviruses that contain RNA (ribonucleic acid) as their genetic material. This class is broken into a subgroup known as lentiviruses, or "slow" viruses, because there is an extended period between initial infection and the onset of serious symptoms.

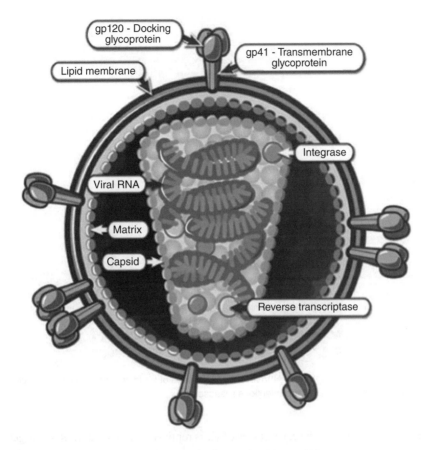

Figure 13.1 An illustrative diagram of a single, infective viral particle of HIV virus.
Courtesy: National Institute of Allergy and Infectious Diseases.

Once HIV enters the body, in the absence of treatment, it rapidly replicates using an enzyme called reverse transcriptase to convert its RNA into DNA (deoxyribonucleic acid) and then proceeds to multiply using the host cell's machinery.

As each day progresses, HIV destroys billions of CD4+ T cells in the infected person, eventually overwhelming the immune system's capacity to regenerate or fight other infections. The virus employs several mechanisms to kill host cells. Cells are killed when a large amount of virus buds from the cell surface and infects the surrounding cells. Or, cells may commit suicide by a process known as programmed cell death or apoptosis when the regulation of a cell's machinery and functions become grossly distorted because of HIV replication. Uninfected cells may die when HIV binds to their surface, making it appear as if the cell is infected, which targets them for death by killer T cells. HIV further suppresses the immune system by effecting the bone marrow and thymus in such a way that they lose the ability to produce precursor or undeveloped cells that are necessary for the development of mature cells with special immune function.

The HIV virus has a diameter of 1/10,000 of a millimeter and is spherical in shape. The envelope or outer coat is coded by the *env* gene and is embedded in a bilayer of glycoprotein lipids (Figure 13.1). These lipids join the viral coat as a newly formed virus buds off an infected host cell (Figure 13.2). The envelope has a spike-like appearance consisting of three molecules of glycoprotein 120 with a stem made up of three gp41 molecules that anchor the structure to the envelope. Between the core and the envelope lies a matrix protein (p17), a structural protein involved in several stages of viral

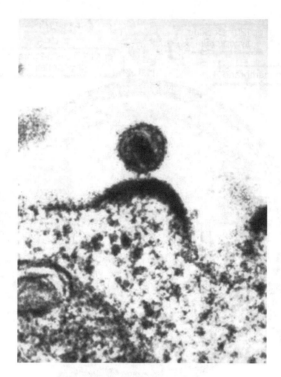

Figure 13.2   Electron micrograph of an HIV virus in the process of budding off from an infected cell. Courtesy: National Institute of Allergy and Infectious Diseases.

development; it participates in the early stages of virus replication as well as in RNA targeting to the cell's plasma membrane, incorporation of the envelope into the virions and virus particle assembly (Fiorentini *et al.* 2006).

The viral core contains an ellipsoid-shaped capsid made of approximately 2000 copies of the protein p24 (Figure 13.1). The core also contains a nucleocapsid protein p7, which like p24 is coded by the *gag* gene, is active in the early steps of retroviral replication, and appears to function largely to facilitate reverse transcription and integration (Thomas and Gorelick 2008). This capsid surrounds two duplicate strands of HIV RNA, each containing a copy of the virus's nine genes (NIAID 2012). Three of these genes *gag, pol,* and *env* code for the proteins needed to produce new virus particles (NIAID 2012). The six other genes, *tat, rev, nef, vif, vpr,* and *vpu* contain the genetic material that controls the virus's ability to infect cells and to reproduce itself (Frankel and Young 1998). The gene *pol* codes for the three enzymes *reverse transcriptase, protease,* and *integrase*. The reverse transcriptase converts the viral RNA into DNA allowing it to insert into the host's genetic material. The viral RNA has a region called the long terminal repeat that can be activated either by the virus or by the host cell and acts as a switch to initiate the production of new virus. The viral DNA is transported to the cell's nucleus, where it is incorporated/spliced into the human genome by the HIV enzyme *integrase*. Using host enzymes, the cell converts the genes into messenger RNA strands. Messenger RNA is transported outside the cell nucleus to the ribosome, which translates it into new HIV protein components. *Protease* cleaves the newly synthesized HIV proteins to yield the mature protein components needed to assemble mature virions. However, proviruses can lie dormant within the host cell for years, but upon activation, these cells will transcribe and translate HIV genes in the same manner as the host's genes. The process of activation of latent provirus is an area of intense research.

Stages of disease progression

Acute primary infection: After the initial exposure, a large number of HIV copies (viral load) circulate throughout the body and accumulate preferentially in lymphoid organs such as the thymus, spleen, and lymph nodes. Initially, the host does not mount an immune response because of lack of specific antibodies directed against the virus. As a result, antibody HIV tests cannot detect an infection at this early stage, and it is a reason why some people remain unaware of their HIV status. However, because of the initial viremia, with high numbers of circulating virus, these individuals are extremely infectious.

The innate immune system: The innate immune system is the first line of defense against infection. It is able to recognize and respond to infections quickly and consists of phagocytic leukocytes, dendritic cells, natural killer cells, circulating plasma proteins, and the body's physical epithelial barrier. HIV, like other viral infections, elicits a strong activation of this system. Two components of the innate immune response contribute to viral control both by killing infected cells and by modulating the development of other immune cells (Chang and Altfeld 2014). Several studies have demonstrated activation of the innate immune system in primary HIV infection, preceding the development of adaptive B-cell and T-cell responses (Chang and Altfeld 2014). This pattern recognition is facilitated by toll-like receptors that can detect double-stranded and/or single-stranded RNA, as well as certain viral proteins (Meier *et al.* 2007; Chang and Altfeld 2014).

The immune response: Approximately 2–4 weeks after the exposure, the adaptive immune system responds with killer T cells (CD8+ T cells) and B cell-produced antibodies. The HIV levels in the blood drop dramatically and the CD4+ T cell counts start to rebound, and for some individuals the number returns to its original level.

Progression to AIDS: If the disease progresses without treatment, in most people, the immune system deteriorates to the point that the human body is unable to fight off OIs such as pneumocystis

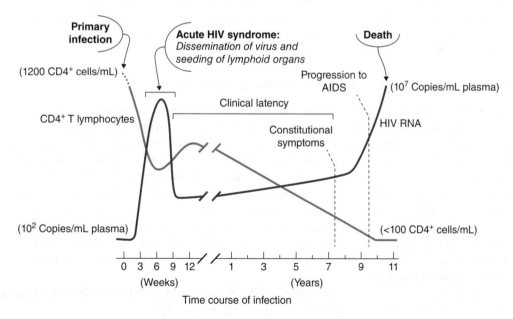

Figure 13.3 Schematic indicating the relationship between the levels of virus and CD4+ T cells, the acute phase, clinical latency, the progression from HIV infection to AIDS, and death.
Credit: Dr. William Abrams. Modified from: http://upload.wikimedia.org/wikipedia/commons/0/0e/Hiv-timecourse_copy.svg Used with permission.

carinii pneumonia or tuberculosis. The HIV load in the blood dramatically increases over time, while the number of infection fighting CD4+ T cells drop to dangerously low levels. An HIV-infected person is diagnosed with AIDS when one or more OIs have been detected and there are fewer than 200 CD4+ T cells per cubic millimeter of blood (Normal CD+T cell levels are between 800 and 1200 CD4+ T cells per mm^3 of blood). Opportunistic infections such as pneumocystis carinii pneumonia, cytomegalovirus (CMV), cryptococcal meningitis, and cryptosporidial diarrheal infection are commonly seen in HIV-positive individuals once the immune system becomes impaired (Slotten 2012). Associated with the disease are the indirect consequences related to T-cell activation, CD4 cell depletion, and inflammation, all of which increase the risk for heart disease, cognitive impairment (dementia), and certain types of malignancies (Slotten 2012).

After possible exposure to the virus, through unprotected sex or needle stick, a person should seek immediate care and advice from a healthcare professional. Signs and symptoms of HIV/AIDS include changes in cognitive abilities; changes in balance; diarrhea and weight loss; fever and night sweats; joint pain; skin rashes; and sores in the mouth, throat, vagina, or rectum. Additional symptoms include chills; sore or enlarged lymph nodes in the neck, jaw, armpit, or groin; lack of energy over an extended period of time; loss of 10 pounds or more in a short period of time; skin bleeding or bruising; cough, shortness of breath or chest tightness; changes in menstrual cycle or flow; or any other body changes that are worrisome.

*Clinical latency: O*nce the virus integrates into the host cell's genetic material, it is shielded from the immune system response and can lie dormant. During this phase, a person infected with HIV may remain free of HIV-related symptoms for several years. People in this symptom-free stage, however, remain infectious and are able to transmit HIV. Even if the individual is receiving antiretroviral medications, which decrease viral load, the individual can still transmit HIV.

It is important to note that there is a small, HIV-positive population that do not progress to AIDS. These individuals have the CCR5 Delta 32 gene (also called Delta 32) that codes for a modified protein CCR5 receptor on the surface of white blood cells, which acts as a nonproductive HIV receptor. The CCR5 Delta 32 gene is mutated such that virus does not bind and consequently does not insert its genetic information into the host cell. This mutation effectively renders the person resistant or immune to HIV (Eugen-Olsen *et al.* 1997).

Opportunistic infections and their relationship to HIV/AIDS

Healthy individuals are frequently exposed to viruses, bacteria, fungi, and parasites and are usually not seriously affected by them. However, PLWHA or other immune-suppressive conditions can face serious health consequences from these pathogens. These illnesses in immune-suppressed individuals are known as "*opportunistic infections*"—which take advantage of a weakened immune system. OIs are indicators of a declining immune system and usually occur when the *CD4 cell count* is below 200 cells/mm^3 and the viral load is >3000 copies/ml. Other factors such as xerostomia, poor oral hygiene, and/or smoking may exacerbate symptoms and may also indicate significant changes in the status of a patient's HIV infection and overall health. Dental healthcare providers may encounter signs and symptoms of immunosuppression and OIs in their patients. Therefore, it is critical that they be familiar with the most common oral pathologies and their manifestations in their immune-suppressed patients.

The CDC has developed a list of more than 20 OIs associated with HIV/AIDS and the most common causes of death caused by these infections (AIDS.gov 2010):

- *Candidiasis of bronchi, trachea, esophagus, or lungs*
- *Invasive cervical cancer*
- *Coccidioidomycosis*

- *Cryptococcosis*
- *Cryptosporidiosis*, chronic intestinal (>1 month duration)
- *CMV* disease (particularly CMV Cytomegalovirus)
- *Encephalopathy*, HIV-related
- *Herpes simplex*, chronic ulcer(s) (>1 month duration); or bronchitis, pneumonitis, or esophagitis
- *Histoplasmosis*
- *Isosporiasis*, chronic intestinal (>1 month duration)
- *Kaposi sarcoma*
- *Lymphoma*, multiple forms
- *Mycobacterium avium complex*
- *Tuberculosis*
- *Pneumocystis carinii pneumonia*
- *Pneumonia*, recurrent
- *Progressive multifocal leukoencephalopathy*
- *Salmonella septicemia*, recurrent
- *Toxoplasmosis* of brain
- *Wasting syndrome* due to HIV

Oral lesions

Oral lesions are classified as infectious—fungal, viral, and/or bacterial; neoplastic—such as Kaposi sarcoma; and nonspecific—aphthous ulcers and salivary gland disease. It is important that all lesions be correctly diagnosed and treated in order to maintain patient's oral health. A complete photo gallery of oral manifestations of HIV can be found at: http://www.hiv.va.gov/provider/image-library/oral.asp?thumbs=999.

Due to the success of HAART in suppressing viral load in HIV-infected individuals, the incidence of oral lesions has decreased over time. And, the type of lesions encountered by oral health providers has changed since the beginning of the epidemic. Since the introduction of HAART, there has been a significant reduction in oral hairy leukoplakia, Kaposi sarcoma, oral candidiasis, and necrotizing ulcerative periodontitis (NUP) (Hodgson *et al.* 2006; Prabhu *et al.* 2013). The effect of HAART on reducing the incidence of oral lesions, other than oral candidiasis, was not as significant (Hodgson *et al.* 2006), and there has been an increase in salivary gland disease (Greenspan and Greenspan 2002; Jeffers *et al.* 2011) and a marked increased incidence of oral warts (Patton 2013). The increased incidence in oral warts and HIV-related salivary gland disease, coupled with a longer life expectancy in HIV patients, strongly supports the need for attention to good oral health care.

Fungal infections (Patton 2013; Preston and Raznik 2013)

The most common fungal infection associated with HIV is oropharyngeal candidiasis or thrush. There are three frequently observed forms:

Erythematous candidiasis   presents as a red, flat, subtle lesion either on the dorsal surface of the tongue and/or on the hard/soft palates. *Typical treatment is administration of topical antifungals such as chlotrimazole troches, nystatin rinse, and nystatin cream or Mycolog-II ointments (nystatin and triamcinolone).*

Pseudomembranous candidiasis   (PC) appears as creamy white, curd-like plaques on the buccal mucosa, tongue, and other oral mucosal surfaces that will wipe away, leaving a red or bleeding underlying surface. PC has declined in patients who are on successful highly active retroviral regimens containing protease inhibitors (PIs). However, it is still one of the most common oral manifestations seen in HIV disease and commonly *treated with topical therapies such as nystatin or chlotrimazole for mild to moderate cases and systemic therapies such as fluconazole, Itraconazole, or ketoconazole for moderate to severe cases for 2 weeks.*

Angular cheilitis,   which may be associated with poor diet and nutritional deficiencies, is an erythematous and/or fissuring lesion affecting the corners of the mouth that can occur with or without the presence of erythematous candidiasis or PC. These lesions are commonly *treated with the application of a topical antifungal cream directly to the affected areas four times a day for a 2-week period.*

Oral candidiasis can be diagnosed in HIV-negative individuals, but it does not cause serious problems for the majority. Signs and symptoms are usually much more severe in those with an immune-compromised system.

Bacterial diseases (Patton 2013; Preston and Raznik 2013)

Three unique presentations are common among persons living with HIV disease: linear gingival erythema, necrotizing ulcerative gingivitis, and necrotizing ulcerative periodontitis. Necrotizing gingivitis describes the rapid destruction of the soft tissue and necrotizing periodontitis describes the rapid destruction of hard tissues. *Typical treatment would be 0.12% chlorhexidine gluconate or 10% povidone–iodine lavage to remove dental plaque, calculus, and necrotic soft tissues.*

Linear gingival erythema   is a periodontal disease that presents as a red band along the gingival margin, which may or may not be accompanied by occasional bleeding or discomfort. It is most frequently associated with anterior teeth but can extend to the posterior teeth. *Typical treatment would include debridement followed by twice-daily rinses with a 0.12% chlorhexidine gluconate suspension for 2 weeks.*

Viral diseases (Patton 2013; Preston and Raznik 2013)

Herpes simplex virus-1 infection is widespread, and oral manifestations of herpes lesions are common. It starts as a small crop of vesicles that rupture to produce small, painful ulcerations, which can merge or coalesce. They are sometimes called cold sores or fever blisters and infect the face or mouth. *Common treatment includes medications such as acyclovir.*

Herpes Zoster is a reactivation of the varicella zoster virus, which causes chickenpox in children and shingles in older adults. It is closely related to the herpes simplex viruses. It can occur along any branch of the trigeminal nerve, and intraoral or extraoral presentation along branches of this nerve is possible. Lesions will start as vesicles, break open, and then crust over. Intraoral lesions will start as vesicles, burst, and then present as oral ulcerations. Patients present complaining of toothache. *Common treatments include acyclovir 800 mg, five times a day for 7–10 days or famciclovir 500 mg, three times a day for 7 days* (Preston and Raznik 2013).

Oral warts due to human papillomavirus have dramatically increased with HAART (King *et al.* 2002). These warts may be related to immune reconstitution (King *et al.* 2002) or medications such as azathioprine or cyclosporin. The lesions may appear cauliflower like, spike or raised with a flat surface. *These lesions tend to recur, and treatment of particularly large and annoying warts can involve several strategies including surgery or cryotherapy.*

Neoplastic diseases (Preston and Raznik 2013)

Kaposi sarcoma (KS) is still the most frequent oral malignancy seen in association with HIV infection, although dramatically decreased in the HAART era. The lesions can appear macular, nodular, or raised and ulcerated, with colors ranging from red to purple. The early lesions tend to be red, flat, asymptomatic, and darken with age.

Non-Hodgkin lymphoma is an AIDS-defining illness that can present in the oral cavity. Lesions tend to present as large, painful, ulcerated masses on the palate or gingival tissues.

Biopsy is required for definitive diagnosis of neoplastic lesions, and patients should be referred to an oncologist for treatment.

Miscellaneous (Preston and Raznik 2013)

HIV–salivary gland disease (HIV-SGD) is AIDS defining in pediatric HIV infection and has increased in the adult HIV population. Salivary gland disease appears as bilateral enlargement of the parotid glands resulting in facial disfigurement, may be associated with pain, and can be accompanied by symptoms of xerostomia—or dry mouth. Histologically, HIV-SGD is characterized by hyperplastic, intraparotid lymph nodes and/or lymphatic infiltrates within the salivary gland tissue (Jeffers *et al.* 2011). Dry mouth is a common complaint among PLWHA. It can be caused by the disease or is a known side effect of many medications. Dry mouth results in irritation and inflammation of the soft tissues in the mouth, which can form a locus for the growth of harmful organisms leading to dental decay. Symptoms can be temporarily alleviated by sucking on sugar-free hard candies, by chewing sugar-free gum or by using oral moisturizers. Patients should be counseled to pay close attention to their oral hygiene and consider the use of a prescribed topical fluoride preparation after consultation with their healthcare professional.

Recurrent aphthous ulcers (RAUs) are a common occurrence, presenting on non-keratinized or non-fixed tissues such as labial and buccal mucosa, floor of the mouth, ventral surface of the tongue, posterior oropharynx, and maxillary and mandibular vestibules (Preston and Raznik 2013). RAUs, also called canker sores, are benign and noncontagious. They typically begin as erythematous macules, or reddened flat areas of mucosa, that develop into ulcers covered with a yellow–gray, fibrous membrane that can be scraped away, characteristically accompanied by an erythematous "halo" of inflammation, which surrounds the ulcer. The ulcers usually last between 7 and 14 days and can recur three to six times per year. In immune-compromised patients, symptoms may be more painful and last longer. *The pain associated with these ulcers should be managed by a healthcare professional with topical anesthetics or systemic analgesics.*

Highly active antiretroviral therapy

*Classes of treatment: U*nfortunately, at present, there is no cure for AIDS. HIV therapeutics are often referred to as antiretrovirals or ARV therapy and are designed to block replication of the virus in the host. No medications are currently available to delete HIV DNA from the host genome and thus eliminate the potential for activation of latent virus. There are many different ARVs approved for HIV treatment (Table 13.1). They are divided into five classes, each working a different mechanism to help fight HIV by interacting at different stages of production (Figure 13.4).

Highly active antiretroviral therapy (HAART) is the combination of three or more medications from at least two different classes of HIV medicine. For HIV-positive individuals initiating HAART treatment, a typical regimen contains two nucleoside reverse transcriptase inhibitors (NRTIs or Nukes) in combination with a non-nucleoside reverse transcriptase inhibitor (NNRTI or non-Nuke), a protease inhibitor (PI), or an integrase inhibitor. The selection of a regimen should be individualized on the basis of efficacy, toxicity, pill burden, dosing frequency, drug–drug interaction potential, resistance testing results, comorbid conditions, general health condition, mental health challenges, and side effects.

Table 13.1   FDA antiretroviral drugs used in the treatment of HIV infection.

Brand name	Generic name	Manufacturer name	Approval date
Multi-class combination products			
Atripla	Efavirenz, emtricitabine, and tenofovir disoproxil fumarate	Bristol-Myers Squibb and Gilead Sciences	Jul 12, 2006
Complera	Emtricitabine, rilpivirine, and tenofovir disoproxil fumarate	Gilead Sciences	Aug 10, 2011
Stribild	Elvitegravir, cobicistat, emtricitabine, and tenofovir disoproxil fumarate	Gilead Sciences	Aug 27, 2012
Nucleoside reverse transcriptase inhibitors			
Combivir	Lamivudine and zidovudine	GlaxoSmithKline	Sept 27, 1997
Emtriva	Emtricitabine, FTC	Gilead Sciences	Jul 2, 2003
Epivir	Lamivudine, 3TC	GlaxoSmithKline	Nov 17, 1995
Epzicom	Abacavir and lamivudine	GlaxoSmithKline	Aug 2, 2004
Hivid	Zalcitabine and dideoxycytidine, ddC (no longer marketed)	Hoffmann-La Roche	Jun 19, 1992
Retrovir	Zidovudine, azidothymidine, AZT, and ZDV	GlaxoSmithKline	Mar 19, 1987
Trizivir	Abacavir, zidovudine, and lamivudine	GlaxoSmithKline	Nov 14, 2000
Truvada	Tenofovir disoproxil fumarate and emtricitabine	Gilead Sciences	Aug 2, 2004
Videx EC	Enteric-coated didanosine, ddI EC	Bristol-Myers Squibb	Oct 31, 2000
Videx	Didanosine and dideoxyinosine, ddI	Bristol Myers-Squibb	Oct 9, 1991
Viread	Tenofovir disoproxil fumarate, TDF	Gilead Sciences	Oct 26, 2001
Zerit	Stavudine, d4T	Bristol Myers-Squibb	Jun 24, 1994
Ziagen	Abacavir sulfate, ABC	GlaxoSmithKline	Dec 17, 1998
Non-nucleoside reverse transcriptase inhibitors			
Edurant	Rilpivirine	Tibotec Therapeutics	May 20, 2011
Intelence	Etravirine	Tibotec Therapeutics	Jan 18, 2008
Rescriptor	Delavirdine, DLV	Pfizer	Apr 4, 1997
Sustiva	Efavirenz, EFV	Bristol Myers-Squibb	Sept 17, 1998
Viramune (immediate release)	Nevirapine, NVP	Boehringer Ingelheim	Jun 21, 1996
Viramune XR (extended release)	Nevirapine, NVP	Boehringer Ingelheim	Mar 25, 2011

(continued)

Table 13.1   *(cont'd)*

Brand name	Generic name	Manufacturer name	Approval date
Protease inhibitors			
Agenerase	Amprenavir, APV (no longer marketed)	GlaxoSmithKline	Apr 15, 1999
Aptivus	Tipranavir, TPV	Boehringer Ingelheim	Jun 22, 2005
Crixivan	Indinavir, IDV	Merck	Mar 13, 1996
Fortovase	Saquinavir (no longer marketed)	Hoffmann-La Roche	Nov 7, 1997
Invirase	Saquinavir mesylate, SQV	Hoffmann-La Roche	Dec 6, 1995
Kaletra	Lopinavir and ritonavir, LPV/RTV	Abbott Laboratories	Sept 15, 2000
Lexiva	Fosamprenavir Calcium, FOS-APV	GlaxoSmithKline	Oct 20, 2003
Norvir	Ritonavir, RTV	Abbott Laboratories	Mar 1, 1996
Prezista	Darunavir	Tibotec Therapeutics	Jun 23, 2006
Reyataz	Atazanavir sulfate, ATV	Bristol-Myers Squibb	Jun 20, 2003
Viracept	Nelfinavir mesylate, NFV	Agouron Pharmaceuticals	Mar 14, 1997
Fusion inhibitors			
Fuzeon	Enfuvirtide, T-20	Hoffmann-La Roche and Trimeris	Mar 13, 2003
Entry inhibitors—CCR5 co-receptor antagonist			
Selzentry	Maraviroc	Pfizer	Aug 6, 2007
HIV integrase strand transfer inhibitors			
Isentress	Raltegravir	Merck & Co., Inc.	Oct 12, 2007
Tivicay	Dolutegravir	GlaxoSmithKline	Aug 13, 2013

U.S. Food and Drug Administration, Page Last Updated: 08/20/2013, accessed January 26, 2014.

Fusion/entry inhibitors

Entry inhibitors block HIV from entering a CD4$^+$ cell. Fusion and entry inhibitors work in a similar manner by targeting receptors on either the HIV or the CD4 cells to block the HIV from entering the cell.

Nukes or NRTIs: Interact with the DNA to block the binding of viral *reverse transcriptase* and prevent the HIV from converting its RNA into host-compatible DNA. When HIV uses a Nuke instead of the actual cell structure, the virus cannot complete the copying process and reproduce itself.

NON-Nukes or NNRTIs: Non-Nukes are very similar to Nukes but work by sticking tightly to the enzyme, *reverse transcriptase*, which HIV uses to replicate itself.

Integrase Inhibitors: Prevent HIV from inserting its viral DNA into the host DNA of CD4-positive cells.

Protease Inhibitors: Block the cleavage of the propeptide containing the enzymes *integrase, protease,* and *reverse transcriptase*.

Chemokine receptor antagonists: Inhibit the entry of the virus into the host cell by blocking the binding to the two chemokine receptors, CXCR4 and CCR5, which are used as co-receptors by the T cell-tropic (X4) and macrophage-tropic (R5) HIV-1 strains.

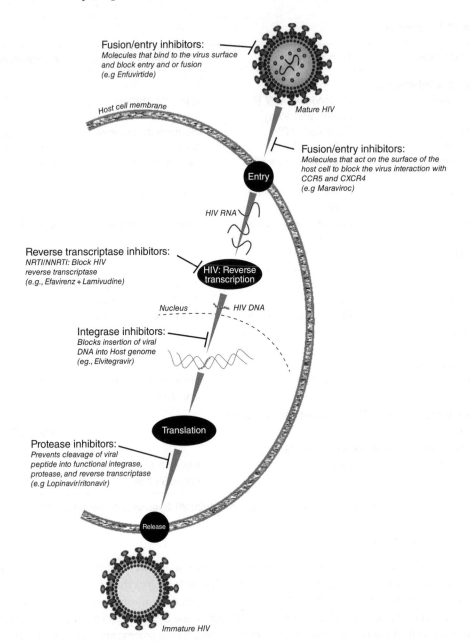

Figure 13.4　Cartoon showing the sites of inhibition for five different AIDS-associated antiretroviral approved for HIV treatment. Credit: Dr. William Abrams.

The current standard of care recommended by healthcare professionals is a HAART treatment plan consisting of a combination of three or more medications from at least two different classes of HIV therapeutics. The combinations of multiple medications provide the greatest potential for controlling the amount of virus in the body, protecting the immune system and preventing viral drug resistance.

Fixed-dose combinations are not a separate class of HIV medications, but combinations of the above classes represent a great advance in HIV therapy. They include antiretrovirals that are combinations of two or more medications from one or more different classes that are combined into one single pill containing specific fixed doses of the medicines (Klein 2006). Table 13.1 shows a list of common HAART drugs, Table 13.2 shows a list of potential drug interactions that should be avoided, and Table 13.3 shows treatment regimens.

There is increasing interest in the potential therapeutic properties of herbal products. Unfortunately, some of these can interact with antiretroviral therapy, such as *Oldenlandia diffusa*, *Allium sativum*, *Codonopsis tangshen*, *Rehmannia glutinosa*, and *Astragalus propinquus*. Some of these herb–drug interactions can lead to induction of CYP3A4 and the reduced efficacy of drugs that are CYP3A4 substrates (Lau *et al.* 2013).The HIV drug classes, PIs and NNRTIs are likely to be decreased in the presence of CYP3A4 inducers; however, their concentrations and ratios will be closely monitored by the healthcare professional.

Unlike prescription medications, natural or herbal products are not closely regulated by the FDA. Therefore, healthcare providers should be consulted before considering their use. In February 2000, the FDA issued a public health advisory for antiretroviral treatment guidelines stating that St. John's wort (*Hypericum perforatum*), a potential CYP3A4 inducer, should not be used with PIs or NNRTIs. New information continues to become available concerning herbs like bitter lemon, green tea, and cat's claw and their ability to provide antiviral and immune support.

Impact of medical treatment on PLWHA

In developed countries, with access to antiretroviral therapy and ongoing supportive treatment, cardiovascular disease (CVD) has become a major cause of death among HIV/AIDS patients. CVD may result from cardiac involvement as a consequence of an OI in the presence of advanced immunosuppression; HIV-induced immune activation; or secondary to dyslipidemia and insulin resistance adverse effects associated with antiretroviral therapy (Thienemann *et al.* 2013) (Palella et al. 2012).

HIV/AIDS patients frequently require additional medications as part of their antiretroviral treatment. A thorough medical history, which includes a review of the over-the-counter medications and prescription drugs, assists the oral healthcare provider in prescribing appropriate additional medications. Prophylactic medications may be advisable to prevent OIs in those at high risk. Evaluation of the periodontal status, in the context of susceptibility to infection, bleeding, potential problems with adverse drug reactions, and drug interactions, provides a basis for developing an appropriate treatment plan. Any known or expected complications related to treatment should be discussed with the patient.

Known adverse effects associated with HIV treatment may necessitate the use of other prescription or over-the-counter medications to prevent or alleviate symptoms such as diarrhea, nausea, or pain. Common, non-communicable diseases, unrelated to HIV, such as high blood pressure or diabetes may also require additional medications that can impact dental treatment. Knowledge of preexisting disease and medications enables the dentist to provide the patient with optimum oral health care.

Dental notes: Dental treatments

Infection control guidelines are available from the Centers for Disease Control and Prevention and the American Dental Association. Compliance with the blood-borne pathogen standards set by Occupational Safety and Health Administration, along with state or local regulations, is critical. Universal precautions should be followed, and HIV patients should be treated as any other patient with a few special considerations.

PLWHA may develop associated skin manifestations and/or cervical lymphadenopathy. Thorough head and neck examination and oral soft-tissue examination should be performed at each dental visit. The cause of lymphadenopathy is frequently uncovered after taking a careful history: such as

Table 13.2 Drug interactions with antiretroviral therapy—antiretroviral drug combinations to avoid.

The drugs below should not be given in combination with protease inhibitors (PIs), non-nucleoside reverse transcriptase inhibitors (NNRTIs), or cellular chemokine receptor-5 (CCR5) antagonists.

Atazanavir (ATV) ± ritonavir (RTV) should not be used in combination with the following (DHHS 2013):
- 3-hydroxy-3-methylglutaryl coenzyme A (HMG-CoA) reductase inhibitors: lovastatin and simvastatin
- Antituberculosis agents: rifampin, rifapentine
- Gastrointestinal drugs: cisapride
- Antipsychotic agents: pimozide
- Benzodiazepines: midazolam, triazolam
- Ergot derivatives: dihydroergotamine, ergonovine, ergotamine, methylergonovine
- Herbal products: St. John's wort
- Antiretroviral agents: nevirapine (NVP), etravirine (ETR)
- Other agents: alfuzosin, irinotecan, salmeterol, sildenafil [for pulmonary arterial hypertension (PAH)]

Darunavir (DRV)/RTV should not be used in combination with the following (DHHS 2013):
- HMG-CoA reductase inhibitors: lovastatin, simvastatin
- Antituberculosis agents: rifampin, rifapentine
- Gastrointestinal drugs: cisapride
- Antipsychotic agents: pimozide
- Benzodiazepines: midazolam, triazolam
- Ergot derivatives: dihydroergotamine, ergonovine, ergotamine, methylergonovine
- Herbal products: St. John's wort
- Other agents: alfuzosin, salmeterol, sildenafil (for PAH)

Fosamprenavir (FPV) ± RTV should not be used in combination with the following (DHHS 2013):
- Antiarrhythmic agents: flecainide, propafenone
- HMG-CoA reductase inhibitors: lovastatin, simvastatin
- Antituberculosis agents: rifampin, rifapentine
- Gastrointestinal drugs: cisapride
- Antipsychotic agents: pimozide
- Benzodiazepines: midazolam, triazolam
- Ergot derivatives: dihydroergotamine, ergonovine, ergotamine, methylergonovine
- Herbal products: St. John's wort
- Antiretroviral agents: ETR
- Other agents: alfuzosin, salmeterol, sildenafil (for PAH)

Lopinavir/ritonavir (LPV/RTV) should not be used in combination with the following (DHHS 2013):
- HMG-CoA reductase inhibitors: lovastatin, pitavastatin, simvastatin
- Antituberculosis agents: rifampin, rifapentine
- Gastrointestinal drugs: cisapride
- Antipsychotic agents: pimozide
- Benzodiazepines: midazolam, triazolam
- Ergot derivatives: dihydroergotamine, ergonovine, ergotamine, methylergonovine
- Herbal products: St. John's wort
- Other agents: alfuzosin, salmeterol, sildenafil (for PAH)

(continued)

Table 13.2 *(cont'd)*

Ritonavir (RTV) should not be used in combination with the following (DHHS 2013):
- Antiarrhythmic agents: amiodarone, flecainide, propafenone, quinidine
- HMG-CoA reductase inhibitors: lovastatin, simvastatin
- Antituberculosis agents: rifapentine
- Gastrointestinal drugs: cisapride
- Antipsychotic agents: pimozide
- Benzodiazepines: midazolam, triazolam
- Ergot derivatives: dihydroergotamine, ergonovine, ergotamine, methylergonovine
- Herbal products: St. John's wort
- Other agents: alfuzosin, sildenafil (for PAH)

Saquinavir (SQV)/RTV should not be used in combination with the following (DHHS 2013):
- Antiarrhythmic agents: amiodarone, dofetilide, flecainide, lidocaine, propafenone, quinidine
- HMG-CoA reductase inhibitors: lovastatin, simvastatin
- Antituberculosis agents: rifampin, rifapentine
- Gastrointestinal drugs: cisapride
- Antipsychotic agents: pimozide
- Benzodiazepines: midazolam, triazolam, trazodone
- Ergot derivatives: dihydroergotamine, ergonovine, ergotamine, methylergonovine
- Herbal products: St. John's wort, garlic supplements
- Other agents: alfuzosin, sildenafil (for PAH)

Tipranavir (TPV)/RTV should not be used in combination with the following (DHHS 2013*)*:
- Antiarrhythmic agents: amiodarone, flecainide, propafenone, quinidine
- HMG-CoA reductase inhibitors: lovastatin, simvastatin
- Antituberculosis agents: rifampin, rifapentine
- Gastrointestinal drugs: cisapride
- Antipsychotic agents: pimozide
- Benzodiazepines: midazolam, triazolam, trazodone
- Ergot derivatives: dihydroergotamine, ergonovine, ergotamine, methylergonovine
- Herbal products: St. John's wort
- Antiretroviral agents: ETR
- Other agents: alfuzosin, salmeterol, sildenafil (for PAH)

Efavirenz (EFV) should not be used in combination with the following (DHHS 2013):
- Antituberculosis agents: rifapentine
- Gastrointestinal drugs: cisapride
- Antipsychotic agents: pimozide
- Benzodiazepines: midazolam, triazolam, trazodone
- Ergot derivatives: dihydroergotamine, ergonovine, ergotamine, methylergonovine
- Herbal products: St. John's wort
- Antiretroviral agents: other NNRTIs

Etravirine (ETR) should not be used in combination with the following (DHHS 2013):
- Antituberculosis agents: rifampin, rifapentine
- Herbal products: St. John's wort
- Antiretroviral agents: unboosted PIs ATV/RTV, FPV/RTV, or TPV/RTV or other NNRTIs
- Other agents: carbamazepine, phenobarbital, phenytoin, clopidogrel

Nevirapine (NVP) should not be used in combination with the following (DHHS 2013):
- Antituberculosis agents: rifapentine
- Herbal products: St. John's wort
- Antiretroviral agents: ATV±RTV, other NNRTIs
- Antifungals: ketoconazole

(continued)

Table 13.2 *(cont'd)*

Maraviroc (MVC) should not be used in combination with the following (DHHS 2013): • Antituberculosis agents: rifapentine • Herbal products: St. John's wort **Alternative recommendations for specific drugs** (DHHS 2013): • Lovastatin, simvastatin: may use pravastatin or fluvastatin, which has the least potential for drug–drug interactions (except for pravastatin with DRV/RTV); may use atorvastatin and rosuvastatin with caution (start with the lowest possible dose and titrate based on tolerance and lipid-lowering efficacy) • Rifampin: may use rifabutin with dosage adjustments • Midazolam, triazolam: may use temazepam, lorazepam, or oxazepam (DHHS 2013):

Panel on Antiretroviral Guidelines for Adults and Adolescents, Department of Health and Human Services, Table 14, Available at http://aidsinfo.nih.gov/ContentFiles/AdultandAdolescentGL.pdf, Table 14. Drugs That Should Not Be Used with Antiretroviral Agents, last updated February 12, 2013, accessed January 26, 2014.

Table 13.3 Highly active antiretroviral therapy—drug classes.

Alternative treatment examples	Non-nucleoside reverse transcriptase inhibitors	Nucleoside reverse transcriptase inhibitors	Integrase inhibitors	Protease inhibitors
Treatment 1	Efavirenz (EFV) +	Tenofovir (TDF) Emtricitabine (FTC)		
Treatment 2		Tenofovir (TDF) Emtricitabine (FTC)		+ Atazanavir/ Ritonavir (ATV/r)
Treatment 3		Tenofovir (TDF) Emtricitabine (FTC)		+ Darunavir/ Ritonavir (DRV/r)
Treatment 4		Tenofovir (TDF) Emtricitabine (FTC)	+ Raltegravir (RAL)	
Fixed-dose combination	Efavirenz (EFV) +	Tenofovir (TDF) Emtricitabine (FTC)		

http://aidsinfo.nih.gov/guidelines—Health & Human Services Panel on Antiretroviral Guidelines for Adults and Adolescents.

upper respiratory tract infection, pharyngitis, periodontal disease, conjunctivitis, lymphadenitis, tinea, insect bites, recent immunization, cat scratch disease, or dermatitis.

Typically, prophylactic antibiotics are prescribed judiciously and microbiological tests, along with sensitivity testing, should be performed only if infections persist. Elective dental procedures are contraindicated in patients with a neutrophil count of <500 cells/mm^3 and a platelet count of <50,000 cells/mm^3. Pre- and postoperative antibiotics, when dental surgery is necessary, should be given in consultation with the patient's physician. Patients with profound neutropenia and thrombocytopenia may require hospitalization in order to receive the necessary care. Because patients with HIV infection may be at increased risk for postoperative bleeding, laboratory tests including platelet count, prothrombin time and/or international normalized ratio, activated partial thromboplastin time, and bleeding time (Table 13.4) should be performed prior to surgery or biopsy.

Table 13.4   Medical assessment of HIV-infected patients.

Significant laboratory tests
The laboratory tests listed below provide important information relative to the HIV-infected patient's overall health. CD4 or T helper cell count measures the number of T helper cells. These cells stimulate the immune system to fight infections. As their numbers go down, the risk of infection goes up.

CD4–CD8 ratios: CD4 cells are T helper cells. CD8 cells are T suppressor cells. As this ratio drops, the risk of infection goes up. A normal ratio is between 1 and 4. *People with viral infections have a decreased ratio.*

Viral load/Plasma HIV-1 RNA: This measurement reveals the number of copies of the virus per milliliter of blood. Ideally, there would be zero detectable copies. As the viral load goes up, indicating the virus is replicating at an increasing rate, the incidence of secondary problems increases. *However, even the highest number of viral copies has no impact on the provided dental care.*

CBC with differential
Platelets:
Platelets are necessary, along with other factors, for blood to clot. An important concern in HIV-infected patients is low platelet count (thrombocytopenia). If this occurs, the risk of bleeding may be so severe as to delay any elective and, at times, even emergency therapy, until the platelets can be replaced.

White count:
The white cells in the body are designed to recognize and fight infections. As the white count decreases (leukopenia), the risk of infection increases.

Absolute neutrophils:
The neutrophils are a special class of white cells, which are also important in fighting infection. If their numbers decrease, the risk of infection increases.

Hematocrit:
Hematocrit (HCT) is the percentage of whole blood, that is, red cells. In most cases of anemia, HCT will decrease.

Hemoglobin:
Hemoglobin (HGB) is the oxygen-carrying component of red blood cells (RBCs). In certain types of anemia, it is possible to have an adequate number of RBCs but inadequate amount of HGB and therefore a decreased capacity for the blood to carry oxygen.

RBC *count:*
RBC count measures the number of RBCs per cubic millimeter of blood. A decrease in their number means an inadequate number of RBCs (anemia). This leads to an inadequate ability to carry oxygen. The patient becomes easily fatigued and is a poor healer. A low RBC count is usually reflected in a low HCT.

Critical laboratory test values
These lab test values represent critical information relative to dental management.

White blood count (total)
<2000 (Granulocytopenia) (normal values: 4,000–10,000 cells/mm^3). Low counts are a cause for concern because the body becomes more susceptible to infection.

Delay elective dental procedures until white blood count improves.

(continued)

Table 13.4 *(cont'd)*

Absolute neutrophils
<1000 (Neutropenia)—Consider therapeutic regimen of antibiotics concurrently with invasive procedures. *Delay elective dental procedures until white blood count improves.*

Platelets
<60,000 (Thrombocytopenia) (Normal values: 150,000–450,000 cells/mm^3). Consult with physician and recommend intervention to boost platelets prior to invasive procedures. *The dentist should receive laboratory confirmation of platelet count immediately (1–2 days) before invasive procedures. Delay elective dental procedures until platelet count improves. Platelets should be above 60–80,000, depending on invasiveness (risk of bleeding) and extent of planned procedure.*

Hematocrit (%)
<10%—Consult with physician (normal values: female 37–47%, male 42–52%). Low values are an indicator of anemia.

Hemoglobin
<10 (normal values: female 12–16 g/dl, male 14–18 g/dl). Consult with physician for invasive procedures.

Red blood cell
<1.0 million/mm^3 (normal values: female 4–5 million/mm^3, male 4–6 million/mm^3). Consult with physician for invasive procedures. Low values are an indicator of anemia.

CD4 T lymphocytes (helper cells) (absolute)

<50 (normal values 590–1120 cells/mm^3)—*Evaluate patient for severe opportunistic disease. There is usually no problem with routine dental care. Dentists may consider delaying elective dental procedures until white blood count improves. Emphasize good oral care and recommend the patient to contact immediately if oral problems appear.*

CD4 above 200—*Obtain a lab report minimally every 6 months, or as performed by primary care physician.*

CD4 < 200—*Obtain a lab report minimally every 3 months, or as performed by primary care physician.*

CD4 count—all other patients—report as performed by primary care physician.

Viral load
Viral load does not have an impact on dental treatment planning. *The number of viral copies is indicative of disease, and modification of the dental treatment plan would be based on the above laboratory test results and not just on the viral load.*

Dental notes: Clinical ramifications for dental treatment

Oral health is an integral part of primary health care for PLWHA because it affects the adherence to HAART treatment. For example, poor oral health can exacerbate nutritional problems when eating is uncomfortable or painful, aggravate psychosocial problems when the appearance of the oral cavity is unpleasant, and signal changes in disease status in relationship to the treatment regimen. As with any other patient, establishing the oral health baseline for PLWHA is an important part of comprehensive oral health care.

The goal in providing oral health care to PLWHA is to help the patient achieve the highest quality of life possible, which includes preserving or restoring healthy teeth and periodontal tissues, avoiding infections in the mouth, preventing and/or treating oral pain, engaging patients in oral health educational programs, and averting the need for cosmetic changes. Viral-induced immune dysfunction can cause many complications, including dental and oral health problems that require monitoring by the dental healthcare professional.

It has been proposed that a solution to improving health care is to increase the utilization of existing healthcare providers, particularly dentists, suggesting that they serve as "oral physicians" who would provide limited preventive primary care, including screening for chronic diseases, while continuing to oversee dental care (Giddon *et al.* 2013). This idea is supported by the fact that dental training already includes the ability to recognize more than 100 manifestations of genetic disorders, systemic disease, and lifestyle problems (Long *et al.* 1998). Key examples of systemic disease groups with oral manifestations include dermatological, inflammatory connective tissue diseases; hematological and inflammatory gastrointestinal diseases; diabetes; as well as neurological and endocrine diseases (Pedersen AM 2010). Periodontitis has been implicated as a factor in diabetes, coronary artery disease, structural heart disease, and preterm delivery (Pedersen and Jensen 2010) though a causative effect has not been proven. Some forms of periodontal disease are more severe in individuals affected with immune system disorders, and people infected with HIV may have especially severe forms of periodontal disease such as necrotizing periodontal diseases (American Academy of Periodontology 2000).Three special considerations for HIV patients with periodontal disease are given as follows:

- Start with a consultation and coordination of treatment with the patient's physician.
- Control for associated mucosal diseases and acute periodontal infections.
- Judiciously administer systemic or local medications (antibiotics) to minimize OIs and adverse drug interactions (Appendix 13.1).

Due to improvements in treatment and health care, HIV-positive individuals have a nearly normal life expectancy, as long as they adhere to their HAART regimen. The side effects of this treatment regimen, however, may result in increased risk of developing other chronic diseases, some of which are secondary to the toxicity of their medications. People living with HIV especially those on HAART can have increased rates of dyslipidemia, smoking, insulin resistance, and metabolic syndrome, all of which are direct or indirect cardiac risk factors. How these risk factors will influence long-term cardiovascular morbidity and mortality is not yet known (Wlodarczyk 2004).

Summary

HIV is now a chronic disease that affects the health of individuals and impacts households, communities, and economic development on national and local levels. Great strides have been made in efforts to reduce the morbidity and mortality associated with HIV/AIDS. Rapid diagnostic tests for HIV and AIDS-related OIs, comprehensive medical care, HAART, and supportive services have improved the quality of lives for PLWHA—who are now able to live longer, productive lives. As compared with the early epidemic, HIV/AIDS is no longer viewed as the "death sentence" it once was. Yet, access to oral health care continues to be one of the primary unmet needs within this community (Fox *et al.* 2012). The dental community could benefit from continuing education about disease transmission, progression, diagnostic tests, treatments, and prevention.

Barriers to dental care include real and perceived stigma, limited oral health literacy, lack of dental insurance, inability to pay for out-of-pocket expenses, pain or discomfort associated with previous dental visits, and fear of dentists. Recent studies indicate that people who have received any form of oral health education, including counseling for nutrition, tobacco cessation, alcohol and substance abuse and simple oral hygiene instruction, were nearly six times as likely to be retained in their HIV healthcare regimen as compared with those who received no oral health education (Tobias *et al.* 2012). This is a compelling reason to stress the importance of retention in dental care. Dentists who spend time talking with and educating their HIV patients about oral health topics are more apt to retain them in both medical and dental treatment. PLWHA should be encouraged to schedule semiannual oral healthcare examinations to monitor the progression of their disease. The benefits of receiving routine dental care treatment are well-known: less tooth decay, sensitivity, bleeding gums, bad breath, loose teeth, and sores. And, the added improvement in overall appearance is a psychosocial benefit not to be underestimated. New collaborative practices are being initiated which allow dentists, physicians, and nurses to work together to promote the complete health of each of their patients.

For uninsured and underinsured PLWHA, limited financing of oral health care remains a significant barrier. Safety nets have been put in place to help PLWHA address these financial barriers, but sustainability of these oral health programs depends on securing ongoing funding to remain viable. The Department of Health and Human Services provides oral health care for PLWHA through the Ryan White HIV/AIDS Program and Medicaid, which provides significant funding for oral health care, but these are a discretionary part of the Federal budget and not an entitlements. Medicaid provides coverage for outpatient physician visits and hospital care, but oral health care is optional. Coverage is determined at the state level, with each state having limitations regarding access to oral health care. Stable financing mechanisms for PLWHA and other vulnerable populations are critically important in achieving and maintaining good oral health, continued overall good health, and the ability to be productive members of society.

Acknowledgments

I would like to thank Dr. Daniel Malamud for his support and encouragement. I would also like to thank Drs. Monica Smiddy and William Abrams who kindly read my work and offered advice and valuable comments and for sharing their knowledge.

References

American Academy of Periodontology (2000) Parameter on periodontitis associated with systemic conditions. *Journal of Periodontology, American Academy of Periodontology*, **71 (5 Suppl.**), 880–883.

AIDS.gov (2010) Staying Healthy with HIV/AIDS: Potential Related Health Problems: Opportunistic Infections. http://www.aids.gov/hiv-aids-basics/staying-healthy-with-hiv-aids/potential-related-health-problems/opportunistic-infections/ [accessed on July 27, 2014].

Altman, L.K. (1982) New homosexual disorder worries health officals. *New York Times*, New York. http://www.nytimes.com/1982/05/11/science/new-homosexual-disorder-worries-health-officials.html [accessed on July 27, 2014].

Anderson, J.R. (2005) *A Guide to the Clinical Care of Women with HIV*. Department of Health and Human Services Health Resources and Services Administration, Rockville, MD.

Barré-Sinoussi, F. (2003) The early years of HIV research: integrating clinical and basic research. *Nature Medicine,* **9 (7)**, 3.

Benjamin, G.M. (2012) Oral health care for people living with HIV/AIDS. *Public Health Reports*, **127 (Suppl. 2)**, 1–2.

CDC (2011) HIV Surveillance Report.23. http://www.cdc.gov/hiv/pdf/statistics_2011_HIV_Surveillance_Report_vol_23.pdf [accessed on July 27, 2014].

CDC (2013) Monitoring selected national HIV prevention and care objectives by using HIV surveillance data—United States and 6 U.S. dependent areas, **18 (5)**. http://www.cdc.gov/hiv/pdf/2011_monitoring_hiv_indicators_hssr_final.pdf [accessed on July 27, 2014].

Chang, J.J. & Altfeld, M. (2014) Innate immune activation in primary HIV-1 infection. *Journal of Infectious Diseases,* **209** (**5**), S297–S301.

Coffin, J., Haase, A., Levy, J.A., *et al.* (1986) What to call the AIDS virus? *Nature,* **321**, 10.

DHHS (2013) Guidelines for the Use of Antiretroviral Agents in HIV-1-Infected Adults and Adolescents. Panel on Antiretroviral Guidelines for Adults and Adolescents, Department of Health and Human Services. http://aidsinfo.nih.gov/ContentFiles/AdultandAdolescentGL.pdf, Table 14. Drugs That Should Not Be Used With Antiretroviral Agents: L5.

Eugen-Olsen, J., Iversen AKN, Garred, P., *et al.* (1997) Heterozygosity for a deletion in CKR-5 gene leads to prolonged AIDS-free survival and slower CD4 T-cell decline in a cohort of HIV-seropositive individuals. *AIDS,* **11**, 305–310.

Fiorentini, S., Marini, E., & Caracciolo, S. (2006). Functions of the HIV-1 matrix protein p17. *The New Microbiologica,* **29**, 1–10.

Fox, J.E., Tobias, C.R., Bachman, S.S., *et al.* (2012) Increasing access to oral health care for people living with HIV/AIDS in the U.S.: baseline evaluation results of the innovations in oral health care initiative. *Public Health Reports,* **127** (**Suppl. 2**), 5–16.

Frankel, A.D. & Young, J.A.T. (1998) HIV-1: fifteen proteins and an RNA. *Annual Review of Biochemistry,* **67**, 1–25.

García-Lerma, J.G., MacInnes, H., Bennett, D., *et al.* (2004) Transmitted human immunodeficiency virus type 1 carrying the D67N or K219Q/E mutation evolves rapidly to zidovudine resistance in vitro and shows a high replicative fitness in the presence of zidovudine. *Journal of Virology,* **78** (**14**), 7545–7552.

Giddon, D.B., Swann, B., Donoff, R.B., *et al.* (2013) Dentists as oral physicians: the overlooked primary health care resource. *The Journal of Prevention,* **34** (**4**), 279–291.

Greene, W.C. (2007) A history of AIDS: looking back to see ahead. *European Journal of Immunology,* **37**, 94–102.

Greenspan, J. & Greenspan D. (2002) The epidemiology of the oral lesions of HIV infection in the developed world. *Oral Disaeses,* **8** (**Suppl. 2**), 34–39.

Harris, C., Small C.B., Klein R.S., *et al.* (1983) Immunodeficiency in female sexual partners of men with the acquired immunodeficiency syndrome. *New England Journal of Medicine,* **308**, 1181–1184.

Hodgson, T.A., Greenspan, D., & Greenspan, J.S. (2006) Oral lesions of HIV disease and haart in industrialized countries. *Advances in Dental Research,* **19** (**1**), 57–62.

Jeffers, L. & Webster-Cyriaque, J.Y. (2011) Viruses and salivary gland disease (SGD). *Advances in Dental Research,* **23** (**1**), 79–83.

King, M.D., Reznik, D.A., O'Daniels, C.M., *et al.* (2002) Human papillomavirus-associated oral warts among HIV-seropositive patients in the era of highly active antiretroviral therapy: an emerging infection. *Clinical Infectious Diseases,* **34**, 641–648.

Klatt, E.C. (2013) *Pathology of AIDS, Version 24.* Savannah, GA.

Klein, R. (2006) *Guidance for industry fixed dose combinations, co-packaged drug products, and single-entityversions of previously approved antiretrovirals for the treatment of HIV.* U.S. Department of Health and Human Services Food and Drug Administration, Atlanta, GA.

Lane, S.D. & Stryker, J. (1993) *Needle Exchange: A Brief History.* A Publication from The Kaiser Forums; Sponsored by The Henry J. Kaiser Family Foundation.

Lau C., Mooiman, K.D., Maas-Bakker, R.F., *et al.* (2013) Effect of chinese herbs on CYP3A4 activity and expression in vitro. *Journal of Ethnopharmacology,* **149** (**2**), 543–549.

Levy, J. (1984) AIDS retrovirus (ARV-2) clone replicates in transfected human and animal fibroblasts. *Nature* **312** (**76**), 763.

Long, R., Hlousek, L., & Doyle, J.L. (1998) Oral manifestations of systemic diseases. *Mount Sinai Journal of Medicine,* **65** (**5–6**), 309–315.

Masur, H., Michelis, M.A., Greene, J.B., *et al.* (1981) An outbreak of community-acquired Pneumocystis carinii pneumonia: initial manifestation of cellular immune dysfunction. *New England Journal of Medicine,* **305** (**24**), 1431–1438.

Meier, A., Alter, G., & Frahm, N. (2007) MyD88-dependent immune activation mediated by human immunodeficiency virus type 1-encoded toll-like receptor ligands. *Journal of Virology,* **81** (**15**), 8180–8191.

MMWR (1982a) Epidemiologic notes and reports: possible transfusion-associated acquired immune deficiency syndrome, AIDS—California. *Morbidity & Mortality Weekly Report*, **31**, 652–654.

MMWR (1982b) Unexplained immunodeficiency and opportunistic infections in infants—New York, New Jersey, California. *MMWR,* **31** (**49**), 665–667.

MMWR (1982c) Update on acquired immune deficiency syndrome (AIDS) among patients with hemophilia A. *MMWR,* **31** (**48**), 644–646.

NIAID (2012) Structure of HIV. HIV virion. National Institute of Allergy and Infectious Diseases. http://www.niaid.nih.gov/topics/hivaids/understanding/howhivcausesaids/pages/howhiv.aspx [accessed on July 27, 2014].

Nikolaitchik, O.A., Dilley, K.A., & Fu, W. (2013) Dimeric RNA recognition regulates HIV-1 genome packaging. *PLOS Pathogens,* **9** (**3**), e1003249.

Palella, F.J. & Phair, J.P., (2012), Cardiovascular Disease in HIV Infection, Current Opinion HIV and AIDS, **6** (**4**), 266–271.

Patton, L.L. (2013) Oral lesions associated with human immunodeficiency virus disease. *Dental Clinics of North America,* **57** (**4**), 673–698.

Pedersen, A.M. & Jensen S. (2010) Oral manifestations in systemic diseases. *Ugeskrift for Laeger,* **172** (**44**), 3033–3036.

Popovic, M.S., Sarngadharan, M.G., Read, E., *et al.* (1984) Detection, isolation, and continuous production of cytopathic retroviruses (HTLV-111). *Science,* **224**, 497–500.

Prabhu, R.V., Prabhu, V., Chatra, L., *et al.* (2013) Oral manifestations of HIV. *Journal of Tropical Diseases*, **1** (**3**), 1–9.

Preston, S. & Raznik, D.A. (2013) *Oral Health Care for the HIV-Infected Patient.* The Mountain Plains AIDS Education and Training Center, Aurora, CO.

Rathbun, R.C., Liedtke, M.D., Lockhart, S.M., *et al.* (2013) Antiretroviral therapy for HIV infection. MedScape. http://emedicine.medscape.com/article/1533218-overview [accessed on July 27, 2014].

Schupbach, J., Popovic, M.,Gilden, R.V., *et al.* (1984) Serological analysis of a subgroup of human T-lymphotropic retroviruses (HTLV-III) associated with AIDS. *Science* **224** (**4648**), 503–505.

Slotten, R. (2012) As therapies improve, how to choose what's right for you. *The HIV Treatment Journal of Test Positive Aware Network* **2012**, 19–22.

Thienemann, F., Sliwa, K., & Rockstroh, J.K. (2013) HIV and the heart: the impact of antiretroviral therapy: a global perspective. *European Heart Journal*, **34** (**46**), 3538–3546.

Thomas, J.A. & Gorelick, R.J. (2008). Nucleocapsid protein function in early infection processes. *Virus Research*, **134** (**1–2**), 39–63.

Tobias, C.R., Fox, J.E., Walter, A.W., *et al.* (2012) Retention of people living with HIV/AIDS in oral health care. *Public Health Reports*, **127** (**Suppl. 2**), 45–54.

UNAIDS (2013) *Core Slides: Global Summary of the AIDS Epidemic.* http://www.unaids.org/en/media/unaids/contentassets/documents/epidemiology/2013/gr2013/201309_epi_core_en.pdf [accessed on July 27, 2014].

Wlodarczyk, D. (2004) Managing medical conditions associated with cardiac risk in patients with HIV. HIV InSite—comprehensive, up-to-date information on HIV/AIDS treatment, prevention, and policy from the University of California, San Francisco, CA.

Yi1, Y., Rana, R., & Turner, J.D. (1998) CXCR-4 is expressed by primary macrophages and supports CCR5-independent infection by dual-tropic but not t-tropic isolates of human immunodeficiency virus type 1. *Journal of Virology*, **72** (**1**), 772–777.

Chapter 14

Radiation and chemotherapy

Introduction	237
Oral signs/symptoms: Head and neck radiation/chemotherapy	239
Laboratory values	241
References	249

Introduction

Patients with malignant cancer that are treated with radiation and/or chemotherapy most likely will experience drug toxicities that can severely affect the entire body including the oral cavity. It is best to perform all necessary dental procedures before the patient undergoes radiation/chemotherapy; however, if the patient has come for the first time to the dental office with a history of radiation/chemotherapy or is currently having radiation/chemotherapy, then dental management becomes a bit more difficult.

Chemotherapy: Since antineoplastic drugs not only are cytotoxic to tumor cells, but they also kill normal cells in the body, many adverse effects are inevitable. Most of these agents affect either the function or the synthesis of DNA and are therefore more active in killing active rapidly proliferating cells such as cancer cells, bone marrow cells, and oral mucosal cells. Cancer cells that are not actively proliferating are more resistant to chemotherapeutic agents.

Chemotherapeutic agents are classified according to the specific phases of the cell cycle. Following mitosis, the phases of the cell cycle are the G_1 or gap phase and a very long phase, the S phase of DNA synthesis, and the G_2 phase (second gap).

Alkylating agents are drugs that do not require working in a specific phase of the cell cycle. These agents consist of cyclophosphamide, triazenes, nitrosoureas, actinomycin D, Adriamycin, daunomycin, 5-fluorouracil, and procarbazine. On the other hand, antimetabolites (e.g., methotrexate, 6-mercaptopurine, thioguanine, and arabinosylcytosine), hydroxyurea and the vinca alkaloids (e.g., vincristine and vinblastine), and bleomycin act at a specific phase of the cell cycle and therefore are more active against rapidly dividing cells.

Doses of chemotherapeutic agents are expressed in terms of surface area rather than weight because there are fewer changes in area during the course of chemotherapy and area is a measure more constant for both children and adults. *One of the most concerning adverse effects of systemic chemotherapy is the development of immunosuppression/myelosuppression (decreased bone marrow activity resulting in less RBCs, WBCs, and platelets) resulting in bacterial, fungal, and viral infections; direct injury or*

The Dentist's Quick Guide to Medical Conditions, First Edition. Mea A. Weinberg, Stuart L. Segelnick, Joseph S. Insler, with Samuel Kramer.
© 2015 John Wiley & Sons, Inc. Published 2015 by John Wiley & Sons, Inc.

cytotoxicity to the oral tissues; loss of tissue-based immune cells; or loss of defensive salivary components (Fleming 1991; National Cancer Institute 2013). The most important issue regarding dental patients who are currently on or who previously had chemotherapy is dental opportunistic infections, which can be so severe that they could actually result in sepsis and death.

Radiation: Radiation to the head and neck region (oral, laryngeal, and nasopharyngeal) is of before concern to the treating dentist; whereas radiation to other parts of the body (e.g., breast and prostate) does not influence dental treatment as much. In other parts of the body, the WBC count can decrease after radiation and should be known for dental treatment. Oral symptoms usually appear with radiation to the head and neck region. While infections resulting from chemotherapy can be severe, immunosuppression with subsequent development of infections is not of as much concern with radiation patients.

High doses of ionizing radiation are directed at the actively dividing tumor cells, damaging their DNA, and are confined to this area as much as possible without going outside the tumor zone; however, unavoidably the salivary glands, oral mucosa, and jaw will be affected (Vissink *et al.* 2003; Weinberg *et al.* 2011). Patients may require radiation therapy before, during, or after surgery, and it may be combined with chemotherapy. The justification for using chemotherapy with radiation for head and neck cancers is to sensitize tumors more than the normal tissues to radiation and to assist in eliminating subclinical distant metastases (Zackrisson *et al.* 2003). For head and neck cancers, the tumor effects of radiation can be increased, as well as adverse effects, by the concomitant administration of chemotherapeutic agents such as cisplatin and 5-fluorouracil (Zackrisson *et al.* 2003).

External beam radiation, where the radiation comes from an external source (e.g., a machine), is used for oral tumors, nasal tumors, soft tissue sarcomas, some bone tumors, and brain tumors. On the other hand, treatment of localized prostate cancer has low–energy-emitting radioactive seeds (brachytherapy or seed therapy) surgically implanted, directly into the prostate gland. Up to 40–100 seeds can be implanted and high doses of radiation slowly reduce over 1 year with most traces being undetectable after 3 months; however, the seeds remain in the body forever (www.wpahs.org/specialties/prostate-cancer/radioactive-seed-implantation). Since some radioactivity may be given off during the treatment, it is important for pregnant women not to be in close contact with the patient for 2 months after the seed implants and children should not sit on the person's lap more than 5 min a day for 2 months after the implant. It is still best to consult with the oncologist when it is safe for the dentist and staff to treat these patients in the dental office (www.wpahs.org/specialties/prostate-cancer/radioactive-seed-implantation).

In breast cancer, after surgery/chemotherapy and depending on the lymph node involvement, radiation can be used to complete the course of treatment and help prevent recurrence.

The amount of ionizing radiation to the tumor cells depends on the sensitivity and rapidity with which the cells divide. Radiation is considered to be local treatment because cells are being destroyed only in the area being treated (Haas 2004). Gray (Gy) is a unit that measures the radiation dose of ionizing radiation that is absorbed by human tissue. Since radiotherapy is a local treatment, the adverse effects seen generally are limited to the tissues exposed directly to the radiation beams. Typically, radiation to the head and neck consists of a total dose of 50–70 Gy administered in fractionated doses of 2.0 Gy/day for 5 days over 5–7 weeks (Jensen *et al.* 2003; Brosky 2007).

Studies have reported that between 50 and 76% of patients are nonadherent to office visits to the dentist even when dental care is available and almost 50% are lost to dental follow-up (Cacchillo *et al.* 1993; Toljanic *et al.* 2002; Brosky 2007). It is an important part of the dental practice to set aside a specific follow-up program for patients that are currently or will be undergoing radiotherapy. Since many patients are nonadherent to oral hygiene care, the dentist should make special requirements for these patients and have a specific staff member call and follow up. It is recommended that after radiotherapy patients be seen at the office every 3 months to monitor adverse effects and oral hygiene (Brosky 2007).

Besides radiation and chemotherapy, bisphosphonates have been prescribed early on in cancer to prevent adverse effects of cancer treatments on bone health, mainly for reducing the loss in bone mineral density (Brown *et al.* 2004; Coleman and McCloskey 2011). Bisphosphonates are indicated for the relief of bone pain due to hypercalcemia in certain cancers (e.g., breast and prostate) that have metastasized (Coleman 2011). Bisphosphonates have been used in conjunction with radiotherapy for bone pain (Brown *et al.* 2004). Refer to Chapter 12 for management of dental patients on bisphosphonates.

Oral signs/symptoms: Head and neck radiation/chemotherapy

Oral adverse effects will affect 100% of patients (Brosky 2007). Complications from cancer therapy can be acute, which are transient and only seen during treatment, and chronic or long-term, lasting months to years after treatment has ended. Oral adverse effects of radiotherapy to the head and neck region are reviewed in Table 14.1. Late oral complications can occur depending on up the radiation dosing (total dose), fraction size, and duration of treatment (National Cancer Institute 2013).

Radiation: The reduced blood flow affects the mandibular teeth more than the maxillary teeth because the only blood supply comes from the inferior alveolar nerve (Oral Cancer Foundation 2013). Oral adverse effects can be attributed to a complex microflora and trauma to oral tissues during normal oral function (Keefe *et al.* 2007). Whether these damaging effects are transient (acute) or long-lasting (chronic) depends on the age of the patient, which tissues are exposed to the radiation beams, the dose of the radiation, fraction size, fractionation, and type of ionizing irradiation (Vissink *et al.* 2003; Lawrence *et al.* 2008). Usually, patients receive external beam radiation in multiple sessions over several weeks. The use of high-energy photon beams with linear accelerator reduces the number of hot spots in normal tissue thereby reducing the incidence and severity of mucositis (Vissink *et al.* 2003). Most epithelial cancers receive radiation at the rate of 1.8–2.2 Gy per fraction for 6–7 weeks for a total dose of 6500–7500 cGy (Epstein and Van Der Waal 2008).

Oral mucositis: Most adverse effects of chemotherapy/radiation will occur anywhere along the gastrointestinal tract, bone marrow, and oral cavity due to a high turnover rate of the cells. Mucositis refers to a painful inflammation or ulceration of the mucous membrane any place along the gastrointestinal tract. Stomatitis specifically refers to mucositis of the oral cavity; stomatitis is oral mucositis or inflammation of the tissues in the oral cavity (O'Brien 2009). If these oral cells/tissues are exposed to radiation therapy, oral mucositis and lowered blood cell count will occur. Stomatitis usually develops with fractions of 180–220 cGy/day by the third or fourth week of radiotherapy and may gradually reduce weeks after completion of radiotherapy (Epstein and Huhmann 2011a). Patients with dental implants, removable appliances, and metal restorations may show more severe mucositis (Epstein and Van Der Waal 2008).

There is a severity scale of mucositis that many oncologists use (adapted from Toth *et al.* 1990; Fleming 1999):

Grade 1 mild mucosal changes: White, red patches, mucosal tissue thinning, no burning or sensitivity, and normal eating.
Grade 2 mild mucosal changes: Localized red and thinning tissue, small local ulceration, slight burning, and normal eating. Pain depends on the amount of tissue with ulceration/damage and the amount of inflammatory mediators released.
Grade 3 moderate mucosal changes: Localized or generalized red and ulcerated tissue, moderate sensitivity and no visible bleeding but clots are evident.
Grade 4 severe mucosal changes: Generalized red and ulcerated tissue, active visible bleeding, extreme pain, and trouble with eating.

Hyposalivation: Radiation-induced xerostomia is unavoidable when in the direct field of radiation. New developments are there in the way radiation is delivered. Intense-modulated radiation therapy (IMRT) is the up-to-date treatment method that delivers high doses of radiation directly to cancer cells in a targeted way, which is more exact than with conventional radiotherapy (Grégoire *et al.* 2007; Oral Cancer Foundation 2013). IMRT uses computer-generated images to plan and deliver tightly focused radiation beams to the cancer cells (Grégoire *et al.* 2007). For head and neck cancer, IMRT permits radiation that will minimize exposure of other parts of the body including spinal cord, optic nerve, and salivary glands to be delivered (Grégoire *et al.* 2007; Oral Cancer Foundation 2013). There needs to be more effective techniques to protect the salivary glands (primarily the parotid glands) during radiation (Brosky 2007).

Hyposalivation or a reduction in saliva production is usually irreversible because of irreparable damage to the salivary glands in doses >25 Gy; however, in low-dose radiation of <25 Gy, it is usually temporary with no permanent changes and recovery of salivary function is within 12–24 months or longer. A clinical study found that 36% of patients continued to experience moderate to severe xerostomia years after the completion of radiotherapy (Wasserman *et al.* 2005; Brosky 2007). In addition, radiotherapy increases salivary viscosity and alters the salivary buffering capacity (Cassolato and Turnbull 2003). Hyposalivation has not been shown to be an adverse effect from just chemotherapy alone; usually, hyposalivation will appear with both radiotherapy and chemotherapy together (Berger *et al.* 2007).

Xerostomia is a debilitating adverse effect and can reduce the patient's quality of life, affecting speech, swallowing, and eating. Treatment is palliative until function is restored (Diriax *et al.* 2006) (Table 14.1). There are significant differences in the treatment protocols for xerostomia primarily because of the lack of proven and well-recognized clinical guidelines (Brosky 2007). Since the introduction of newer IMRT, the incidence of hyposalivation has diminished (Epstein and Huhmann 2011b). The most important palliative treatment starts with oral home care/plaque control. Supplemental care includes nonalcoholic oral rinses (e.g., chlorhexidine, alcohol free—GUM) and fluoride applications. As a result of hyposalivation, candidiasis infections may occur and remain localized without systemic involvement unless the patient is immunocompromised (Epstein and Van Der Waal 2008). Wearing dentures and smoking are two contributing factors for the development of fungal infections (Epstein and Van Der Waal 2008). Examples of common antifungal medications used in dentistry are nystatin suspension or pastilles, miconazole troches (Note that these products contain sucrose so caution used in high caries risk), and miconazole 2% (20 mg/g) oral gel (Daktarin® oral gel; not available in USA). In patients that have residual salivary glands that continue to function, massaging the area has shown to be beneficial (Ngeow *et al.* 2006a).

Radiation caries: Radiation caries, due to a decreased salivary production secondary to radiation, clinically appears as spotty demineralization on the buccal and lingual cervical thirds of the tooth. Caries can begin as early as 3 months after the start of radiation, so early prevention is the key (Chai *et al.* 2006). Weekly applications of fluoride in office as well as custom trays for home (daily application) are recommended, as tolerated. Neutral sodium fluoride is recommended as acidulated phosphate fluoride is too irritating to the tissues.

Chemotherapy: The oral cavity is highly sensitive to the toxic effects of both radiation and chemotherapy, which can be due to either immunosuppression leading to opportunistic infections (e.g., bacterial, viral, and fungal) or the direct action on the damaged epithelial cells. Table 14.1 reviews oral complications of chemotherapy and its dental management.

Oral mucositis: The severity of oral mucositis increases with combination chemotherapy and radiation (Carl 1995). Oral mucositis develops from epithelial cell thinning which leads to ulceration, which is a portal for oral bacteria to enter and cause secondary infection. Oral mucositis seems to be more severe in patients with poor oral hygiene, older age, smoking, and hyposalivation in the beginning of treatment (Epstein and Van Der Waal 2008).

Most treatment of mucositis, induced by radiation or chemotherapy, has not been effective, and there are no published specific guidelines (Sonis 2004; Ngeow *et al.* 2006b). Treatment of mucositis is different when due to site-specific radiation or systemically administered chemotherapy (Sonis 2004). It should be noted that mucositis can occur in the mucous membranes of the stomach or intestines as well as the oral cavity. Chemotherapy-induced mucositis occurs rather quickly, usually within 1 week after the start of chemotherapy and disappears in 2 weeks (Epstein and Huhmann 2011). Radiation-induced oral mucositis takes on a more chronic course after multiple small fractions are administered over a few weeks, starting at doses of 15 Gy and reaching a plateau at 30 Gy. Both radiation- and chemotherapy-induced oral mucositis undergo stages of development, which will affect their treatment. Candidiasis infections may increase the discomfort of mucositis. It is important to frequently exam and monitor oral mucosal tissues especially if the patient has mucositis. Table 14.1 reviews the treatment for oral mucositis. In addition to local therapy, amifostine has been used for the prevention of oral mucositis from radiation and chemotherapy; however, there are conflicting results and insufficient data (Nicolatou-Galitis *et al.* 2012).

Nausea/vomiting: Nausea and vomiting are other effects of chemotherapy that the dentist needs to be concerned. Nausea and vomiting can be caused by the cancer itself or due to treatment (Warr 2008). Nausea can affect the patient's desire to eat prompting diet counseling. Antiemetics can help to reduce the incidence of nausea. Benzodiazepines (e.g., lorazepam) are prescribed to help the patient with anticipated nausea and vomiting (Epstein and Huhmann 2011b). Promethazine, prochlorperazine, or metoclopramide are indicated to reduce nausea primarily within 24 h of chemotherapy. To treat nausea after 24 h of chemotherapy, 5-hydroxytryptamine 3 (5-HT$_3$) antagonists (e.g., ondansetron, placed on tongue, and tropisetron) or corticosteroid combination and neurokinin 1 (NK$_1$) receptor antagonists [e.g., aprepitant (Emend)] are prescribed (Jordan 2006; Billio *et al.* 2010; Epstein and Huhmann 2011b). In spite of the use of 5-HT$_3$ receptor antagonists and other drugs, chemotherapy-induced nausea and vomiting still remain a concern (Warr 2008). As an adjunctive use to standard therapy, the NK$_1$ receptor antagonist, aprepitant reduces the incidence of vomiting (Warr 2008).

Laboratory values

The most current lab values (actually, it should be of the day before the dental procedure) should be known (American Academy of Pediatrics 2013):

a. WBC count, which should be >2000/mm^3
b. Absolute neutrophil count (ANC)
　　i. Should be >2000/mm^3 (no antibiotic prophylaxis required).
　　ii. If 1000–2000, use clinical judgment; some sources use prophylaxis (Hong *et al.* 2010; National Cancer Institute 2013)
　　iii. If <1000/mm^3, postpone and dental treatment.
c. Platelets should be >75,000/mm^3 for dental treatment.
　　i. 40,000–7,500: Platelet transfusion may be required before/after dental procedure; consult with oncologist
　　ii. <40,000: Postpone dental treatment; consult with oncologist.

Table 14.1 Oral adverse effects after radiation to head and neck or chemotherapy (Fleming 1991; Guggenheimer and Moore 2003; Ngeow *et al.* 2006c; Ramli *et al.* 2006; Brosky 2007; Keefe *et al.* 2007; Epstein and Van Der Waal 2008; Hsiung *et al.* 2008; O'Brien 2009; Epstein and Huhmann 2011a, b; American Academy of Pediatrics 2013; Connolly *et al.* 2013; Elad *et al.* 2013; National Cancer Institute 2013; Oral Cancer Foundation 2013).

Oral lesion	Causes	Dental management
Hyposalivation (mouth and lips), fissured tongue with atrophic filiform papillae	Radiation: Acute xerostomia: acute inflammatory reactions, temporary Chronic (late) xerostomia (after radiation): fibrosis of salivary glands, loss of cells, reduced blood flow Chemotherapy: toxic to salivary glands	Stepwise approach: • Coating agents such as bismuth salicylate or sucralfate • Water-soluble lubricants for mouth and lips • For thick/ropy saliva: guaifenesin (Organidin NR) as a liquid or a tablet (a mucolytic drug; 200–400 mg, 3–4 times a day) • Topical analgesics (benzocaine and lidocaine viscous) for temporary pain relief. Not recommended. • Xylitol-containing chewing gum, sugar-free candies, moisturizing products (e.g. Biotene), alcohol-free rinses (e.g., chlorhexidine), frequent sips of water, rinsing with club soda, sucking on ice cubes. • Prescribe pilocarpine (Salagen) (5 and 10 mg doses) or cevimeline (Evoxac). May show some improvement but reviews are mixed. • Topical antifungal agents for *Candida albicans* infections
Oral mucositis (stomatitis)	Chemotherapy: due to the death of epithelial basal cells with thinning of the oral epithelium resulting in mucositis (oral inflammation and ulcers) and oral ulceration that can result in secondary infection and sepsis due to the presence of oral bacteria that invade the oral open ulcers. Most commonly seen on lips, tongue, floor of mouth, buccal mucosa, and soft palate. The hard palate and gingiva are not as affected. Radiation: acute effect/temporary First visible sign of mucositis is either a white appearance of the mucosal tissues or a red appearance due to epithelial thinning. Thereafter, a pseudomembrane forms due to ulceration with a fibrinous exudate with bacterial and oral debris	Severity of stomatitis goes from mild changes to severe. The same treatment is indicated if palliative or curative. Only localized therapy, not systemic

Table 14.1 (*cont'd*)

Oral lesion	Causes	Dental management
		Key to treatment is pain control: • Debilitating condition affecting swallowing, speech, and sleep • Can lead to dehydration and malnutrition. Nutritional counseling is important • Optimal oral home care: brushing teeth and tongue 2–3 times a day with soft nylon bristled brush or electric toothbrush (Caution must be taken during use because it can cause tissue trauma). Use non-fluoride paste if burning occurs. Flossing • Water-soluble lubricating jelly or lanolin for lips • Fluoride in office/home application • Chlorhexidine (alcohol free) rinses; salt/sodium bicarbonate rinses; for severe mucositis use a 1:4 hydrogen peroxide rinse for 1–2 days followed by a salt/bicarbonate rinse; ice chips, frequent water rinses. • Analgesics: viscous lidocaine 2% solution; benzocaine 20% (Orajel); benzocaine in Orabase • Mucosal coating agents: diphenhydramine (Benadryl) elixir mixed with Kaopectate (50% mixture by volume); nystatin (1 ml) mixed with Maalox (120 ml): swish with 5 ml for 30 s. • Xylitol-containing gums to stimulate saliva • IV amifostine Once the WBC count returns to normal, the mucositis disappears. It takes about 3–6 weeks after radiation therapy for healing to occur
Pain (neurotoxicity— nerve damage)	Chemotherapy: pain in tooth that mimics a toothache. Especially seen with plant alkaloids (e.g., viscristine and vinblastine). Due to tooth hypersensitivity from decreased saliva and lowered salivary pH, tumor invasion of neural tissues and neuronal damage by surgery, chemotherapy, and radiation therapy	Tooth pain is transient and will usually disappear soon after reducing or stopping chemotherapy. Severe pain managed by the oncologist with analgesics

(*continued*)

Table 14.1 *(cont'd)*

Oral lesion	Causes	Dental management
Taste alterations (hypogeusia)	May be due secondary to mucosal infections Radiation: changes start about 1 week into radiotherapy and persist till 3–6 weeks after the end of therapy. Chemotherapy: with therapy taste changes (sour/bitter) may stay for months	Changes are transient or permanent. Foods may taste metallic. Reduce the intake of spicy foods. Eat soft foods
Bleeding	Chemotherapy: may be due to thrombocytopenia (decrease in platelets) and/or coagulation factors resulting in bleeding and bruising	Consultation from oncologist regarding platelet count
Secondary infections (herpes simplex virus and candidiasis)	Chemotherapy: decreased WBC count can result in infections but more common with radiation. Radiation: can be severe and life-threatening. Bone marrow cells show decreased turnover resulting in neutropenia and sepsis and secondary systemic infections. Candidiasis is common especially in the oropharyngeal region	Consultation from oncologist regarding WBC count. Herpes simplex virus may present as mucosal burning or ulceration. Evaluate the patient's dentures to verify retention; ill-fitting dentures can cause chronic atrophic candidiasis (denture sore mouth). Monitor the patient for angular cheilitis around the commissures of the lips; due to candida infection and loss of vertical dimension Topical antifungal agents are used because the infection is localized to the oral cavity without systemic involvement • Nystatin oral suspension (contains sucrose; caution is required in patients with caries) • Clotrimazole 10 mg troche • Nystatin or clotrimazole cream (apply to inside of denture) (Note that creams are not labeled for internal use and some pharmacists will not fill a prescription written for internal use) • In addition, chlorhexidine rinse can be prescribed Herpes simplex viral infections can be treated with topical acyclovir
Mandibular dysfunction	Radiation: musculoskeletal problems secondary to radiotherapy and surgery including soft-tissue fibrosis, surgically induced mandibular discontinuity, and stress-induced parafunctional habits. If not treated can lead to trismus	Evaluate and stabilize occlusion, physical therapy (mandibular muscle–stretching exercises) to reduce the fibrosis, pain- and stress- relief regimens including muscle relaxants

Table 14.1 *(cont'd)*

Oral lesion	Causes	Dental management
Trismus	Radiation to masticatory muscles involving the temporal mandibular joint; chronic/long-lasting; fibrosis of tissues. Incidence of trismus is related to the dose of radiation	Physical therapy starting before radiation therapy and continuing during therapy includes: exercises, analgesics, moist heat, muscle relaxants, and trigger point injections
Osteonecrosis	High-dose radiation: blood vessel compromise and necrosis of bone do not allow bone healing when traumatized Radiation; chronic/long-lasting; also from antiresorptive drugs indicated for hypercalcemia	Treatment of osteonecrosis may require referral to a maxillofacial oral surgeon
Radiation caries	Radiation: secondary to damage to salivary glands resulting in decreased saliva with loss of mineral (demineralization) from the gingival one-third of the tooth (by the CEJ) and the incisal/cuspal area. Caries can start within 3 months after completing radiotherapy.	Fluoride in office and home applications. Recommend daily use of 1.1% sodium fluoride (custom application). Monitor patient carefully. Do not eat or drink for at least 30 min after fluoride application.
Periodontal disease	Radiation/chemotherapy: decreased salivary protective proteins and alteration in buffering capacity	Monitor plaque control and for gingivitis/periodontitis; if necessary referral to a periodontist
Nausea/vomiting	Chemotherapy/radiation: due to many factors including medications (high-dose cisplatin), radiation therapy, effect of cancer itself, infection, gastritis, bowel obstruction, and hypercalcemia	Anticipatory nausea: lorazepam <24 h after chemotherapy (acute): promethazine, prochlorperazine, metoclopramide, and dexamethasone >24 h after chemotherapy (delayed): ondansetron, granisetron, and aprepitant (Emend) Monitor for enamel erosion

Information from the patient

When interviewing a patient that will begin chemotherapy shortly after visiting the dentist, has had radiation/chemotherapy in the past, or is currently on a regimen, it is important to ask the following questions:

1. What type of cancer are you diagnosed with?
2. Are there any other medical conditions?
3. Are you undergoing radiation, chemotherapy, or both?
4. What is the chemotherapy regimen? What is the drug? How many cycles have been administered? What is the route of administration?
5. What is the current WBC count (with differential, platelet)?

Treatment plan

Prevention of oral complications from high-dose chemotherapy, radiation, or stem-cell transplant is accomplished by regular dental visits and optimal oral hygiene. Dental care depends on the radiation dose and duration of the treatment, the body part that was treated, and any complications that occurred. Pre-radiotherapy/pre-chemotherapy dental screening is of utmost importance in the overall treatment of cancer patients (Mealey *et al.* 1994; Andrews and Griffiths 2001).

Before the patient is scheduled for radiation/chemotherapy, the dentist needs to get them ready for anticipated oral complications (Mealey *et al.* 1994; Vissink *et al.* 2003; National Cancer Institute 2013):

1. Consult with oncologist team; discuss time required to perform all necessary dental procedures.
2. Review medical history; know the patient's current lab values.
3. Full mouth series of radiographs.
4. Diagnostic casts.
5. Review past dental history and dental habits (tooth brushing, flossing, and fluoride use). Start the patient on fluoride supplementation (office/home applied). To prevent demineralization, a high-potency fluoride gel with custom trays (all tooth structure is covered while keeping away from the gingiva) is recommended. Fluoride therapy should begin a few days before radiation therapy begins. (Initially a, 10 min application of a 1.1% neutral pH sodium fluoride gel or a 0.4% stannous fluoride gel, preferably unflavored.) Use neutral fluoride if patients have porcelain/resin crowns or glass ionomer restorations. Acidulated phosphate fluoride should not be used because it is irritating to the tissues (Mealey *et al.* 1994). As an alternative to custom trays, the fluoride can be brushed on the teeth for 2–3 min (Shiboski *et al.* 2007; National Institute of Health 2014a, b).
6. Review patient's nutritional profile to help prevent dehydration and nutritional deficiencies and dental caries.
7. From the oncologist, know the locations of radiation portals so that location of complications can be anticipated. For example, radiation to the nasopharyngeal and posterior soft palate regions will most likely result in hyposalivation and caries rather than osteonecrosis; whereas, radiation to the mandible most likely will result in osteonecrosis. Radiation to the salivary glands most likely results in hyposalivation and caries (Mealey *et al.* 1994).
8. Initial treatment plan: Elimination of active/acute dental infections in order to prevent systemic infections and extractions of teeth with hopeless prognosis. Treat periodontal conditions; perform periodontal debridement. Eliminate any sources of tissue irritation (e.g., dentures and orthodontic appliances). Evaluate third molars; some recommend to extract all partially erupted third molars before cancer therapy starts. Extractions should be performed at least 7–10 days before the start of cancer therapy. If there is time before the patients start radiation/chemotherapy, then the secondary treatment plan is started. Get a prosthodontic consultation.
9. Secondary plan: Carious lesions (even small incipient caries), endodontics, replace any faculty restorations.
10. Evaluate prosthodontic and orthodontic appliance; remove all irritating edges (Epstein and Huhmann 2011c).

During the time the patient is having cancer therapy, it is primarily important to maintain oral hygiene and manage oral adverse effects of therapy (National Institute of Health 2014a, b).

1. Continual consultation with oncologist team.
2. Need for antibiotic prophylaxis.

3. Known current lab values for patients undergoing chemotherapy: delay dental treatment if platelet count is <75,000/mm^3 or abnormal coagulation factors and ANC is <1,000/mm^3; discuss with oncologist about antibiotic prophylaxis.
4. If the patient has a central venous catheter, consult with the oncologist whether to prescribe antibiotic prophylaxis.
5. See the patient as often to maintain oral health, with more frequent intervals if the patient has ongoing oral symptoms.
6. Prevent and/or minimize oral complications and tissue trauma, which can lead to systemic infections and even death.
7. Extraction of teeth is not recommended *during* head and neck radiotherapy because of risk of osteo-radionecrosis. Extractions disturb large blood vessels entering the bone leaving the smaller vessels, which are more susceptible to be affected by radiation and developing osteoradionecrosis (Mealey *et al.* 1994).If extractions are an emergency, use antibiotic coverage before and after extractions and possibly hyperbaric oxygen therapy. Instituting optimal oral hygiene can be beneficial (Atri *et al.* 2007). A minimum of 14–21 days is recommended after extractions *before* radiotherapy is started (National Institute of Health 2014b). Also, the risk for osteonecrosis is minimal if there is a waiting time of a minimum of 21 days between extraction and the start of radiotherapy (Atri *et al.* 2007). If the radiation dose to the mandible is <5000 cGy there is minimal risk of osteonecrosis *after* radiotherapy is finished (National Institute of Health 2014b). There is no specific "safe" time to wait *after* completion of head and neck radiation to perform extractions. Tooth extractions should be avoided for many years after head and neck radiation (Vissink *et al.* 2003; Atri *et al.* 2007).
8. Once saliva becomes thick and ropy or reduced in volume, it becomes extremely important to pay attention to oral hygiene.
9. For chemotherapy, know the current lab values (WBC, ANC, and platelets); if the patient is immunosuppressed, dental procedures should be deferred.
10. Review tooth brushing and flossing gently. See section on "Patient Instructions."
11. Continue with fluoride supplementation.

After cancer therapy: Dental considerations of the patient that has finished cancer therapy (Vissink *et al.* 2003; Rahman *et al.* 2006; Epstein and Huhmann 2011b; National Cancer Institute 2013; National Institute of Health 2014a) are as follows.

1. If all oral complications have resolved, instruct patient to maintain and stabilize oral health.
2. Reinforce oral home care: brushing and flossing.
3. Continue with fluoride supplementation.
4. To treat any dental conditions that were not treated before or during chemotherapy unless the patient is still immunocompromised, especially if the patient has had stem-cell transplantation. Many patients may be taking an antiresorptive drug.
5. After the patient has finished radiation therapy and all oral adverse effects are eliminated (Sometimes, oral complications can remain for a time afterward.), the patient should be evaluated and monitored every 4–8 weeks for the first 6 months. Afterward, a schedule can be designed for each patient.
6. After radiation therapy, there can be long-term caries risk, xerostomia, and osteonecrosis. Continuously monitor patient.
7. Maintain nutritional and dietary changes; may require diet supplementation.
8. Reevaluate dentures and refabricate if there is any source of continual tissue irritation. Old dentures should not be worn. New dentures are recommended for at least 1 year after radiation. It is imperative to minimize trauma to the tissues. It is recommended to fabricate overdentures or implant supported dentures to lessen the masticatory load of the denture.

Patient instructions (National Cancer Institute 2013)

1. It is emphasized that there are no evidence-based protocols regarding the optimal approach for oral hygiene in cancer patients. Most patients that undergo either high-dose chemotherapy or extended-field radiation therapy have similar maintenance care.
2. Be in contact with the oncologist/radiotherapist.
3. Maintain meticulous oral hygiene. Routine oral home care is important to reduce prevalence and severity of oral effects of cancer therapy: use ultrasoft or soft nylon-bristled brush (softened in hot water); Bass technique (2–3 times a day) with light pressure, fluoride toothpaste, frequent rinsing (every 2–4 h) with a 0.9% saline, sodium bicarbonate rinse/water or saline mixed. Use of electric toothbrush should be discouraged because it could cause tissue trauma/laceration. Rinse the toothbrush after every use with chlorhexidine and then rinse with water and allow drying. Floss once a day. There may be bleeding if platelets <30,000. Rinse with antimicrobial rinses (e.g., nonalcoholic rinses such as chlorhexidine 0.12%—GUM® Paroex™) or bicarbonate solution at least two to four times a day. Alcohol-containing rinses can dehydrate the oral tissues. Avoid tartar control toothpastes and whitening products.
4. For lip dryness/cracking, use petrolatum- or lanolin-containing products.
5. Meticulous oral care will help reduce mucositis, but it will be still difficult to treat.
6. Monitor for oral ulcers or infections.
7. Monitor for periodontal diseases because their development will increase the prevalence of bleeding and infection.
8. Care of dentures and orthodontic appliances: Wear denture only when eating. Clean at night and soak in an antimicrobial solution. Any orthodontic appliance should be removed before therapy.
9. Do not wear appliances or dentures when mucositis is present.
10. Smoking cessation is important for patients with head and neck cancer.
11. Nausea causing vomiting and its effect on the dentition must be addressed during radiotherapy. Monitor for tooth erosion.
12. Monitoring the patient after radiotherapy is a long-term process; initially, see the patient every 4–8 weeks during the first 6 months after radiotherapy; thereafter, have a special schedule set up for each patient (National Institute of Health 2014b).

Summary: Dental notes

1. There are no specific published guidelines or protocol regarding dental treatment. When is the ideal time to proceed with dental treatment in a patient that is currently on chemotherapy?
2. First of all, a consult from the oncologist is required before, during, and immediately after cancer therapy.
3. For chemotherapy patients, find out chemotherapy regimen including the number of cycles, the chemotherapeutic agent, the route of administration, and lab values.
4. For radiation patients, find out the parts of the body that will have radiation, the size of the area getting the radiation, and the total dose.
5. Patients that have had head and neck radiation may have a reduced alveolar bone quality and may not be suitable for extractions, implant or periodontal surgery. Consult with the patient's oncologist.
6. Oral complications of chemotherapy: oral mucositis, severe infections (sepsis), bleeding, and nerve damage (pain).
7. Oral complications of radiation therapy: dental caries, periodontal disease, bone and tissue destruction in the area of radiation, and fibrosis of tissue and muscle in the area of radiation, trismus.

8. Oral complications of chemotherapy or radiation therapy: oral mucositis, taste changes, tooth pain, xerostomia, changes in dental growth in children, caries, and periodontal disease.

9. Secondary opportunistic infections including candidiasis are common if the patient has mucositis or xerostomia due to a change in the normal oral flora, poor oral hygiene and lack of salivary lubrication (Ngeow *et al.* 2006c).

10. Consult if antibiotic prophylaxis is needed.

11. Oral mucositis is one of the more commonly encountered adverse effects of both chemotherapy and radiation to the head and neck area as well as other parts of the body. The severity of the inflammation depends on the patient's oral hygiene, age of the patient and the amount of radiation administered.

12. In patients having chemotherapy for other cancers (e.g., breast) and including head and neck cancer, their WBC, ANC, and platelet counts must be known before dental procedures are started.

13. In patients having radiation for head and neck cancer or other cancers, a current WBC and ANC is required.

14. An initial oral examination is important before as well as during and after cancer therapy. Prevention is the key to minimizing oral complications. (American Academy of Pediatrics 2013).

15. Set up a special program for patients that will be undergoing radiation/chemotherapy that will increase patient adherence to routine office visits and oral hygiene.

16. It has been recommended that the best time to administer dental treatment during chemotherapy is by the next cycle of chemotherapy. For a patient that has already had chemotherapy, there is no specific time recommended to treat the patient.

17. If invasive dental surgery is planned, it is important to know the radiation dose that has been given.

18. Clinical studies have documented that patients who stopped head and neck radiation and had a new denture insertion in 180 days or less had the same number of complications when compared with patients who received their dentures in 181–365 days and longer than 1 year (Gerngross *et al.* 2005). However, most clinicians prefer to wait 6 months to a year before inserting new dentures.

19. Precautions should be taken with male patients that have had radioactive seed implants for prostate cancer. Pregnant dentists and staff should not be in close contact with the patient for 2 months after the seed implants. Consult with oncologist and radiologist regarding when it is safe to treat patients as the dentists will be required to enter a certain distance while treating these patients.

References

American Academy of Pediatrics (2013) *Guideline on dental management of pediatric patients receiving chemotherapy, hematopoietic cell transplantation, and/or radiation*. http://www.aapd.org/media/Policies_Guidelines/G_Chemo.pdf [accessed on January 13, 2014].

Andrews, N. & Griffiths, C. (2001) Dental complications of head and neck radiotherapy. *Australian Dental Journal*, **46**, 174–182.

Atri, R., Dhull, A.K., Dhankhar, R., *et al.* (2007) Orodental care related to radiotherapy for head and neck cancer. *Journal of Oral Health & Community Dentistry* **1**, 59–62.

Berger, A.M., Shuster, J.L., & Von Roenn, J.H. (2007) Symptoms and syndromes. Part C: Gastrointestinal symptoms and syndromes. In: A.M. Berger, J.L. Shuster, & J.H. Von Roenn (eds), *Principles and Practice of Palliative Care and Supportive Oncology*, 3rd ed. Lippincott William & Wilkins, Philadelphia.

Billio, A., Morello, E., & Clarke, M.J. (2006) Serotonin receptor antagonists for highly emetogenic chemotherapy in adults. *Cochrane Database of Systematic Reviews*, **2010** (**10**), CD006272.

Brosky, M.E. (2007) The role of saliva in oral health: strategies for prevention and management of xerostomia. *The Journal of Supportive Oncology*, **5**, 215–225.

Brown, J.E., Neville-Webbe, H., & Coleman, R.E. (2004) The role of bisphosphonates in breast and prostate cancers. *Endocrine-Related Cancer*, **11**, 207–224.

Cacchillo, D., Barker, G.J., & Barker, B.F. (1993) Late effects of head and neck radiation therapy and patient/dentist compliance with recommended dental care. *Special Care Dentist*, **13**, 159–162.

Carl, W. (1995) Oral complications of local and systemic cancer treatment. *Current Opinion in Oncology*, **7**, 320–324.

Cassolato, S.F. & Turnfull, R.S. (2003) Xerostomia: clinical aspects and treatment. *Gerodontology*, **20**, 64–77.

Chai, W.L., Ngeow, W.C., Ramli, R. *et al.* (2006) Managing complications of radiation therapy in head and neck cancer patients: Part II. Management of radiation-induced caries. *Singapore Dental Journal*, **28**, 4–6.

Coleman, R. (2011) The use of bisphosphonates in cancer treatment. *Annals of the New York Academy of Sciences*, **1218**, 3–14.

Coleman, R.E. & McCloskey, E.V. (2011) Bisphosphonates in oncology. *Bone*, **49**, 71–76.

Connolly, I., Zaleon, C., & Montagnini, M. (2013) Management of severe neuropathic cancer pain: an illustrative case and review. *The American Journal of Hospice & Palliative Care*, **30**, 83–90.

Diriax, P., Nuyts, S., & Van den Bogaert, W. (2006) Radiation-induced xerostomia in patients with head and neck cancer: a literature review. *Cancer*, **107**, 2525–2534.

Elad, S., Bowen, J., Zadik, Y. *et al.* (2013) Development of the MASCC/ISOO Clinical Practice Guidelines for Mucositis: considerations underlying the process. *Supportive Care in Cancer*, published online. 10.1007/s00520-012-1593-6. http://link.springer.com/article/10.1007/s00520-012-1593-6/fulltext.html [accessed January 20, 2014].

Epstein, J. & Van Der Waal, I. (2008) Chapter 7: Oral cancer. In: M.S. Greenberg, M. Glick, & J.A. Ship (eds). *Burket's Oral Medicine*, 11th ed, pp. 153–189. BC Decker Inc., Lewiston, NY.

Epstein, J.B. & Huhmann, M.B. (2011a) Dietary and nutritional needs of patients undergoing therapy for head and neck cancer. *Journal of the American Dental Association*, **142**, 1163–1167.

Epstein, J.B. & Huhmann, M.B. (2011b) Dietary and nutritional needs of patients after therapy for head and neck cancer. *Journal of the American Dental Association*, **143**, 588–592.

Fleming, P. (1999) Dental management of the pediatric oncology patient. *Current Opinion in Dentistry*, **1**, 577–582.

Gerngross, P.J., Martin, C.D., Ball, J.D. *et al.* (2005) Period between completion of radiation therapy and prosthetic rehabilitation in edentulous patients: a retrospective study. *Journal of Prosthodontics*, **14**, 110–121.

Grégoire, V., De Neve, W., Eisbruch, A. *et al.* (2007) Intensity-modulated radiation therapy for head and neck carcinoma. *The Oncologist*, **12**, 555–564.

Guggenheimer, J. & Moore, P.A. (2003) Xerostomia: etiology, recognition and treatment. *Journal of the American Dental Association*, **134**, 61–69.

Haas, M. (2004) Radiation therapy. In: C.G. Varricchio (ed). *A Cancer Source Book for Nurses*, 8th ed, pp. 131–147. Jones and Barlett, Sudbury, MA.

Hong, C.H., Allred, R., Napenas, J.J. *et al.* (2010) Antibiotic prophylaxis for dental procedures to prevent indwelling venous catheter-related infections. *American Journal of Medicine*, **123** (**12**), 1128–1133.

Hsiung, C.Y., Huang, E.Y., Ting, H.M. *et al.* (2008) Intensity-modulated radiotherapy for nasopharyngeal carcinoma: the reduction of radiation-induced trismus. *British Journal of Radiology*, **81**, 809–814.

Jensen, S.B., Pedersen, A.M., Reibel, J. *et al.* (2003) Xerostomia and hypofunction of the salivary glands in cancer therapy. *Support Care Cancer*, **11**, 207–225.

Jordan, K. (2006) Neurokinin-1-receptor antagonists: a new approach in antiemetic therapy. *Onkologie*, **29** (**1–2**), 39–43.

Keefe, D.M., Schubert, M.M., Elting, L.S. *et al.* (2007) Updated clinical practice guidelines for the prevention and treatment of mucositis. *Cancer*, **109**, 820–831.

Lawrence, T.S., Ten Haken, R.K., & Giaccia, A. (2008) Principles of radiation oncology. In: V.T. Jr. DeVita, T.S. Lawrence, S.A. Rosenberg (eds). *Cancer: Principles and Practice of Oncology*, 8th ed. Lippincott Williams & Wilkins, Philadelphia.

Mealey, B.L., Semba, S.E., & Hallmon, W.W. (1994) The head and neck radiotherapy patient: Part 2—management of oral complications. *Compendium*, **15**, 442, 444, 446–452.

National Cancer Institute (2013) *PDQ® Oral complications of chemotherapy and head/neck radiation*. Bethesda, MD: National Cancer Institute. Date last modified August 11, 2013. http://www.cancer.gov/cancertopics/pdq/supportivecare/oralcomplications/HealthProfessional/page4/AllPages [accessed January 10, 2014].

National Institute of Health, National Institute of Dental and Craniofacial Research. (2014a) *Oral complications of cancer treatment: what the dental team can do*. Last updated January 6, 2014. http://www.nidcr.nih.gov/OralHealth/Topics/CancerTreatment/OralComplicationsCancerOral.htm [accessed January 20, 2014].

National Institute of Health, National Institute of Dental and Craniofacial Research. (2014b) *Dental provider's oncology pocket guide*. Last modified January 6, 2014. www.nidcr.nih.gov/OralHealth/Topics/CancerTreatment/ReferenceGuideforOncologyPatients.htm [assessed February 14, 2014].

Ngeow, W.C., Chai, W.L., Rahman, R.A., *et al.* (2006a) Managing complications of radiation therapy in head and neck cancer patients: Part I. management of xerostomia. *Singapore Dental Journal*, **28**, 1–3.

Ngeow, W.C., Chai, W.L., Rahman, R.A., *et al.* (2006b) Managing complications of radiation therapy in head and neck cancer patients: Part V. Management of mucositis. *Singapore Dental Journal*, **28**, 16–18.

Ngeow, W.C., Chai, W.L., Rahman, R.A., *et al.* (2006c) Managing complications of radiation therapy in head and neck cancer patients: Part VI. Management of opportunistic infections. *Singapore Dental Journal*, **28**, 19–21.

Nicolatou-Galitis, O., Sarri, T., Bowen, J., *et al.* (2012) Systematic review of amifostine for the management of oral mucositis in cancer patients. Supportive Care in Cancer, Published online. October 3, 2012. 10.1007/s00520-012-1613-6. Htpp://link.springer.com/article/10.1007/s005520-012-1613-6/fulltext.html [accessed January 20, 2014].

O'Brien, P.C. (2009) Management of stomatitis. *Canadian Family Physician*, **55**, 891–892.

Oral Cancer Foundation. (2014) Last updated June 8, 2013. www.oralcancerfoundation.org/dental/dental-complications.htm [accessed January 16, 2014].

Rahman, R., Ngeow, W.C., Chair, W.L. *et al.* (2006) Managing complications of radiation therapy in head and neck cancer patients: Part III. Provision of dentures. *Singapore Dental Journal*, **28**, 7–10.

Ramli, R., Ngeow, W.C., Rahman, R.A., *et al.* (2006) Managing complications of radiation therapy in head and neck cancer patients: Part IV. Management of osteoradionecrosis. *Singapore Dental Journal*, **28**, 11–15.

Shiboski, C.H., Hodgson, T.A., Ship, J.A. *et al.* (2007) Oral complications. In: K.G. Blume & S.J. Forman (eds). *Thomas' Hematopoietic Cell Transplantation*, 3rd ed, pp. 911–928. Blackwell Science Inc., Malden, MA.

Sonis, S.T. (2004) A biological approach to mucositis. *The Journal of Supportive Oncology*, **2**, 21–32.

Toljanic, J.A., Heshmati, R.H., & Bedard, J.F. (2002) Dental follow-up compliance in a population of irradiated head and neck cancer patients. *Oral Surgery Oral Medicine Oral Pathology Oral Radiology Endodontology*, **93**, 35–38.

Toth, B.B., Martin, W.W., & Fleming, T.J. (1990) Complications associated with cancer therapy. *Journal of Clinical Periodontology*, **17**, 508–515.

Vissink, A., Burlage, F.R., Spijkervet, F.K.L., *et al.* (2003) Prevention and treatment of the consequences of head and neck radiotherapy. *Critical Reviews of Oral Biology and Medicine*, **14**, 213–225.

Warr, D.G. (2008) Chemotherapy-and cancer-related nausea and vomiting. *Current Oncology*, **15** (**Suppl. 1**), S4–S9.

Wasserman, T.H., Brizel, D.M., Henke, J., *et al.* (2005) Influence of intravenous amifostine on xerostomia, tumor control, and survival after radiotherapy for head-and-neck cancer: 2-year follow-up of a prospective, randomized, phase III trial. *International Journal of Radiation Oncology Biology Physics*, **63**, 985–990.

Weinberg, M.A., Segelnick, S.L., & Kye, W. (2011) Dental complications of head and neck cancer radiotherapy. *US Pharmacist*, **36** (**Oncology Suppl.**), 3–7.

Zackrisson, B., Mercke, C., Srander, H., *et al.* (2003) A systematic overview of radiation therapy effects in head and neck cancer. *Acta Oncologica*, **42**, 443–461.

Antibiotic prophylaxis of the dental patient

Although its incidence is rare, infective endocarditis (IE) is a critical and potentially lethal condition that can be caused by microorganisms other than bacteria. Endocarditis most often is an infection of the valves of the heart. The heart valves are made of avascular tissue. In a healthy heart, the cusps of each valve are washed as blood passes over them with each heartbeat. However, when one of the valves is functioning abnormally, the individual may be susceptible to infection. The avascular nature of the valve tissue enables foreign microorganisms to colonize and literally hide from the immune system. Once bacteria have colonized the valve(s), they proliferate and affect the function of the valve(s). The valve affected most often is the mitral valve or bicuspid valve, on the left side of the heart. Some medical conditions create a higher risk of IE than others. In April 2007, the American Heart Association (AHA) changed the guidelines, which were last published in 1997, for patients required to take prophylactic antibiotics. These most recent guidelines are published in *Circulation* April 23, 2007. The new guidelines are aimed at patients who have the greatest risk of a serious infection if they developed a heart infection. For patients requiring antibiotic prophylaxis, the same antibiotics and dosing as stated in the previous guidelines are to be followed. Table A.1 lists the patients that are recommended to have antibiotic prophylaxis.

According to the new guidelines, patients who have taken prophylactic antibiotics in the past but no longer need them include patients with:

- Mitral valve prolapse
- Rheumatic heart disease
- Bicuspid valve disease
- Calcified aortic stenosis
- Congenital heart conditions such as ventricular septal defect, atrial septal defect, and hypertrophic cardiomyopathy.

Other conditions possibly requiring premedication prior to invasive dental treatment include the following (Lockart *et al.* 2007):

- Hemophilia
- Renal transplants/dialysis
- Shunts
- Immunosuppression secondary to cancer and cancer chemotherapy
- Systemic lupus erythematosus

The Dentist's Quick Guide to Medical Conditions, First Edition. Mea A. Weinberg, Stuart L. Segelnick, Joseph S. Insler, with Samuel Kramer.
© 2015 John Wiley & Sons, Inc. Published 2015 by John Wiley & Sons, Inc.

Table A.1 Conditions recommended for prophylaxis antibiotics: 2007 guidelines (Wilson *et al.* 2007)

---

1. Artificial heart valves
2. A history of IE
3. Certain specific, serious congenital (present from birth) heart conditions, including the following:
   - Unrepaired or incompletely repaired cyanotic congenital heart disease, including those with palliative shunts and conduits
   - A completely repaired congenital heart defect with prosthetic material or device, whether placed by surgery or by catheter intervention, during the first 6 months after the procedure.
   - Any repaired congenital heart defect with residual defect at the site or adjacent to the site of a prosthetic patch or a prosthetic device.
4. A cardiac transplant that develops a problem in a heart valve.

Cardiac conditions associated with the highest risk of adverse outcome from IE for which antibiotic prophylaxis is indicated (Wilson *et al.* 2007) are as follows:

- Prosthetic cardiac valve or prosthetic material used for cardiac valve repair.
- Previous IE.
- Congenital heart disease (CHD)
- Unrepaired cyanotic CHD, including palliative shunts and conduits.
- Completely repaired congenital heart defect with prosthetic material or device, whether placed by surgery or by catheter intervention, during the first 6 months after the procedure.
- Repaired CHD with residual defects at the site or adjacent to the site of a prosthetic patch or prosthetic device (which inhibit endothelialization).
- Cardiac transplantation recipients who develop cardiac valvulopathy.

Table A.2 lists the prophylactic antibiotic regimens for oral and dental procedures.

In 2003, the American Academy of Orthopedic Surgeons (AAOS) and the American Dental Association (ADA) Advisory Statement recommended antibiotic prophylaxis for all patients within the first 2 years after total joint replacement surgery only. After 2 years, the recommendation for antibiotic prophylaxis was limited to high-risk or medically compromised/immunosuppressed patients, which might place them at increased risk for total joint infection. In 2009, recommendations for antibiotic prophylaxis were updated by the AAOS. The AAOS recommended that clinicians consider antibiotic prophylaxis of all total joint replacement patients prior to any invasive procedure that may cause bacteremia. Finally, the most clinical practice current guidelines were published in 2012. The American Dental Association and the AAOS published the first co-developed evidence-based guideline on the Prevention of Orthopaedic Implant Infection in Patients Undergoing Dental Procedures. This review published found no direct evidence that dental procedures could cause orthopaedic implant infections and the dental practitioner should consider that it may not be necessary to routinely prescribe antibiotics for dental procedures in patients with joint implants. Additionally, it was noted in the 2012 guidelines that the development of periprosthetic joint infections were not depended upon whether antibiotics were prescribed or not. The guidelines recommend that patients with prosthetic joint implants maintain good oral hygiene to prevent orthopaedic implant infection in patient undergoing invasive dental procedures. (http://www.ada.org/sections/professionalResources/pdfs/PUDP_guideline.pdf). *It is advisable to obtain a medical consult from the patient's orthopedic surgeon.*

Table A.2   Prophylactic antibiotic regimens for oral and dental procedures (Wilson *et al.* 2007)

Situation	Drug	Regimen (single dose taken 30–60 min before dental procedure)
Standard general prophylaxis	Amoxicillin	Adults: 2.0 g orally; children: 50 mg/kg orally
Unable to take oral medication	Ampicillin	Adults: 2.0 g intramuscularly (IM) or intravenously (IV); children: 50 mg/kg IM or IV
	OR	Adults: 1 g IM or IV; children: 50 mg/kg IM or IV
	Cefazolin* or ceftriaxone*	
Allergic to penicillins—oral	Cephalexin*	Adults: 2 g; children: 50 mg/kg
	OR	
	Clindamycin	Adults: 600 mg; children: 20 mg/kg
	OR	
	Azithromycin or clarithromycin	Adults: 500 mg; children: 15 mg/kg
Allergic to penicillin and unable to take oral medications	Cefazolin*	Adults: 1.0 g; children: 25 mg/kg IM or IV
	OR	
	Clindamycin	Adults: 600 mg; children: 20 mg/kg IV

*Cephalosporins should not be used in patients with immediate-type hypersensitivity reaction (urticaria, angioedema, or anaphylaxis) to penicillins.

Suggested (ADA) antibiotic prophylaxis regimens in patients at potential increased risk of hematogenous total joint infection

Situation	Drug	Regimen
Standard general prophylaxis	Cephalexin or amoxicillin	2 g orally 1 h before dental procedure
Patients unable to take oral medications	Cefazolin or ampicillin	1 g IM or IV 1 h before procedure 2 g IM or IV 1 h before procedure
Allergic to penicillin	Clindamycin	600 mg orally 1 h before procedure
Allergic to penicillin and unable to take oral medications	Clindamycin	600 mg IV 1 h before procedure

References

Gross L. AAOS, ADA release CPG for prophylactic antibiotics. New Guideline includes shared decision-making tool, implications for practice. AAOS Now. January 2013 Issue. http://www.aaos.org.news/aaosnow/jan13/cover1.asp (Accessed September 8, 2014).

Little, J.W., Jacobson, J.J., & Lockhart, P.B. (2010) The dental treatment of patients with joint replacements. *Journal of the American Dental Association*, **141** (**6**), 667–671.

Lockart, P.B., Loven, B., Brennan, M.T. *et al.* (2007) The evidence base for the efficacy of antibiotic prophylaxis in dental practice. *Journal of the American Dental Association*, **138** (**4**), 458–474.

Wilson, W., Taubert, K.A., Gewitz, M. *et al.* (2007) Prevention of infective endocarditis. Guidelines from the American Heart Association Rheumatic Fever, Endocarditis and Kawasaki Disease Committee, Council on Cardiovascular Disease in the Young, and the Council on Clinical Cardiology, Council on Cardiovascular Surgery and Anesthesia, and the Quality of Care and Outcome Research Interdisciplinary Working Group. *Circulation*, **116**, 1736–1754.

Appendix B

Common dental drug interactions

An increasing number of episodes of adverse drug reactions are linked to drug interactions. Some drug interactions are beneficial, for example, when the clinician administers synergistic combination of drugs to enhance the therapeutic response of the drugs. During World War II, with short supplies of penicillin, probenecid, an antigout drug, was administered with penicillin to prolong the action of penicillin by inhibiting its elimination. However, since most drug interactions are harmful and even deadly, the dentist must be cognizant when prescribing any medications to patients. A thorough medical and drug history of all prescription, OTC, and herbal products must be taken and documented and reviewed at every dental visit.

Table B.1 reviews the different types of drug interactions. Once ingested, a drug interaction can occur at any point along the pathway of the drug through the body, from absorption to elimination. Knowing the type of drug interaction can assist in predicting, detecting and avoiding them.

Types of drug interactions (Table B.1) and ratings of drug interactions (Table B.2) describe the mechanism of a drug interaction and how severe it can be. Metabolism-type drug interactions occur primarily due to metabolism of drugs. Few drugs are eliminated from the body unchanged in the urine. Most drugs are metabolized or chemically altered to a less lipid-soluble compound, which is more easily eliminated from the body. One way of metabolizing drugs involves alteration of groups

Table B.1 Types of drug interactions.

There are five main types of interactions:	
Interaction	**Definition**
Pharmacokinetic	A change in the pharmacokinetics of one drug caused by the interacting drug
Pharmacodynamic	Interactions in which one drug induces a change in a patient's response to a drug without altering the drug's pharmacokinetics
Addition	The effect of two or more drugs when administered together is the same as when the drugs are given separately
Synergism	The effect of two or more drugs when administered together is greater than when the drugs are given separately; may produce responses equivalent to over dosage
Antagonism	The effect of two or more drugs when administered together is less than when the drugs are given separately

The Dentist's Quick Guide to Medical Conditions, First Edition. Mea A. Weinberg, Stuart L. Segelnick, Joseph S. Insler, with Samuel Kramer.
© 2015 John Wiley & Sons, Inc. Published 2015 by John Wiley & Sons, Inc.

Table B.2　Rating of drug interactions.

Severity rating	Documentation rating
Major: Potentially life-threatening or causing permanent body damage	Established: Proven with clinical studies to cause an interaction
Moderate: Could change the patient's clinical status and require hospitalization	Probable: Very likely to cause an interaction
Minor: Only mild effects are evident or no changes are seen	Suspected: Supposed to cause an interaction, but more clinical studies are required Possible: Limited data proven Unlikely: Not certain to cause an interaction

on the drug molecule via the **cytochrome P450 enzymes** (Table B.3). These enzymes are found mostly in the liver, but can also be found in the intestines, lungs, and other organs. Each enzyme is termed an isoenzyme, because each derives from a different gene. There are more than 30 cytochrome P450 enzymes present in human tissue.

A *substrate* is a drug that is metabolized by a specific CYP450 isoenzyme. An *inhibitor* is a drug that inhibits or reduces the activity of a specific CYP450 isoenzyme. An *inducer* is a drug that increases the amount and activity of that specific CYP450 isoenzyme.

Drug interactions can occur when a drug that is metabolized and/or inhibited by these cytochrome enzymes is taken concurrently with a drug that decreases the activity of the same enzyme system (e.g., an inhibitor). The result is often increased concentrations of the substrate. Another scenario is when a substrate that is metabolized by a specific cytochrome enzyme is taken with a drug that increases the activity of that enzyme (e.g., an inducer). The result is often decreased concentrations of the substrate.

Some substrates are also inhibitors for the same enzyme, probably due to competitive inhibition of enzyme activity. Some inhibitors affect more than one isoenzyme and some substrates are metabolized by more than one isoenzyme.

Table B.4 describes clinically significant drug–drug, drug–food, and drug–disease interactions in dentistry and possible ways to avoid or manage an interaction (Tables B.5 and B.6).

Table B.3 Common cytochrome P450 drug interactions in dentistry.

Enzyme	Substrate drug*	Inhibitor drug§	Inducer drug¶	Management
CYP1A2	Caffeine **Theophylline** Tacrine (Cognex) **Tricyclic antidepressants**: Amitriptyline (Elavil) Imipramine (Tofranil) **SSRIs**: fluvoxamine (Luvox); **Antipsychotics:** Clozapine (Clozaril) Haloperidol (Haldol)	Fluvoxamine (Luvox) Ciprofloxacin (Cipro)	Tobacco (smoking) Omeprazole (Prilosec) Phenytoin (Dilantin)	If possible, do not give a substrate with an inducer or inhibitor if they will interact; if necessary, give and then observe the therapeutic and adverse effects.
CYP3A4	Lidocaine Erythromycin Clarithromycin (Biaxin) **Calcium channel blockers:** Amlodipine (Norvasc) Diltiazem (Cardizem) Felodipine (Plendil) Nifedipine (Adalat, Procardia) Verapamil (Calan, Isoptin) **Antidepressants:** Sertraline (Zoloft), trazodone (Desyrel), nefazodone (Serzone) **Benzodiazepines:** Diazepam (Valium) Midazolam (Versed) Triazolam (Halcion) **Cholesterol-lowering drugs (statins):** Atorvastatin (Lipitor) Lovastatin (Mevacor) Simvastatin (Zocor) Warfarin (Coumadin) Fexofenadine (Allegra)	**Grapefruit juice** (lasts about 24 h) Erythromycin Clarithromycin **Antifunguals:** Ketoconazole (Nizoral) fluconazole (Diflucan) itraconazole (Sporanox) **Antidepressants:** Fluvoxamine (Luvox) Nefazodone (Serzone) **H2 receptor blocker:** Cimetadine (Tagamet)	**Trigeminal neuralgia/ antiseizure:** Carbamazepine (Tegretol) Phenytoin (Dilantin) Phenobarbital **Antituberculosis:** Rifampin (Rifadin, Rimactane)	

Table B.3 *(cont'd)*

Enzyme	Substrate drug*	Inhibitor drug§	Inducer drug¶	Management
	Corticosteroid: Hydrocortisone			
	Antidiabetics: Glyburide (Glynase, Micronase)			
	Antirejection drugs: Cyclosporine			
	Hormones: Estradiol Progesterone			
	HIV protease Inhibitors: Ritonavir (Norvir) Saquinavir (Invirase) Indinavir (Crixivan) Nelfinavir (Viracept)			
	Antigout: Colchicine			
CYP2C9	**Nonsteroidal anti-inflammatory drugs:** Ibuprofen (Motrin, Advil) Naproxen sodium (Aleve) Celecoxib (Celebrex)	**Antibiotics:** Metronidazole (Flagyl) **Antifungals:** Fluconazole (Diflucan) Ketoconazole (Nizoral)	**Antituberculosis:** Rifampin	If possible, do not give a substrate with an inducer or inhibitor if they will interact; if necessary, to give and then observe the therapeutic and adverse effects
	Antiseizure: Phenytoin (Dilantin)			
	Anticoagulant: Warfarin (Coumadin)			

* *Substrate*: A drug that is metabolized by an enzyme system.
§ *Inhibitor*: A drug that decreases the activity of the enzyme which may decrease the metabolism of the substrate and generally lead to increased drug effect.
¶ *Inducer*: A drug that will stimulate the synthesis of more enzymes enhancing the enzyme's metabolizing actions. Inducers increase metabolism of substrates, generally leading to decreased drug effect.

Table B.4 Clinically significant drug–drug interactions in dentistry.

Antibiotics			
Drug	Interacting drug	Effect	What to do?
Doxycycline (including doxycycline 20 mg, Atridox)	Antacids (magnesium hydroxide/ aluminum hydroxide), iron (ferrous sulfate)	Decreased doxycycline absorption into the blood	Take doxycycline 1 h before or 2 h after the antacid
	Penicillins	Interferes with bactericidal effect of penicillins	Do not take at the same time; take penicillin a few hours before the doxycycline
	Oral contraceptives	May interfere with contraceptive effect	May not be clinically significant; some sources say to use alternative methods of birth control
	Phenytoin (Dilantin)	Decreased serum doxycycline levels	Either switch to another antibiotic or monitor
Minocycline (including Arestin)	Warfarin	Increased anticoagulant effect	Minimal risk; monitor patients for enhanced anticoagulant effects; warfarin dosage may need adjustments.
	Oral contraceptives	May interfere with contraceptive effect	May not be clinically significant; some sources say to use alternative methods of birth control
	Antacids (magnesium hydroxide/aluminum hydroxide), calcium- containing products, iron (ferrous sulfate)	Decreased *amount* of tetracycline absorption into the blood	Do not take concurrently. Take minocycline 1 h before or 2 h after the antacid
	Phenytoin (Dilantin)	Decreased serum doxycycline levels	Either switch to another antibiotic or monitor
Tetracycline	Antacids (magnesium hydroxide/aluminum hydroxide), calcium-containing products, iron (ferrous sulfate)	Decreased *amount* of tetracycline absorption into the blood	Do not take concurrently. Take tetracycline 1 h before or 2 h after the antacid
	Warfarin	Increased anticoagulant effect	Minimal risk; monitor patients for enhanced anticoagulant effects.

(continued)

Table B.4 (cont'd)

Antibiotics

Drug	Interacting drug	Effect	What to do?
	Penicillins	Interferes with bactericidal effect of penicillins	Do not take at same time; take penicillin a few hours before the tetracycline
	Digoxin	Digoxin is partially metabolized by bacteria in intestine; increased digoxin blood levels	Either switch antibiotic or monitor for increased serum digoxin levels
	Oral contraceptives	May interfere with contraceptive effects	May not be of clinical significance; some sources recommend to use alternative birth control
Penicillins	Erythromycin, tetracyclines	Decreased effectiveness of penicillin	Do not take at the same time; give the penicillin a few hours before the tetracycline
	Probenicid (Benemid): drug for gout	Inhibits penicillin excretion	Can take together; make sure penicillin levels are not excessive
	Oral contraceptives (including ampicillin)	May interferes with contraceptive effects	May not be clinically significant; some say to use alternative birth control methods
Erythromycins Clarithromycin	Theophylline	Increased theophylline levels	Avoid together; contact physician; reduce theophylline dosage to avoid toxicity
	Carbamazepine (Tegretol)	Increased carbamazepine levels	Avoid concurrent use.
	Statins: atorvastatin (Lipitor); simvastatin (Zocor)	Increases statin levels (increased myopathy, including muscle pain)	Switch either to azithromycin or to another statin drug like lovastatin (Mevacor) or pravastatin (Pravachol)
	Oral contraceptives	Interfere with contraceptive effects	Some sources recommend alternative birth control
	Digoxin	Increased digoxin levels (see increased salivation and visual disturbances) Increased	Switch antibiotic to penicillin. Monitor for signs of digoxin toxicity or switch antibiotic
	Cyclosporine	Cyclosporine toxicity	Cyclosporine doses may need reduction
	Ergot alkaloids [e.g., ergotamine (Bellergal-S, Cafergot)] (for migraine headache)	Toxic ergot levels (ergotism; pain, tenderness, and low skin temperature of extremities)	Use azithromycin or another antibiotic

Drug	Interacting drug	Effect	What to do?
	Midazolam (Versed)	Increased sedation	Avoid combination; use alternative drugs
	Disopyramide (Norpace)	Prolongation of QTc interval	Switch to another antibiotic or monitor for development of arrhythmias
	Warfarin	Increases anticoagulant effect	Switch to azithromycin (Zithromax) or monitor for anticoagulant effects; contact physician. Switch to azithromycin (Zithromax)
Fluoroquinolones [ciprofloxacin (Cipro)]	Antacids, iron (decrease absorption of the drug)	Decreases fluoroquinolone effect	Do not take concurrently. Take fluoroquinolone 1 h before or 2h after the antacid
	Caffeine	Increases caffeine effects	Do not take together
Clindamycin (Cleocin)	Neuromuscular blockers (succinylcholine)	Increased neuromuscular blocking effect	Since most dental patients are not taking these drugs, there are no special precautions
Metronidazole (Flagyl)	Alcohol	Severe disulfiram-like reaction with headache, flushing and nausea	Avoid alcohol
	Warfarin	Inhibits warfarin metabolism; increased anticoagulant effect	Contact physician; adjust warfarin dosage or select different antibiotic
	Lithium	Lithium excretion inhibited resulting in toxic levels	Contact physician

Analgesics

Drug	Interacting drug	Effect	What to do?
Aspirin and nonsteroidal anti-inflammatory drugs (NSAIDs) (ibuprofen, naproxen)	Warfarin	Synergistic anticoagulant effects (increased bleeding)	Avoid concurrent use/contact patient's physician
	Angiotensin-converting enzyme (ACE) inhibitors (e.g., enalapril and captopril); beta-blockers; angiotensin II receptor blockers (ARBs)	Decrease antihypertensive response (lowers blood pressure). Short-term course (5 days) may not significantly increase blood pressure	Interaction causes lowering of blood pressure. Monitor blood pressure. Use alternative analgesic such as acetaminophen or narcotic after 5 days or more of use of NSAIDS. Note: NSAIDS cancel out the cardioprotective effect of low-dose aspirin

(continued)

Table B.4 *(cont'd)*

Analgesics

Drug	Interacting drug	Effect	What to do?
	Lithium oral antidiabetic drugs (occurs with aspirin)	Inhibits renal clearance of lithium Increases hypoglycemic effects	Decrease lithium dosage. Limited importance
	Furosemide (Lasix)	Decreased diuretic effect	Monitor patient
	Venlafaxine (Effexor)	Possible serotonin syndrome	Avoid concurrent use
	Phenytoin (Dilantin)	Decreased hepatic phenytoin metabolism (increased serum levels)	No special precautions
Acetaminophen	Alcohol Phenytoin Phenobarbital Carbamazepine Isoniazid	Increase risk of hepatotoxicity	Contraindicated in alcoholics; avoid taking together
	Warfarin	Increased anticoagulant effect	Avoid concurrent use or adjust warfarin dosage

Sympathomimetics

Drug	Interacting drug	Effect	What to do?
Epinephrine (contained in local anesthetics)	Beta-blockers, nonselective ($\beta_1\beta_2$) such as propranolol (Inderal), nadolol (Corgard), timolol (Blocadren), and sotalol (Betapace)	Elevated blood pressure	Epinephrine should be used cautiously. Limit the amount used to 0.04 mg (two cartridges of 1:100,000)
	Selective beta-blockers (β_1, such as atenolol (Tenormin), metoprolol (Lopressor), acebutolol (Sectral), and betaxolol (Kerlone)	No elevation in blood pressure	No concerns.
	Tricyclic antidepressants	Hypertension (enhances sympathomimetic effects)	Treat similar to the cardiac patient; maximum amount is two cartridges of EPI 1:100,000

Drug	Interacting drug	Effect	What to do?
Levonordefrin (contained in mepivacaine)	Cocaine	Increased heart contraction leading to death	Do not use epinephrine if the patient used cocaine within 24 h
	Digoxin	Increase cardiac excitation and arrhythmias	Use caution when administering epinephrine
	Nonselective beta-blockers (e.g., propranolol and nadolol)	Stimulates alpha-receptors on heart tissue, causing an increase in blood pressure; limit use of vasoconstrictor	Minimize the amount of levonordefrin
	Tricyclic antidepressants (e.g., imipramine and amitriptyline)	Enhanced sympathomimetic effects	Avoid the use of levonordefrin

Antianxiety drugs (benzodiazepines)

Drug	Interacting drug	Effect	What to do?
Diazepam (Valium), alprazolam (Xanax)	Grapefruit juice+midazolam (Versed) or triazolam (Halcion)	Inhibits CYP3A4 enzyme, decreasing metabolism of these drugs thus increasing blood levels	Do not take juice while on these drugs
	Cimetadine (Tagamet)	Inhibits diazepam elimination	Little clinical importance
	Opioids (narcotics; codeine, hydrocodone)	Increases CNS depression	Avoid taking together
		Increases CNS depression	
	Clarithromycin with midazolam (Versed)	Increased sedation	Avoid combination; use alternative drugs

Note: Most drug–drug or drug–food interactions occur when two or more drugs are taken at the same time. To avoid these interactions, most drug dosings are spaced so as not to administer them concurrently. If in doubt, the patient's physician should be contacted.

Table B.5 Clinically significant drug–food interactions in dentistry.

Dental drug	Food	What to do?
Tetracycline	Dairy products, (e.g., milk and yogurt) (forms a calcium/tetracycline complex that inhibits tetracycline absorption)	Space 1 h before or 2 h after meal.
Doxycycline (Vibramycin), minocycline (Minocin)	Dairy products (only 30% decrease in bioavailability)	No special management, can take with dairy products.
Ciprofloxacin (Cipro)	Caffeine (decreases absorption of the drug) Food (e.g. orange juice fortified with calcium) and dairy products (decreases absorption of the drug)	Space 1 h before or 2 h after the calcium containing supplement or food
Erythromycins	Food (decreases absorption of the drug)	Take drug 1 h before or 2 h after meals.
Azithromycin (Zithromax)	Food (decreases absorption of the drug)	Take 1 h before or 2 h after meals.

Table B.6 Clinically significant drug–disease interactions in dentistry.

Dental drug	Condition	What to do?
Clindamycin (Cleocin)	Ulcerative colitis, Crohn's disease, pseudomembranous enterocolitis	Do not give clindamycin; remember that this antibiotic is given for infective endocarditis prophylaxis if patient is allergic to penicillins.
Tetracyclines (doxycycline, minocycline)	Pregnant and lactating women Children under 8 years	Do not give to these patients.
Clarithromycin (Biaxin)	Prolonged QT interval Ventricular arrhythmias	Do not give to these patients.
Erythromycins	Cardiac arrhythmias Liver disease Prolonged QT interval	Do not give to these patients.
Penicillins	Infectious mononucleosis Pseudomembranous enterocolitis Renal disease	Do not give to these patients. Do not give to these patients. Reduce dosage or do not give depending on severity.
Metronidazole (Flagyl)	Central nervous system disorder, epilepsy, lactating mother	Do not give; substitute another antibiotic.
Ciprofloxacin (Cipro)	Achilles tendonitis, pseudo- membranous enterocolitis	Do not give; substitute another antibiotic.
NSAIDs (e.g., naproxen and ibuprofen) Aspirin	Gastrointestinal bleeding (ulcers), nasal polyps with asthma, blood coagulation disorder, pregnancy	Do not give; give acetaminophen.
Epinephrine	Narrow-angle glaucoma, dilated cardiomyopathy Hypertension, diabetes, hyperthyroidism	Do not give to these patients. Use with caution; limited quantities.

Selected References

Anastasio, G.D., Cornell, K.O., & Menscer, D. (1997) Drug interactions: keeping it straight. *American Family Physician* **56**, 883–894.

Aronson, J.K. (2004) Classifying drug interactions. *British Journal of Clinical Pharmacology*, **58**, 343–344.

Brown, C.H. (2000) Overview of drug interactions.*U.S. Pharmacist* **25 (5)**, HS-3–HS-30.

Cupp, M.J. & Tracy, T.S. (1998) Cytochrome P450: new nomenclature and clinical implications. *American Family Physician* **57**, 107–114.

Haas, D.A. (1999) Adverse drug interactions in dental practice: interactions associated with analgesics—Part III in a series. *Journal of the American Dental Association*, **130**, 397–406.

Hansten, P.D. & Horn, J.R. (2005) *The Top 100 Drug Interactions:A Guide to Patient Management*. H& H Publications, Edmonds, WA.

Hersh, E.V. (1999) Adverse drug interactions in dental practice: interactions involving antibiotics—Part II of a series. *Journal of the American Dental Association*, **130**, 236–251.

Hersh, E.V. & Moore, P.A. (2004) Drug interactions in dentistry: the importance of knowing your CYPs. *Journal of the American Dental Association*, **135**, 298–311.

Hulisz, D. (2007) Food–drug interactions. Which ones really matter? *US Pharmacist* **32 (3)**, 93–98.

Marek, C. (1966) Avoiding prescribing errors: a systematic approach. *Journal of the American Dental Association*, **127**, 617–623.

Moore, P.A. (1999) Adverse drug interactions in dental practice: interactions. *Journal of the American Dental Association*, **130**, 541–554.

Weinberg, M.A., Westphal Thiele, C., & Fine, J.B. (2013) Drug Interactions. In: *Oral Pharmacology*. Pearson Publications, Upper Saddle River, NJ.

Appendix C

Summary of tables/boxes

Chapter 1

Table 1.1   Medications for peptic ulcer disease and gastroesophageal reflux disease.
Box 1.1   Therapy for *H. pylori* management.
Table 1.2   Dental drug–drug interactions (www.rxlist.com; Peters *et al.* 2010).
Table 1.3   Dental drug–drug interactions (www.drugs.com; www.rxlist.com).

Chapter 2

Table 2.1   Step-by-step treatment of asthma in adults.
Box 2.1   Common dental drug–drug interactions.
Table 2.2   Rescue and long-term control medications for asthma.
Table 2.3   Drug regimens for latent tuberculosis infection (prophylaxis): Patients with positive purified protein derivative but negative chest X-ray and no symptoms; was exposure but the patient did not develop the infection.
Table 2.4   Drug regimens for active tuberculosis (two or more drugs are needed to treat active TB to reduce emergence of resistant bacteria).

Chapter 3

Table 3.1   Chronic kidney disease: severity and staging (National Kidney Foundation).
Table 3.2   Common dental drugs that require dose adjustment (dosing or dosing interval) in end-stage renal disease.
Table 3.3   Dental drug–drug interactions in chronic kidney disease patients.
Table 3.4   Dental drug–drug interactions in the kidney transplant patient.

Chapter 4

Table 4.1   Fasting/oral glucose tolerance test goals set by AACE and ADA.
Table 4.2   Guidelines for patients taking systemic corticosteroids.

The Dentist's Quick Guide to Medical Conditions, First Edition. Mea A. Weinberg, Stuart L. Segelnick, Joseph S. Insler, with Samuel Kramer.
© 2015 John Wiley & Sons, Inc. Published 2015 by John Wiley & Sons, Inc.

Chapter 5

Table 5.1   JNC-VIII classification of blood pressure for adults.
Table 5.2   Major risk factors for hypertension.
Table 5.3   Summaries of antihypertensive medications and management of patients taking these medications in the dental office .
Table 5.4   Dental management of patients on antianginal drugs.
Table 5.5   Drugs in the treatment of heart failure.
Table 5.6   Anti-arrhythmic drugs.
Table 5.7   Prophylactic antibiotic regimens for oral and dental procedures (Wilson *et al.* 1997).
Table 5.8   Antibiotic prophylaxis recommendations for dental procedures (Wilson *et al.* 1997).
Table 5.9   Recommendations when to start dental treatment after cardiac surgery.
Box 5.1   International normalized ratio (INR) guidelines for dental treatment.

Chapter 6

Table 6.1   FDA pregnancy categories.
Table 6.2   List of drugs used in pregnancy and lactating women.

Chapter 7

Table 7.1   Child–Pugh classification of risk assessment for chronic liver disease.
Table 7.2   Dental drugs metabolized in the liver.
Table 7.3   Serologic tests and interpretation for viral hepatitis.
Table 7.4   Dental drug–hepatitis B drug interactions.
Table 7.5   Serological and virological tests and interpretation for hepatitis C.
Table 7.6   Drug therapy for hepatitis C.
Table 7.7   Dental drug–drug interactions in the liver transplant patient.
Table 7.8   Oral adverse reactions of drugs taken by liver transplant candidates.

Chapter 8

Table 8.1   Dental drug–drug interactions.
Table 8.2   Dental adverse effects of Parkinson's disease.
Table 8.3   Dentally related effects of multiple sclerosis.
Table 8.4   Medications for multiple sclerosis.
Table 8.5   Dental treatment modifications in the MS patient.
Table 8.6   Anti-epileptic drugs.
Table 8.7   Common oral adverse effects of AEDs.
Table 8.8   Dental drug–antiepileptic drug interactions.
Table 8.9   Dental concerns in the epileptic patient and their management.
Box 8.1   Common oral features in the epileptic patients.

Chapter 9

Table 9.1   More commonly prescribed typical antipsychotics.
Table 9.2   Commonly prescribed atypical antipsychotics.
Table 9.3   Clinically available monamine oxidase inhibitors.
Table 9.4   Common tricyclic antidepressants.
Table 9.5   Common selective serotonin reuptake inhibitors.

Chapter 10

Table 10.1   Common bleeding disorders and screening tests.
Table 10.2   Classification of platelet disorders.
Table 10.3   International normalized ratio (INR) guidelines for dental treatment.
Table 10.4   Medications and products used in preventing oral bleeding events.
Table 10.5   Medical/drug management of patients with bleeding disorders.
Table 10.6   Dental management of the patient with bleeding disorders.

Chapter 11

Table 11.1   CBC with differential.
Table 11.2   Common causes of anemia.
Table 11.3   Acute leukemia: Common oral complications and their management.
Table 11.4   Dental management of WBC disorders.

Chapter 12

Table 12.1   Bisphosphonates.
Table 12.2   Staging criteria for ARONJ.
Table 12.3   Drugs used to treat rheumatoid arthritis (RA) and dental management.
Table 12.4   Dental drug–drug interactions with medications for gout.
Table 12.5   Dental drug–fibromyalgia drug interactions.
Table 12.6   Common medications for systemic lupus erythematosus (SLE) and their dental implications.
Table 12.7   Signs and symptoms of Sjögren's syndrome (SS) and its management.
Table 12.8   Drugs for Sjögren's syndrome (SS).

Chapter 13

Table 13.1   FDA antiretroviral drugs used in the treatment of HIV infection.
Table 13.2   Drug interactions with antiretroviral therapy—antiretroviral drug combinations to avoid.

Table 13.3   Highly active antiretroviral therapy—drug classes.
Table 13.4   Medical assessment of HIV-infected patients.

Chapter 14

Table 14.1   Oral adverse effects after radiation to head and neck/chemotherapy.

Appendix D

Interpretation of common laboratory values

	Therapeutic range	"High" value	"Low" value
Whole blood			
Hematocrit (HCT)	38–54% (men) 36–47% (women)	High-altitude areas, chronic smoker, dehydration (false positive), polycythemia vera, erythropoietin (Epogen)	Anemia, blood loss, nutritional deficiency (iron, vitamin B_{12}, and folate), chemotherapy, cancer (bone marrow), kidney failure
Hemoglobin (Hb)	14–18 g/dl (men) 12–16 g/dl (women) 12–14 g/dl (children) 14.5–24.5 g/dl (newborns)	High-altitude areas, dehydration (false positive), chronic smoker, polycythemia vera, emphysema, erythropoietin (Epogen)	Loss of blood (injury, surgery, ulcers, and cancer); chemotherapy; iron, vitamin B_{12}, or folate deficiency; thalassemia; sickle cell anemia; bone marrow complications
Complete blood count (CBC)			
Erythrocytes (RBCs)	$4.5–6 \times 10^4$ (men) $4.3–5.5 \times 10^4$ (women)	Dehydration, polycythemia vera, kidney cancer, kidney transplant, heart failure, chronic obstructive pulmonary disease (COPD), congenital heart disease, carbon monoxide poisoning, sleep apnea	Anemia; bone marrow complications; bleeding; multiple myeloma; copper, folate, and vitamin B_6 and B_{12} deficiency; leukemia; pregnancy; RBC destruction
Reticulocytes	0–1% of RBCs	Kidney disease producing erythropoietin, hemolytic anemia, erythroblastosis fetalis	Bone marrow failure; liver disease (cirrhosis); vitamin B_{12}, iron, or folate deficiency; kidney disease; radiation therapy
Leukocytes, total	5,000–10,000 cells/mm^3	Bacterial infection, smoking, inflammatory diseases (e.g., rheumatoid arthritis), leukemia, tissue damage, some drugs (e.g., albuterol, lithium, and corticosteroids)	Some drugs (e.g., chemotherapeutics, clozapine, antibiotics, and diuretics), bone marrow problems, autoimmune diseases (e.g., systemic lupus erythematosus), liver or spleen disease, radiotherapy, viral infections

The Dentist's Quick Guide to Medical Conditions, First Edition. Mea A. Weinberg, Stuart L. Segelnick, Joseph S. Insler, with Samuel Kramer.
© 2015 John Wiley & Sons, Inc. Published 2015 by John Wiley & Sons, Inc.

	Therapeutic range	"High" value	"Low" value
Myelocytes	0; 0% of leukocytes	Eosinophils, neutrophils, and basophils: chronic myeloid leukemia	
Juvenile neutrophils	0–100; 0–1% of leukocytes		
Band neutrophils	0–500; 0–5% of leukocytes		
Segmented neutrophils Lymphocytes	2500–6000; 40–60% of leukocytes		
Eosinophils Basophils	1000–4000; 20–40% of leukocytes		
Monocytes	50–300; 0–5% of leukocytes		
	0–100; 0–1% of leukocytes		
	200–800; 4–8% of leukocytes		
Platelets	150,000–400,000 cells/mm^3	Hemolytic anemia, iron-deficiency anemia, splenectomy, cancer, von Willebrand disease	Chemotherapy/radiation, cancer of bone marrow
RBC Measurements			
Mean corpuscular volume (MCV)	80–94 µm^3	Pernicious anemia, alcoholism, vitamin B_{12} or folate deficiency	Iron-deficiency anemia, blood loss, thalassemia, chronic disease
Mean corpuscular hemoglobin (MCH)	27–32 pg	Macrocytic anemia	Chronic blood loss, microcytic anemia
Mean corpuscular hemoglobin concentration	33.4–35.5 g/dl	Sickle cell anemia	Microcytic and macrocytic anemias
Electrolytes			
Bicarbonate (carbon dioxide) (total)	18–30 mEq/l	Metabolic alkalosis	Metabolic acidosis (kidney disease, liver failure, diarrhea)
Calcium (total)	9–11 mg/dl; 4.5–5.5 mEq/l	Hyperparathyroidism (tumor), sarcoidosis, multiple myeloma, excessive vitamin D intake, Paget's disease	Hypothyroidism, osteomalacia
Chloride	98–106 mEq/l	Metabolic acidosis, renal tubular acidosis	Addison's disease, heart failure, syndrome of inappropriate diuretic hormone secretion (SIADH)

(*continued*)

	Therapeutic range	"High" value	"Low" value
Magnesium	1.8–3.6 mg/dl; 1.5–3.0 mEq/l	Addison's disease, chronic renal failure, dehydration, diabetic acidosis	Alcoholism, chronic diarrhea, hypoparathyroidism, ulcerative colitis, liver cirrhosis
Phosphorus	3–4.5 mg/dl; 1.8–2.3 mEq/l (adults) 4–6.5 mg/dl; 2.3–3.8 mEq/l (children)	Liver disease, renal failure, hypoparathyroidism	Hyperparathyroidism
Potassium	3.5–5.5 mEq/l	Kidney failure, Addison's disease, angiotensin-converting enzyme inhibitors (ACEIs; anti-hypertensive), diuretics, drug abusers, type 1 diabetes	Eating disorders (bulimia—vomiting), sweating, chronic diarrhea
Sodium	135–147 mEq/l	Cushing's syndrome, hyperaldosteronism, increased fluid loss (vomiting, diarrhea), excessive dietary salt, NSAIDs, corticosteroids, laxatives, lithium, oral contraceptives	Heart failure, burns, vomiting, dehydration, liver cirrhosis, syndrome of inappropriate diuretic hormone secretion (SIADH), diuretics
Enzymes			
Alkaline phosphatase	50–160 U/l	Paget's disease, biliary obstruction, osteoblastic bone tumors, hyperparathyroidism	Protein deficiency
Amylase	53–123 U/l	Acute pancreatitis, pancreatic cancer, intestinal/bile duct blockage, perforated ulcer	Toxemia of pregnancy
creatine kinase (CK) or creatine phosphoki-nase (CPK)	38–174 U/l (males); 96–140 U/l (females)	Bowel obstruction, duodenal ulcer, pancreatic cancer	Crohn's disease, celiac disease, cystic fibrosis
Lipase	10–150 U/l	Liver cirrhosis, hepatitis, infectious mononucleosis, acute myocardial infarction, alcoholism	Normal results
ALT (SGPT)	0–30 U/l		
AST (SGOT)	0–40 U/l	Recent myocardial infarction, liver disease, hepatitis, skeletal muscle trauma	Normal results

	Therapeutic range	"High" value	"Low" value
Others			
Albumin	3.5–5.5 g/dl	Dehydration, high protein diet	Liver disease, kidney disease
Bilirubin	0.1 mg/dl	Cirrhosis, hepatitis, pancreatic cancer	No concerns
Total cholesterol (depends on age)	<200 mg/dl	Hereditary, diet, risk of heart disease	Normal results
Creatinine	0.5–1.4 mg/dl	Chronic kidney disease	Normal results
Glucose, fasting serum	65–99 mg/dl	Diabetes	Normal results
Triglycerides	40–200 mg/dl	Risk of heart disease	Normal results
Blood urea nitrogen (BUN)	6–20 mg/dl	Severe dehydration, kidney disease, heart failure, GI bleeding	Low protein diet, malnutrition, over-hydration
Uric acid	2.0–4.0 mg/dl	Diabetes, alcoholism, renal failure, lead poisoning	Syndrome of inappropriate diuretic hormone (SIADH), Wilson's disease, Fanconi syndrome

Data from: http://www.fda.gov/downloads/ICECI/Inspections/IOM/UCM135835.pdf; http://www.nlm.nih.gov/medlineplus/ency/

Note: The normal ranges in each laboratory depend on the local population, test methodology and conditions of assay, units, and a variety of other circumstances. The ranges above are typical, but the normal values established for each laboratory should be used for most purposes.

Index

acetaminophen
  in asthmatic patients, 23, 26
  in kidney disease, 33, 34, 41
  in liver disease, 93, 97, 99
  interaction with warfarin, 158
acid-peptic disorders *see* peptic ulcer disease
acquired immunodeficiency syndrome (AIDS) *see* AIDS
acute adrenal insufficiency *see* adrenal crisis
acute lymphoblastic leukemia (ALL), 183–185
acute myeloid leukemia (AML), 183–185
acute pancreatitis, 12–13
acute renal disease, 30
adalimumab (Humira) *see* Anti-tumor necrosis factor (Anti-TNF) drugs
Addison's disease, 54
adrenal crisis, during dental treatment, 55
adrenal gland disorders
  clinical synopsis, 53, 54
  dental notes of, 54–56
  physiology of adrenal gland, 54
aggrenox *see* antiplatelet drugs
agranulocytosis
  clozapine, 130
  definition, 130
  significance in dentistry, 131
AIDS *see* human immunodeficiency virus (HIV)
alcohol
  association with periodontal disease, 142
  handling a patient, 142
  interaction with metronidazole, 142
alcoholic liver disease, 98, 99
Aleve *see* nonsteroidal anti-inflammatory drugs
aminocaprioic acid (Amicar)
  hemophilia A and B, 155
  managing intraoral bleeding, 160–162

amlodipine (Norvasc) *see* calcium channel blockers
analgesics
  acetaminophen, 97, 99
  aspirin, 154
  during pregnancy/lactation, 84–87
  in kidney disease, 33
  in liver disease, 97
  nonsteroidal anti-inflammatory drugs (NSAIDs), 35, 41
ANA test *see* antinuclear antibody test
anemia(s)
  dental management of, 181
  diagnosing, 174, 175
  folic acid deficiency, 178
  glucose-6-phosphate dehydrogenase (G6PD) deficiency, 178
  in liver disease, 177
  iron deficiency, 175, 176
  oral signs and symptoms of, 180
  pernicious, 177
  sickle cell, 179
  thalassemia, 176
  types of, 175–178
  vitamin B_{12}, 177
angina
  clinical synopsis, 68
  dental management of, 69, 70
  dental notes for, 69, 70
  medications prescribed for, 8
  use of epinephrine, 70
angioplasty
  dental treatment scheduling, 79
angiotensin II receptors blockers (ARBs)
  treatment for hypertension, 65
angiotensin converting enzyme inhibitors (ACEIs)
  treatment for hypertension, 65

The Dentist's Quick Guide to Medical Conditions, First Edition. Mea A. Weinberg, Stuart L. Segelnick, Joseph S. Insler, with Samuel Kramer.
© 2015 John Wiley & Sons, Inc. Published 2015 by John Wiley & Sons, Inc.

antacids
  interactions with tetracyclines, 4
  treatment for GERD, 3, 5
antianxiety drugs *see* benzodiazepines
antibiotic(s)
  in kidney disease, 33
  in liver disease, 97
  in peptic ulcer disease, 3
  in pregnancy, 85
  interactions with oral contraceptives, 90
  interactions with psychiatric drugs, 137
  interactions with warfarin, 158
  QT interval prolongation, 76, 131, 264
antibiotic prophylaxis
  American Heart Association(AHA) Guidelines
    for, 252
  antibiotic regimens for oral and dental
    procedures, 253
anticoagulants *see also* warfarin
  apixaban (Eliquis), 159
  dabigatran (Pradaxa), 159
  dental procedures, 163–165
  heparin, 159
  international normalized ratio (INR), 151, 157,
    158
  low-molecular-weight heparin (LMWH), 159
  rivarixaban (Xarelto), 159
  warfarin, 157, 158
antidepressants
  monoamine oxidase inhibitors, 133
  selective serotonin norepinephrine reuptake
    inhibitors (SNRIs),
  selective serotonin reuptake inhibitors (SSRIs), 135
  tetracyclic antidepressants, 134
  tricylic antidepressants, 134
    cardiac risks, 138
    drug interactions, 134
    epinephrine, 134
antinuclear antibody test (ANA)
  positive, in SLE, 198
antiplatelet drugs
  actions of, 153, 154
  dental management of patients on, 153, 154, 164
  effects of, 154
antipsychotics
  atypical, 127
    associated with periodontal disease, 132
    elevated cholesterol and/or triglycerides, 132
    glucose control, 132
  QT prolongation, 131, 138, 144, 145
  typical, 126
antiresorptive therapy

antiresorptive osteonecrosis of the jaw (ARONJ)
    due to, 195
  dental management of ARONJ, 196
  dental notes for, 197
  for cancer bone pain, 194
  for multiple myeloma, 187
  for osteoporosis, 194
  mechanism of action, 194
anti-tumor necrosis factor (Anti-TNF) drugs
  treatment in Crohn's disease, 8
  treatment in rheumatoid arthritis, 200
  treatment in ulcerative colitis, 8, 9
ARONJ *see* antiresorptive osteonecrosis of the jaw
arrhythmias
  anti-arrhythmic drugs, 76, 77
  clinical synopsis, 75, 76
  dental treatment scheduling, 77
  dental management of patients with, 77
  pacemakers, 77
aspirin
  antiplatelet effect, 154
  for prevention of myocardial infarction, 70
  management of patients, 153, 154
  mechanical valves, 79
asthma
  aspirin sensitivity, 21
  clinical synopsis, 17–18
  dental notes, 18–22
  diagnostic lab values, 18
  drug interactions, 21
  features of, 17
  Guidelines for the Diagnosis and Management
    of Asthma, 17
  medications prescribed, 18–20
  nitrous oxide use, 22
  nonsteroidal anti-inflammatory prescribing, 21
  triggers of, 18
  use of epinephrine, 21, 22
  xerostomia with inhalers, 23
azathioprine (Imuran) *see also* immunomodulator drugs
  adverse effects of, 103
  liver transplantation, 103
azithromycin *see* also macrolide antibiotics
  cytochrome P450 enzymes/drug-drug interactions, 104
  in liver disease, 97
  in kidney disease, 33
  interaction with warfarin, 159

benign prostatic hypertrophy (BPH), 42–43
benzodiazepines (antianxiety)
  dental drug interactions, cytochrome P450
    enzymes, 257, 263

beta-blockers
  cardioselective beta-blockers, 69
    epinephrine use, 79
  noncardioselective beta-blockers, 69
    epinephrine use, 79
bisphosphonate-associated osteonecrosis of the jaw
    (BONJ) *see* antiresorptive osteonecrosis of
    the jaw
bipolar disorder *see* mood stabilizers
bisphosphonates *see* antiresorptive therapy
Bleeding, intraoral
  bleeding disorders, 151, 155
  chronic kidney disease, 31, 35, 37, 38, 39, 41
  management of, 160–163
  platelet disorders, 151
bleeding disorders
  dental notes, 163–167
  lab values, 150
bleeding time, 151
blood dyscrasias
  CBC with differential, 171–173
bronchitis, chronic *see* chronic obstructive
    pulmonary diseases

calcium channel blockers
  gingival enlargement, 69
  use in cardiac conditions, 64, 69, 75
  use in organ transplant patients, 104
carbamazepine see mood stabilizers
cardiac arrhythmias see arrhythmias
cardiac conditions
  dental treatment scheduling, 79
  INR values, 71
cardiac stent
  antibiotic prophylaxis, 72
  dental treatment scheduling, 79
  INR, 71
celiac spruce, 13
chemotherapy
  dental notes, 248
  dental treatment planning, 246
  in cancer treatment, 237
  laboratory values, 241
  oral complications, 240
    nausea/vomiting, 241
    oral mucositis, 240
  oral complications, management, 242
chronic kidney disease (CKD)
  alterations of drug dosing in, 33–35
  antibiotics prescribed, 36
  bleeding tendencies, 35
  clinical synopsis, 30–31

  dental notes for, 35–36, 41–42
  diabetes, 36
  diagnostic lab tests, 32
    creatinine clearance (CrCl), 32
    glomerular filtration rate (GFR), 30, 32
  hypertension, 36
  infection, increased risk of, 36
  iron-deficient anemia, 34, 35, 36, 172
  medications prescribed, 33–35
  oral features of, 32
  relationship to periodontal diseases, 36
  staging and severity of, 31
chronic obstructive pulmonary disease (COPD)
    (emphysema and bronchitis)
  clinical synopsis, 23
  dental drug interactions, 24
  dental notes for, 24
  diagnostic lab values, 23
  medications prescribed, 23
  nitrous oxide use, 24
  types of, 23
cirrhosis of the liver, 93, 95, 97, 98, 100
clarithromycin *see also* macrolide antibiotics
  cytochrome P450 enzymes/drug interactions,
    257, 260
clindamycin
  dose adjustment in liver disease, 97
  in kidney disease, 33, 36, 41
  prolong QT interval (torsades de pointes), 40, 76,
    131, 264
clopidogrel (Plavix) *see* antiplatelet drugs
Clostridium difficile infections
  in ulcerative colitis, 10
  pseudomembranous colitis, 13, 14
  C. difficile, 8, 10, 11, 13, 14
Clostridium difficile associated diarrhea (CDAD) *see*
    Clostridium difficile infections
clozapine (Clozaril)
  agranulocytosis, 130, 131
coagulation cascade, 149, 150
coagulation disorders *see* von Willebrand's disease
    (vWD), hemophilias
cocaine, 145
codeine, 137
  drug-drug interactions, 263
  in kidney disease, 33
coronary artery bypass graft (CABG)
  dental treatment scheduling, 79
corticosteroids, inhaler
  oral candidiasis, 23, 34
corticosteroids, systemic
  Addison's disease, 54

anti-inflammatory, asthma, 20–22
  drug interactions, 21, 49
  guidelines for dental patients taking systemic
    corticosteroids, 54–56
  systemic lupus erythematous (SLE), 207
  treatment of Crohn's disease, 8
  ulcerative colitis, 11
creatinine clearance
  kidney function, 32
cyclosporine *see also* immunomodulator drugs
  adverse effects, 104, 105
  drug-drug interactions, 40, 200
  gingival enlargement, 105, 200
  liver transplantation, 40, 104
cytochrome P450 enzymes
  drug-drug interactions, 257–258
  drug metabolism, 256
Crohn's disease (CD)
  dental notes, 9–10
  lab tests, 8
  medical synopsis, 7
  oral features of, 8
  treatment of, 8
  use of corticosteroids, 8–10
cystatin C, 32

dental caries
  radiation head and neck, 240, 245
desmopressin acetate (DDAVP)
  hemophilia A and B, 155
  management of intraoral bleeding, 163–165
diabetes
  chronic kidney disease, 36
  clinical synopsis, 46–47
  dental management
    blood pressure, 49, 50
    drug interactions, 49
    epinephrine, 50
    periodontal disease, 50
  diagnostic criteria, 48
  hemoglobin A1c (HbA1c), 48, 50
  management of, 48–49
  oral features, 49
dialysis *see* kidney dialysis
diflunisal (Dolobid)
  in kidney disease patients, 33
diuretics
  for hypertension, 61, 62, 65
  for heart failure, 74
  loop diuretics, 74
  potassium-sparing, 62
  potassium-sparing/thiazide, 63

  thiazides, 61, 62, 68
diverticular disease
  clinical synopsis, 11
  dental notes for, 12
  diagnostic lab values, 12
  treatment for, 12
doxycycline *see also* tetracyclines
  drug-drug interactions, 40, 259, 260, 264
  in kidney disease, 33, 41
drug-disease interactions in dentistry
  clindamycin, 264
  prolonged QT interval, 76, 131, 264
  tetracyclines, 264
drug-drug interactions in dentistry
  analgesics, 261, 262
  anti-anxiety drugs, 263
  antibiotics, 259–261
  cytochrome P450 enzymes, 137, 257, 258
  epinephrine, 263
  levonordefrin, 263
  types of, 255, 256
drug-food interactions in dentistry, 264
duodenal ulcer *see* peptic ulcer disease

enamel defects
  celiac spruce, 13
emphysema *see* chronic obstructive pulmonary diseases
epinephrine
  drug-drug interactions, 262–264
  in asthmatic patients, 20–22, 26
  in cardiac patients, 79
  in diabetic patients, 50
  in pregnancy, 83
end stage renal disease (ESRD), 30
erythropoietin
  for chronic kidney disease, 34, 36, 38

fentanyl
  use in kidney disease, 34
fibromyalgia syndrome, 203
furosemide (Lasix) *see* diuretics

gallstones, 105
gastric ulcer *see* peptic ulcer disease
gastroesophageal reflux disease (GERD)
  clinical synopsis of, 5
  complications of, 5
  dental notes for, 5
  oral symptoms of, 5
  treatment of, 5
GERD *see* gastroesophageal reflux disease
gingival enlargement, drug induced, 67, 105, 200

glucocorticoids *see* corticosteroids, systemic
glomerular filtration rate (GFR), 30–32
gout, 201
graves disease *see* thyroid gland diseases,
        hyperthyroidism
Guidelines for the Diagnosis and Management
        of Asthma *see* asthma

HAART *see* highly active antiretroviral therapy
heart arrhythmias *see* arrhythmias
heart failure
    clinical synopsis, 73
    dental management of, 73, 74
    epinephrine use, 73
    medications prescribed for, 74, 75
    nitrous oxide, use of, 73
    NSAID use, 73, 74
heart valve replacement *see* valvular heart disease
Helicobacter pylori
    dental biofilm, 3
    peptic ulcer disease, 2, 3
hemoglobin, 171, 172, 177, 181
hemoglobin A1c, 48
hematocrit, 171, 172
hemophilias
    clinical synopsis, 155
    dental notes for, 163–165
    hemophilia A, 155
    hemophilia B, 155
heparin, in dialysis, 153
hepatitis, viral
    dental notes, 100
    hepatitis B
        diagnostic lab values, 99
        FDA approved medications, 99
        drug interactions, 100
    hepatitis C
        serologic tests 100, 101
        medications, 101, 102
        drug treatment guidelines, 102
        adverse drug reactions, 102
        dental notes for, 102
    lab values, 99
highly active antiretroviral therapy (HAART)
    for HIV/AIDS, 216, 221–223, 226, 230
histamine 2-receptors antagonists (H2RAs),
        for PUD, 2, 4
HIV *see* human immunodeficiency virus (HIV)
human immunodeficiency virus (HIV)
    biology of, 216
    dental notes for, 227
    medical assessment of HIV-infected patients, 231

opportunistic infections, 220
oral lesions, 221
prevalence of, 215
progression to AIDS, 219
hydrochlorothiazide *see* diuretics
hypercoagulable state, 71
hyperparathyroidism
    kidney function, 30, 31, 35, 37
hypertension
    2014 classification of, 59, 60
    clinical synopsis, 59–61
    dental notes for, 64–68
    diuretics, 62, 63, 65
    epinephrine, 67
    in kidney disease, 36
    in pregnancy, 89
    medications for, 61–65
    mepivacaine, 67
    nitrous oxide, 64
    medication management in dental patient,
        64–68
    risk factors for, 60
    target blood pressure for dental treatment, 61
hyperthryoidism
    causes of, 51
    clinical synopsis, 51
    dental guidelines for, 52, 53
    oral features of, 52
    treatment of, 51
    use of epinephrine, 53
hypothyroidism
    clinical synopsis, 51
    dental guidelines for, 52, 53
    oral features of, 51, 52
    treatment of, 51

ibuprofen *see* nonsteroidal anti-inflammatory drugs
immunomodulator drugs *see also*
        immunosuppressant drugs
    treatment in Crohn's disease, 8
    treatment in ulcerative colitis, 11
immunosuppressant drugs *see* immunomodulator
        drugs
infliximab (Remicade) *see* anti-tumor necrosis factor
        (Anti-TNF) drugs
INR, *see* international normalized ratio
international normalized ratio (INR)
    acceptable range, 71
    guidelines for dental treatment, 71
    in cardiac conditions, 71
    in liver disease, 94
    with warfarin, 71

irritable bowel disease (IBD) *see* Crohn's disease;
    ulcerative colitis
  types of, 7
irritable bowel syndrome (IBS)
  clinical synopsis, 6
  dental notes for, 7
  treatment of, 6
isoniazid (INH), for TB 26

kidney diseases
  acute renal injury, 30
  chronic kidney disease *see* chronic kidney
    disease (CKD)
kidney dialysis
  antibiotics dialyzable, 38
  bleeding, 38
  clinical synopsis, 37–38
  dental notes for, 38
  infection, 38
  medications prescribed, 37
  premedication with antibiotics, 38
  scheduling for dental appointment, 38
kidney transplant
  clinical synopsis, 39
  dental notes for, 41–42
  drug-drug interactions, 40
  medications prescribed, 39–40

lactation *see* pregnancy
lasix *see* furosemide
leukemia(s)
  acute lymphoblastic (ALL), 183
  acute myeloid (AML), 183
  chronic, 183
  dental notes for, 184, 185
  laboratory values, 183
  oral implications of, 183, 184
lithium *see* mood stabilizers
liver disease
  altered drug metabolism, 96, 97
  blood abnormalities/tendencies, 94, 98, 156
  classification, 93
  dental notes for, 96, 97
  diagnostic lab values, 93, 94
  oral features, 95
  prognosis
    Child–Pugh Classification, 95
liver transplant
  antibiotic prophylaxis, 105
  bleeding tendencies, 105
  dental notes for, 105
  medications, 103

MELD score, 103
  oral adverse effects of medications, 104, 105
  post-transplantation, 105
  pre-transplantation, 105
local anesthetics
  in liver disease, 97
  in pregnancy, 83, 86
  renal clearance in kidney disease, 34
long QT syndrome
  definition, 76
  drug-induced
    "azole" antifungal agents, 76, 135, 264
    ciprofloxacin, 76, 131, 264
    clarithromycin, 76, 131, 264
    erythromycin, 76, 131, 264
    torsades de pointes, 76
low-dose aspirin *see* aspirin
low-molecular-weight heparin (LMWH), 79, 159
lymphoma
  Hodgkin's, 186
  non-Hodgkin's, 186

macrolide antibiotics (e.g., erythromycin; azalides:
    clarithromycin, azithromycin)
  cytochrome P450 enzymes/drug interactions, 260
mepivacaine (with levonordefrin)
  use in hypertensive patient, 67
  use in pregnant patient, 83, 84, 86
mesalamine, 8, 11
metronidazole
  interaction with alcohol, 261
  interaction with warfarin, 261
  interactions with lithium, 261
  treatment for *clostridium difficle* infection, 11
  treatment in Crohn's disease and ulcerative colitis, 11
mood stabilizers
  carbamazepine, 141
  lithium
    bipolar disorder, 139
    interaction with metronidazole and
      tetracyclines, 139
    interaction with NSAIDs, 139
  valproic acid
    thrombocytopenia, 140
MS *see* multiple sclerosis
mucositis *see* oral mucositis
multiple myeloma
  clinical synopsis, 187
  dental notes, 188
  laboratory values, 187
  oral and general signs/symptoms, 187
  treatment, 187

multiple sclerosis
  categories of, 113
  clinical synopsis, 113
  dental notes for, 114
  dental related effects, 114
  diagnostic lab values, 113
  medications for, 113–116
myocardial infarction
  clinical synopsis, 70
  dental management of, 72–73
  dental treatment scheduling, 79
  international normalized ratio (INR), 71
  medications management, 70–72
  risk for second episode, 72
  use of epinephrine, 72
mycophenolate mofetil (cellcept), 42

naproxen *see* nonsteroidal anti-inflammatory drugs
narcotics *see* opioids
nifedipine (Adalat, Procardia) *see* calcium
      channel blockers
nitrates
  use in angina, 69, 70
nitroglycerin *see* nitrates
nonsteroidal anti-inflammatory drugs (NSAIDs)
  drug-drug interactions, 261
  implication in peptic ulcer disease, 2, 5
  in patients taking warfarin, 72
  interaction with anti-hypertensive medications, 65,
      66, 68
  prescribing in asthmatic patients, 21, 23
  prescribing in kidney disease patients, 35, 41
  risk of cardiovascular events, 73

obstructive sleep apnea (OSA)
  clinical synopsis, 27
  dental notes for, 27
  medications prescribed, 27
opioids
  dependence, 143
  drug interactions, 263
oral contraceptives
  antibiotic use, 84, 85, 90
  drug-drug interactions, 82, 89, 90
oral mucositis
  chemotherapy and radiation treatment, 239–241
  management of, 241, 242
orthostatic hypotension
  antidepressants, 135
  antihypertenisves, 62, 65–67, 69, 70, 72, 74, 75
osteoarthritis, 197, 198
osteonecrosis of the jaw (ONJ) *see* antiresorptive
      osteonecrosis of the jaw

osteoporosis
  antiresorptive agents
    antiresorptive osteonecrosis of the jaw (AONJ),
        194–196

pacemaker
  dental treatment scheduling, 79
  use with ultrasonic devices, 77
Parkinson's disease
  clinical synopsis, 109
  dental adverse effects of, 111, 112
  dental drug interactions, 110
  dental notes, 111, 113
  diagnostic lab values, 110
  medications, 110
partial prothrombin time (PTT), 151
peptic ulcer disease (PUD)
  causes of, 2
  clinical synopsis, 1–2
  dental drug-drug interactions, 3–4
  dental notes for, 5
  lab tests, 2
  oral adverse effects, medications, 3
  treatment of, 2–3
  types of, 1–2
periodontal diseases
  in chronic kidney disease, 36, 39
  in diabetes, 48–50
platelet count
  in liver disease, 94, 96, 98
  laboratory values, 151
  platelet transfusion required, 165
platelet disorders *see* thrombocytopenias;
      thrombocytopathies
Plavix *see* clopidogrel
polycystic kidney disease, 39
polycythemia vera, 181, 182
prednisone *see* corticosteroids, systemic
pregnancy
  analgesics prescribed during, 84–87
  anti-fungal/antiviral agents prescribed during, 87,
      88
  antibiotics prescribed during, 84, 85
  clinical synopsis, 82
  consultation with obstetrician, 89
  dental notes for, 88, 89
  drug dosing, 84
  drug interactions, 90
  drug safety during
    FDA category A,B,C,D,X, 82, 83
    intravenous sedation, 83
    nitrous oxide, 83
    epinephrine, 83

gestational diabetes, 89
gingivitis, 88
hypertension, 89
local anesthetics, 86
nitrous oxide, 86
oral effects of, 88
radiographs during, 89
sedative/hypnotic/anti-anxiety drugs prescribed
  during, 87, 88
probiotics, 6
prostatic hypertrophy (BPH) *see* benign prostatic
  hypertrophy
prothrombin time (PT), 151
proton pump inhibitors (PPIs), for PUD, 2
psychiatric disorders *see* specific conditions
psuedomembranous colitis *see also* clostridium
  difficile infections
  antibiotics associated with, 14
  clinical synopsis, 13
  treatment of, 14
pulmonary tuberculosis
  clinical synopsis, 24–25
  dental drug-drug interactions, 26
  dental notes for, 26–27
  diagnostic lab values, 25
  medications prescribed, 25–26

QT interval prolongation *see* long QT syndrome

radiation/radiotherapy, 238
  head and neck radiation, 238
    dental notes, 248
    dental treatment planning scheduling, 246
    lab values, 241
    management of oral complications, 242
    oral signs and symptoms, 239
rescue medication *see* asthma
rheumatoid arthritis
  clinical synopsis, 198
  dental notes, 201
  lab values, 198
  treatment, 199

samter's triad, 21
schizophrenia/psychosis
  antipsychotics
    atypical antipsychotics, 127
    drug interactions/adverse side effects, 257
    typical antipsychotics, 126
  periodontal disease, 129
sedative hypnotics, 143
seizure disorders
  classification of, 117

clinical synopsis, 116
  dental drug-drug interactions, 118–120
  dental notes for, 122, 123
  diagnostic lab values, 117
  medications, 117, 118
selective serotonin reuptake inhibitors (SSRIs)
    see also antidepressants
  list of, 136
  use of epinephrine, 145
serotonin syndrome, 134, 136, 137
Sjögren's syndrome, 208
  oral signs and symptoms of, 208
SSRIs *see* selective serotonin reuptake inhibitors
sulfasalazine, 8, 11
systemic lupus erythematosus (SLE)
  positive ANA test, 206

tacrolimus (Prograf) *see also* immunomodulator
    drugs
  adverse effects, 105
  drug interactions, 104
  liver transplant, 39
tetracyclines
  FDA category, 84, 85
  use in kidney disease, 33
  use in pregnancy, 84, 85
thyroid gland diseases
  cancer of thyroid, 51
  dental notes for, 52
  diagnostic lab values, 52
  epinephrine use in, 53
  hyperthyroidism, 50, 51
  hypothyroidism, 50
  oral manifestations of, 52
torsades de pointes *see* Long QT syndrome
tricyclic antidepressants
  cardiac risks, 138
  interactions with dental epinephrine, 134
  use in irritable bowel syndrome, 6
thrombocytopaties, 153
thrombocytopenias, 152
tuberculosis *see* pulmonary tuberculosis

ulcerative colitis (UC)
  clinical synopsis, 10
  dental drug-drug interactions, 11
  laboratory tests, 10–11
  medications for, 11
  oral features of, 11
ulcerative colitis (UC) *see* irritable bowel
    disease (IBD)
uremia, 31, 41
uremic syndrome, 31

valproic acid *see* mood stabilizers
valvular heart disease (heart valve replacement)
    antibiotic prophylaxis, 78
    clinical synopsis, 78
    dental management of heart valve replacement,
        79
    dental treatment scheduling, 79
vitamin D
    deficiency in kidney disease, 31
    periodontal disease, 37
von Willebrand's disease (vWD)
    clinical synopsis, 154
    dental notes, 155
    medications, 155
    orofacial findings, 155

warfarin
    anticoagulant, 157, 158
    dental drug-drug interactions, 158
    international normalized ratio (INR), 157, 158
    management of dental patient on, 157, 158
white blood cells (WBCs)
    disorders of, 182
    in chemotherapy, 241, 243

xerostomia
    in diabetes, 49
    in fibromyalgia, 203
    in hypertension (drug-induced), 65, 67, 74
    in radiation therapy, 240, 242, 248
    in Sjörgen's syndrome, 209